Building a Profitable Nutrition Practice

Building a Profitable Nutrition Practice

D. Katie Wiedman, M.Ed., R.D.
ARA/Healthcare Nutrition Services

Dorothy J. Page
ARA/Healthcare Nutrition Services

With contributions by ARA/Healthcare Nutrition Services

VAN NOSTRAND REINHOLD
New York

Library of Congress Catalog Card Number 91-31916
ISBN 0-442-00914-3

Printed in the United States of America.

Van Nostrand Reinhold
115 Fifth Avenue
New York, New York 10003

Chapman and Hall
2-6 Boundary Row
London, SE1 8HN, England

Thomas Nelson Australia
102 Dodds Street
South Melbourne 3205
Victoria, Australia

Nelson Canada
1120 Birchmount Road
Scarborough, Ontario MIK 5G4, Canada

16 15 14 13 12 11 10 9 8 7 6 5 4 3 2 1

Library of Congress Cataloging-in-Publication Data

Building a profitable nutrition practice / D. Katie Wiedman, Dorothy J. Page.
p. cm.
Includes bibliographical references and index.
ISBN 0-442-00914-3
1. Dietetics—Practice. I. Wiedman, D. Katie. II. Page, Dorothy J.
RM218.5.B85 1992 91-31916 91-31916
613.2'023—dc20 CIP

Contents

Preface ix

Part 1 Introduction **1**

Chapter 1 An Enabling Perspective **3**

ADJUSTING CURRENT PERCEPTIONS 3

THE CHANGING AND INTENSIFYING DEMAND FOR NUTRITION SERVICES 5

PLACING A VALUE ON NUTRITION SERVICES 8

EXPANDING UPON CURRENT CAPABILITIES TO MEET CONSUMER DEMANDS 9

INTRAPRENEURSHIP AND BUSINESS MANAGEMENT SKILLS 15

SUMMARY 17

Part 2 The Planning Process **19**

STRATEGIC PLANNING 20

OUTLINE STRATEGIC PLANNING PROCESS 21

Chapter 2 Gathering Data for Strategic Planning **23**

DEFINE YOUR MISSION 23

SELECT SERVICES, PRODUCTS, AND MARKET SEGMENTS 24

MARKET ANALYSIS 32

Chapter 3 **Key Action Strategies 60**

FINALIZE SELECTION OF SERVICES AND PRODUCTS FOR SPECIFIC TARGET MARKETS 60

SET GOALS 62

DETERMINE KEY STRATEGIES 63

TRANSLATE YOUR PLANS INTO DOLLARS AND CENTS 79

Chapter 4 **Case Study—Strategic Plan 95**

ABOUT THE CASE STUDY 95

BACKGROUND OF THE INSTITUTION 95

SELECTING SERVICE AND PRODUCTS AND TARGET MARKETS 97

ANALYZING THE MARKET 99

FINALIZING SELECTION OF SERVICES AND TARGET MARKETS 106

DETERMINING GOALS 107

DETERMINING KEY ACTION STRATEGIES 108

FINANCIAL PROJECTIONS 114

Chapter 5 **Gaining the Approval of Administration 130**

HELPFUL SUGGESTIONS 131

THE WRITTEN WORD 133

Part 3 **The Planning Process 145**

Chapter 6 **Administrative Considerations in Establishing the Practice 147**

DEVELOPING GUIDERULES 147

LEGAL AND ETHICAL CONSIDERATIONS 177

REIMBURSEMENT FOR NUTRITION SERVICES 184

Chapter 7 Executing Business and Marketing Plans 194
EXECUTING PLANS 194
PROMOTING YOUR PRACTICE 208
MAXIMIZING RETURNS ON YOUR PROMOTIONAL EFFORTS 226

Chapter 8 Worksite Nutrition Programs—Planning and Promoting
LEARNING ABOUT WORKSITES 246
PROMOTING TO WORKSITES 253

Part 4 Administration 303

Chapter 9 Monitoring Performance 305
TRACKING RESULTS 305
MONITORING AND ADAPTING TO CHANGING DEMANDS 317

Chapter 10 Conclusion 318

Glossary 320
FURTHER READINGS 322

References 324

Index 327

Preface

ON THE THRESHOLD OF RADICAL CHANGE

The profession of dietetics is on the threshold of a radical change that will influence both how we see ourselves and how we are seen by others. Many of our younger members have taken the lead in bringing about this change. They learn skills that get results in the marketplace, take advantage of career opportunities in fields where nutrition counselors previously feared to tread, and speak out on behalf of their programs and ideas. They have proved that dressing for success works, that networking is not exclusive to the old girls and old boys, and that money is not a dirty word. (Mary Abbott Hess, M.S., R.D. 1988)

Whether you agree with Mary Abbott Hess or not, comments like this, describing some aspect of the changing role of nutrition counselors, appear in every nutrition journal every month. Their essence is the excitement that surrounds the evolution of outpatient nutrition services.

In the early 1980s prophecies abounded about the inevitable downfall of many health care professionals if they did not make drastic changes in their approach and delivery of services. Changes in the industry placed many nutrition careers in jeopardy. Consumers were beginning to scrutinize the performance of health care providers and make choices in the services they purchased. Nutrition services, like all other health services, were evaluated on the basis of the financial contribution they made to the health care institution.

OUTPATIENT SERVICES EMERGE

As a result of these changing demands, one of the largest expanding nutrition careers is that of outpatient nutrition counselors. At the onset, nutrition counselors in health care institutions were expected to counsel outpatients as a part of their daily routine, usually in a crowded office, in the cafeteria, or, worse yet, in the kitchen of the facility. Braver dietary managers were willing to relinquish only part of one dedicated nutrition counselor's time to outpatient services until the business grew. Juggling a workload of inpatient and outpatient needs has not been conducive to focusing on the demands of starting up a successful outpatient practice. The pressures of a heavy workload left some counselors wondering what to wish for—clients who would return or clients who would not. Many counselors decided that the institutions with which they were affiliated were not committed to developing these practices, so they ventured into private practice.

The opportunity to turn a bleak prophecy into a whirlwind of growth and activity has arrived. Today, outpatient nutrition counselors know that they must be marketers and business planners, as well as counselors. They are learning to "sell" themselves. The nutritional needs and wants of the "well" consumer are a primary focus. Standardized approaches have been abandoned, in favor of counseling approaches that take needs, preferences, and lifestyles into account. Nutrition practitioners are venturing out of traditional health care settings into fitness centers, worksites, restaurants, and grocery stores. They are using their creativity to market everything from computer programs to food shopping tours.

As the need for quality outpatient services continues to change and intensify, many institutions and individuals are searching for the tools to provide high-quality, profitable nutrition services. The new demands require new skills. Specifically, nutrition professionals need advanced training in marketing, business planning, management, and counseling skills.

Outpatient nutrition practitioners are taking responsibility for aggressively seeking ways to improve their own skills. Also, they are venturing into new areas of opportunity, conscientiously striving to build the skills they need along the way. The pioneering approach has its advantages. Laying back and waiting until new skills are fully developed may cost their practices the competitive edge in the marketplace.

BUILDING MARKETING AND MANAGEMENT SKILLS

Purpose and Commitment

This book aims to help outpatient nutrition practitioners succeed. Venturing into the consumer-oriented mode of marketing nutrition, meeting the needs of clients, and delivering the profit expectations for the practice are what *Building a Profitable Nutrition Practice* is all about.

Building a Profitable Nutrition Practice was developed out of ARA Healthcare Nutrition Services' commitment to promote the dietitian as the "nutrition expert" and to help the nutrition industry grow and change. The organization has marketed nutrition services for over 30 years, and the management team felt that they had much to offer outpatient nutrition practitioners endeavoring to build profitable practices. This book does not document the status quo, but challenges nutrition managers and practitioners to apply new and sound business approaches in order to establish their practices.

Target Audience

"You" is used throughout the text to address those who will plan and manage the outpatient nutrition practice. *Building a Profitable Nutrition Practice* is written for clinical nutrition managers, food service directors, and nutrition practitioners who expect to establish a profitable nutrition practice or improve the profitability of an existing outpatient nutrition practice.

An attempt has been made to look at the specific needs, advantages, and problems of both clinical managers and practitioners of outpatient nutrition practices supported by health care institutions. No attempt is made to cover every topic related to outpatient nutrition services. Instead, particular emphasis is lent to topic areas that are unfamiliar to nutrition professionals.

Content Overview

After a brief review of the radical changes affecting the increasing demand for and delivery of outpatient nutrition services, this text focuses on the step-by-step method of researching the market. Analyzing business potential, writing business and marketing plans, and presenting to administration are detailed in the text and exemplified in the case study. To aid in establishing and growing a profitable nutrition practice, the last few chapters deal with start-up issues, promotional efforts, and monitoring results. A section on analyzing financial opportunity provides basic accounting principles essential to the survival of a practice. Other topics reviewed are meeting the changing and intensifying client demands, setting goals, determining key action strategies, and third-party reimbursement.

While marketing and business management are the focus of this book, they are careers in themselves, and justice cannot be given to these subjects in a few chapters. Each practice will be unique, as will be the variables affecting individual practices. Consumer needs, competition, and economic status of the community will vary from market to market. These factors and the mission of the institution will influence the goals of the practice and determine the necessary resources.

There is *not* one "right way" to manage a nutrition practice. Human factors complicate the issues. Also, information on "what really works" is difficult to obtain (Kotler, 1971). You are encouraged to use this book as a valuable resource and to explore the specific needs of your practice with marketing, financial, and legal experts.

Uniqueness of the Book

This book is unique in:

- The strong profit orientation;
- The practical, methodical approach that provides the road map enabling the nutrition practitioner to act;
- The valuable tools provided, including forms, surveys, a proposal, an observer critique sheet, advertisements, and correspondence; and
- The reference tables, case studies, charts, scripts, examples, and illustrations, which provide added dimension to the text.

Content Resources/Contributors

More than 50 contributors provided insight, and a committee of executive managers, marketing experts, training specialists, food service directors, clinical managers, and experienced outpatient nutrition practitioners reviewed the work. Focus groups were conducted with physicians, food service directors, and managers in business and industry. Over 100 personal interviews were conducted with outpatient nutrition care providers, and over 100 actual educational and counseling sessions were observed.

As is customary, a list of references appears at the back of the book. Because much of the valuable advice contained in this book grew out of the personal experiences of contributors, you will not find references for some of the content.

Part 1

Introduction

Chapter 1

An Enabling Perspective

ADJUSTING CURRENT PERCEPTIONS

In order to build a profitable nutrition practice, your attitudes and perspectives must "enable" you to succeed.

Our ability to market dietetics, along with opportunities and jobs, is the key to our future—as individual practitioners and as a profession. How we fare will depend on our attitude, our self-esteem, and our competency, as well as on how well we track and manage the explosive changes in health care.

Susan Calvert Finn, Ph.D., R.D. (Ross Laboratories) and Wolf Rinke, Ph.D., R.D. (Wolf Rinke Associates, Inc.) (1989)

Building profitable nutrition practices requires a willingness on the part of nutrition care providers to change current perceptions. Calvert and Rinke encourage nutrition professionals to widen their perspectives and to develop a marketing mentality. In the health care field, marketing is often considered a "bad-word." For some, it conjures images of the classic "snake oil" salesman capitalizing on poor health, or billboards plastered with names, smiling faces, and phone numbers.

Developing a marketing mentality means more than advertising and promoting products for the purpose of making money. Marketing is a process of meeting the needs and desires of consumers, while fulfilling the goals and objectives of business (in this case, nutrition practices). Because consumers are demanding new approaches, nutrition practitioners are establishing themselves in places they have never been before—corporations, restaurants, fitness centers, rehabilitation facilities, and more. And the timing for these increasing demands couldn't be better, since inpatient nutrition career opportunities are shrinking, primarily due to legislative changes in reimbursement. The bulk of this book prepares the nutrition practitioner to successfully and profitably manage nutrition practices that are leading the explosive changes in the nutrition field.

This chapter addresses the attitudes and perceptions that Calvert and Rinke suggest are key to nutrition practitioners' futures. Since the marketing mindset is so critical to an enabling perspective, it's a good place to begin.

To develop a marketing mindset, the nutrition care provider must eliminate the perceptions that:

- Marketing focuses on the gains of the business, neglecting the humanitarian aspect of health care.
- Physicians control the services that can be offered by an outpatient nutrition practice.
- Nutrition care providers must provide services for a large population with a myriad of medical conditions.
- Nutrition services are of low value to consumers, physicians, and health care administrators.
- Making the public aware of nutrition services (advertising) is unethical.

These perceptions must be replaced with the confidence that a marketing mentality will build a profitable nutrition practice. Clearly, nutrition practitioners must enter the business with an understanding that:

- As the demand for nutrition services among consumers, physicians, and health care administrators changes and intensifies, the value of quality nutrition services increases, and current approaches must be abandoned for approaches that more directly meet the needs of clients.
- Nutrition services are only of low value if they are offered in ways that do not meet clients' needs.
- Marketing is consumer-oriented; therefore, meeting the needs of consumers is the most important concern of the practice. Profitability does not compromise quality of nutrition care. In fact, it may actually improve the quality of care, as practitioners strive for excellence in satisfying consumers.
- Since client needs are changing and clients are demanding more, nutrition practitioners must expand upon current capabilities to meet client needs.
- A spirit of intrapreneurship and a set of business, marketing, management, and counseling skills are requisite to an effective practice.
- It is an advantage for a practice to be affiliated with an institution.

Each of these six concepts will be reviewed on the following pages. First, nutrition practitioners must understand how the demand for nutrition services is changing and intensifying, in order to feel the value of them.

THE CHANGING AND INTENSIFYING DEMAND FOR NUTRITION SERVICES

The demand for outpatient services is growing among consumers. As referral agents (physicians), worksite benefit providers, and health care administrators are recognizing this demand, they realize that meeting the nutritional needs of the community meshes well with the missions and financial objectives of most health care providers and institutions. The reasons for the increasing demand for outpatient nutrition services stem from the changing needs of potential clients, referral agents (physicians), worksite benefit providers, and health care administrators. The concerns of each group deserve close examination.

The Changing Concerns of Potential Clients

Following are some of the strongest concerns raised by outpatient nutrition clients:

- Increased interest in nutrition—Nutrition care is a recognized need of "well" and "sick" clients. Nationally, the wave of interest in fitness and good nutrition continues to swell. It is important to note, however, that the increasing interest in nutrition among the well population appears to be for the enhancement of appearance, increased energy, and a more satisfying social life, as often as it is for health benefits.
- The decreased length of hospital stay—The decrease in length of hospital stay often means that patients are discharged before nutrition services are even ordered by the physician. In other cases, they are discharged on short notice, and the inpatient dietitian does not reach the patient before the discharge. These patients are now seeking help on an outpatient basis.
- Clients want more than education—As clients have become more informed about nutrition, they have found that changing eating patterns isn't easy. They want help. Depending on clients' needs, education may or may not be accomplished in the inpatient setting. Unquestionably, counseling needs and needs for ongoing support cannot be addressed in the inpatient setting.
- The behavior change process demands time and involvement—Research shows that behavior change occurs over a long period of time, even with the guidance of trained professionals. Lasting change comes from gradual change (Zifferblatt and Wilbur, 1977). This means that one-time nutrition consultations have little impact. The atmosphere of a hospital room and the shock of illness often prevent patients from being receptive to education and counseling during their hospital stay. As nutrition counselors explore the possibilities of providing outpatient services to clients in a stepwise series, they realize the need to reduce the amount of information given to the patient upon hospital discharge and to follow up with outpatient nutrition services.

- The changing lifestyles of consumers—The changing role of women in the work force, the familial issues arising from two-income or single-parent families, and the increased pace of life are just a few of the societal changes that affect eating habits and health behaviors. These lifestyle changes make it increasingly difficult for people to change eating habits. The business world has capitalized on these factors by promoting convenient and time-saving products and services.
- Research on adult learning—Research suggests that active involvement is prerequisite to adult learning. Adults need to have some control over the learning situation, with ample opportunity to practice new behaviors. Adults need help to integrate nutrition plans into their personal lifestyles. They want ongoing support for behavior change. Whether seeking information on disease prevention or on specific dietary recommendations, clients want guidance on how to change food-related behaviors. They need to be reinforced for positive steps, have the opportunity to share experiences, and examine information from different perspectives so that change may take place.

The Changing Concerns of Physicians

In focus groups with physicians addressing the need for outpatient nutrition services, the following concerns were surfaced:

- Concern for low compliance rates of their patients—Physicians are appealing to nutrition counselors for more effective approaches to changing eating behaviors. They expect counselors to help their patients with applied nutrition.
- A better feedback and follow-up system—As a group, physicians feel the need for a better feedback and ongoing follow-up system when they refer their patients to nutrition counselors outside of their own practice. As adequate feedback becomes the rule rather than the exception, physicians have indicated that they would relinquish control of their patients' nutritional care more often.
- Physicians' desire to differentiate their practices—As competition for health care services increases, physicians need to differentiate their practices in order to maintain an adequate patient load. An outpatient nutrition service is one method of accomplishing this. Physicians find that offering nutrition services to their patients creates the image of comprehensive health care.

The Changing Concerns of Health Care Institutions

Changing concerns of health care institutions that affect nutrition care include:

- Health care institutions need additional sources of revenue—Financial pressures facing health care institutions today are encouraging administrators to expect nutrition services departments to offset as much of their costs as possible and to generate profits.

- The rising need for continued treatment after hospital discharge—As the length of hospital stay has decreased, methods of treating patients have evolved to limit the necessity for "round-the-clock" care. Health care experts project that 90 percent of diagnostic tests and 70 percent of treatments will soon be performed in an outpatient setting. The role of nutrition care in these outpatient services will become increasingly important (Goldsmith, 1989).
- Health care institutions must market themselves to survive—As health care institutions are now forced to market their services, community exposure has become tremendously important. Outpatient programs are very effective services for promotion of the hospital in the community.

The Needs and Desires of Nutrition Practitioners

The needs and desires of nutrition care providers are also changing, and these changing needs and desires provide even more impetus for new approaches to providing nutrition care. Their changing needs and desires follow:

- New career opportunities—As the number of inpatient nutrition career opportunities has receded, primarily due to the changes in reimbursement legislation, nutrition counselors have had to seek additional opportunities. Through marketing efforts, nutrition practitioners can establish themselves in places they have never been before—corporations, restaurants, fitness centers, rehabilitation facilities, and more. They find themselves dealing with a "well" population in addition to a "sick" population and are recognizing that their approach to each must be clearly different.
- Desire to distinguish themselves from unqualified, self-proclaimed "nutritionists," diet gimmicks, and commercial nutrition programs—A growing concern has developed among nutrition professionals over the large amount of money being spent for fraudulent or suspect nutrition products and services. The American Dietetic Association representatives deserve credit for their efforts to influence the public's recognition of the registered dietitian as the nutrition expert. Some states have even passed licensure bills to affirm their recognition of dietitians as nutrition experts. However, the true test comes from the individual nutrition counselor's ability to draw business from the less reliable sources and to compete effectively in the marketplace.
- The need for support and teamwork in developing nutrition counseling as a process—As nutrition counselors explore the possibilities of providing outpatient services to clients in a stepwise series, they realize the need to reduce the amount of information given to the patient upon hospital discharge and work

more closely with the inpatient nutrition counselor in developing a referral system.

PLACING A VALUE ON NUTRITION SERVICES

As the demand for nutrition services changes and intensifies, the value of the services increases. Pioneers in outpatient nutrition practices found that placing a high value on nutrition services benefits the consumer, as well as the physician and health care institution. In the past, health care institutions offered outpatient nutrition services at little or no charge, considering them "good public relations" with physicians, patients, and the community. Besides the fact that health care institutions can no longer absorb the expenses of such lavish public relations campaigns, limiting the value of outpatient nutrition services has caused many outpatient dietitians to question their own worth. Placing a fair value on nutrition services provides revenues for the institution and job satisfaction for the nutrition practitioner. Also, a prosperous practice may ultimately enhance the institution's public relations more than offering free services. The benefits to the institution of charging for nutrition services are fairly easy to understand. How charging aids the individual is more difficult.

The old adage "nothing worth having is free" holds true for health care services. People begin to question the quality of services offered at low or no charge. They assume that they will get more from a program that costs more. This factor may drive consumers to purchase nutrition scams and programs offered by businesses with no qualified nutrition experts. It's important to note that consumers pay a premium for many of these alternatives to sound nutrition care. For nutrition care providers to draw consumers away from these sensationalists requires that they place a fair value on services.

Consumers are often more serious about services for which they pay. One of the biggest problems that nutrition counselors have had with ongoing counseling is gaining a commitment from clients to continue. "No shows" have been common in outpatient nutrition practices. When people are paying for services, they are more likely to attend sessions. How often have you heard, "I'm paying for this, and I intend to get my money's worth"? In the case of nutrition services, clients must make a commitment of time and interest to gain a return on their investment; they must make a commitment.

Does this then mean that those who cannot afford nutrition services will not receive them? Services to the indigent do not cease to exist when a practice becomes profit-oriented. However, the practice will be forced to account for such activities, or profits will be limited. Those who wish to be profitable and choose the indigent population as their primary market will find it necessary to actively seek funding through grants and third-party reimbursement.

Once nutrition practitioners feel they are competing with self-proclaimed nutritionists, they work harder to meet the needs of their clients. However, the price alone will not draw clients. The nutrition services must fit the needs and desires of consumers. That is the key to marketing.

EXPANDING UPON CURRENT CAPABILITIES TO MEET CONSUMER DEMANDS

Wise practitioners realize that they need clients in order to survive and that consumers have many choices in purchasing nutrition care. Therefore, nutrition practices must be consumer-oriented to be successful. Successful nutrition practitioners build upon their current capabilities by expanding their skills and their repertoire of techniques and approaches. The traditional approaches must be examined for their appropriateness to the changing needs of the client, referring agents, and the health care institution. No longer can nutrition counselors simply depend on physician referrals.

Why Consumers Seek Nutrition Services

What do consumers want in terms of nutrition care? Pioneers of outpatient nutrition care have found that, in general, consumers seek a nutrition expert for three primary reasons:

1. Knowledge of what and how to eat—They want to know specific menu planning, food selection, and preparation techniques.
2. Help to incorporate new eating behaviors into their lifestyle—They want new eating habits to mesh with their current occupational, familial, and social activities.
3. Ongoing support—They want counselors to:
   a. Guide them to self-sufficiency;
   b. Facilitate the change process;
   c. Help them track progress or regression; and
   d. Reinforce progress.

Not only do consumers want knowledge, guidance, and support, they also want it tailored to their medical condition, culture, environment, personal food preferences, motivation, and social influences. They want convenience and time-saving measures. Obviously, this places the demand on today's practitioners to go beyond education and become effective counselors, facilitating and supporting behavior change. The need for these new counseling skills are obvious, yet the development of these skills will demand much time, commitment, and practice. A high priority must be assigned to counseling skill development.

Preparing Referral Agents for Change

Traditionally, health care products and services have been dictated by physicians and health care administrators (Halling, 1986). Although the physician still offers a wealth of information about what patients want and need, to be aware of the true needs and desires of consumers requires that practitioners confront the consumer.

Meeting the needs of consumers may first require reeducating physicians and other health care providers, as they are the primary referral agents for nutrition services. Health care professionals have, for the most part, been trained in the medical model, which implies that knowledge will evoke behavior change. They may need to be convinced that new approaches to outpatient nutrition care will be more effective. Therefore, nutrition care providers must listen to physicians' needs and their perceptions of patient needs in order to develop appropriate services. Also, health care professionals must be educated with regard to new approaches and services and the benefits of these approaches and services to their clients.

Specializing vs. Generalizing

Generalized practices attempt to be all things to all people. It isn't possible. Too often, generalizing means that nothing that is done can be deemed notable or outstanding. Consequently, generalized practices rarely grab the attention of physicians or consumers.

Establishing specific services targeted at specific groups of people creates benefits for the consumer, the physician, and the nutrition practice. Specialized practices are more beneficial to consumers and physicians because they:

- Offer programs and services that best affect their specific clientele;
- Are recognized as "expert" in specific areas of nutrition care;
- Have the time and funds to develop expertise, resources, and programs that revolve around the clients they serve;
- Are able to network with the select group of physicians and organizations who deal with these select clients, increasing rapport, feedback, follow-up, and referrals;
- Use marketing tools that are most likely to reach specific sectors of the population, increasing the chances that potential clients will realize that nutrition services that meet their particular needs exist;

- Are able to schedule programs and office hours that fit into the schedules of their clients; and
- Offer group programs in which all participants have similar needs and lifestyles, increasing the support network.

Specializing does not necessarily mean hiring specialist dietitians and/or catering to people with just one specific medical condition. Instead, current practices may need to reevaluate their business, and new practices must begin by determining and understanding the groups of people they can best serve. Market research will be essential to determine the needs of specific groups of people, and innovative ways to meet these needs must be developed. Then and only then do nutrition care providers realize the alternatives they possess for offering services. Outpatient nutrition practitioners' capabilities are quite unique when compared to traditional nutrition care.

Outpatient vs. Inpatient

Nutrition practitioners often feel that outpatient services will be easy to establish and provide. They believe that they can continue to do on an outpatient basis what they have done on an inpatient basis. Quite the contrary is true. Not only do your clients want and need different things in each of these settings, but your ability to service those needs is different, too. Capabilities are affected by time, resources, and the patient/client's state of mind in each setting.

A difficult transition to make is from the mindset of an inpatient dietitian to that of an outpatient nutrition counselor. Their roles are similar in that they provide nutrition care, but the differences are dramatic. Perhaps Table 1-1 will help you understand a few of the differences.

Obviously, inpatient and outpatient nutrition service providers have the potential for an effective team, a point that will be discussed later. However, pioneers have found that successful outpatient practitioners must make the transition from the behaviors listed in the first column to the behaviors listed in the second column.

The challenge in making this transition lies in the fact that new skills and capabilities must be developed to meet the changing client needs and to market services. Consider the question: "How can I alter services to better meet the needs of today's clients?"

Counseling vs. Education

Because most outpatient nutrition services offer more education than counseling, a practice can be set apart from the rest by marketing its nutrition counselors as change agents. Granted, more training may be required to nurture effective coun-

TABLE 1-1 Differences Between Inpatient and Outpatient Nutrition Providers

Inpatient providers	Successful outpatient providers
Generally have only one encounter with the patient	Have the opportunity to establish a relationship with the client over time
Consider themselves educators	Consider themselves counselors or facilitators of change
Measure success based on number of patients seen and patient understanding	Measure success based on business developed, profitability, and a track record of client behavior change
Spend less than 50 percent of their time educating/counseling	Educate/counsel 80 percent of the day
Provide services to those who have medical conditions and their families	Provide services to both sick and well populations
React to the institution's patient load	Continuously market their services to develop and maintain a clientele
See patients during those hours between breakfast and dinner because patients are "in-house"	Offer services during flexible hours that conveniently fit into clients' schedules
Are forced to work with the patients referred by physicians	Can select target markets and deal with only selected clients
Communicate with physicians through charting, direct contact, and nurses	Determine effective ways to communicate with and market to referring agents
May not be expected to generate revenue, in most cases	Must, for the most part, generate revenue to survive
Have preset charting and record-keeping procedures	Develop their own charting and record-keeping systems
Are not usually required to travel to provide services	May be required to travel to various locations to provide services
Are not responsible for obtaining third-party reimbursement	Aid clients in filing for third-party reimbursement
Advise or provide information or guidelines on diets	Guide clients to resolve own problems and incorporate information into their nutrition plans
Pace information according to amount of material	Pace information according to individuals' accomplishments

selors; however, pursuing further skill development offers great rewards. In fact, successful clients could eventually become the practice's best promoters.

Traditionally, nutrition counselors have focused on providing information to their clients. Most nutrition counselors were trained in the "medical model," which assumes that, if clients know what is good for them, they will change their behavior. Thus, nutrition educators came to believe that imparting knowledge would result in behavior change. "Education" is imparting knowledge.

"Counseling," on the other hand, considers environment, culture, social influences, personal preferences, and motivation in assisting clients to incorporate new eating behaviors into their lifestyles. Today's nutrition counselor targets behavior change by using many different skills, techniques, and strategies. Effective counselors are now viewed as supporters and facilitators of change. Recommending dietary changes is just the tip of the iceberg. Nutrition education is a part of nutrition counseling, but "nutrition counselors" need to become expert at helping individuals solve problems and make changes.

Another way to encourage learning and facilitate change is through group educational and counseling programs. Group programs can afford greater profits than individual counseling and will actually benefit clients as well.

Group vs. Individual Counseling

Nutrition practitioners often hold the misconception that individual counseling sessions are more effective than group sessions because clinical dietitians traditionally meet with patients on an individual basis. Many dietitians believe that group programs are beneficial only to the over-booked outpatient counselor. They feel that clients want the personal attention that individual sessions afford. In actuality, clients seeking nutrition counseling for education, counsel, and support (the three reasons consumers seek a nutrition expert) may have a better chance of meeting these needs through group rather than individual sessions.

In fact, individual counseling is only a must in a few specific instances. When a personalized nutrition plan has not been established, individualized counseling allows the counselor to tailor plans and activities to the client. Sometimes a client is only willing to accept individual services or is not well suited to a group, due to unique needs or disruptive behaviors. Clients who are unable to accommodate a regular schedule of sessions at designated times or would be unable to work at the pace of the group for any reason are prime candidates for individual counseling.

Additional knowledge can be provided in a group forum. Adult learning theory suggests that many adults learn best in groups where experiences are shared. Sharing ideas and experiences provides a process that enables clients to integrate new information with old beliefs. Other group members ask questions that clarify information and fulfill the needs of timid participants. Therefore, integrating nutrition recommendations into lifestyle is often accomplished most successfully in groups. Also, of course, group members can provide ongoing support. Psychologists have successfully counseled in groups for many years for these same reasons. The advantages of group programs to the practice are increased profits, reduced waiting lists, and an increased referral base.

Community outreach can be expanded through group programs, improving image. Through group programs, the counselor is afforded more time and flexibility. Also, variety enriches the counselor's work life and reduces the monotony of individual counseling. Success in establishing counseling and group programs will depend greatly on the ability to influence consumers, referral agents and administrators. Successful programs depend heavily on the nutrition practitioner's enthusiasm, communicative skills, and business savvy.

Creating vs. Responding to Customer Flow

Because health care professionals have in the past responded to the clients/patients who seek them out, recognizing your capability to create your own customer traffic may stretch the imagination. Potential clients are both "sick" and "well." They are in organizations, worksites, community activities, and malls, as well as health care institutions.

Your capability to go to clients, instead of hoping or trying to get them to come to you is a primary advantage. You even have the opportunity to alter how inpatient services are delivered in lieu of an effective outpatient practice. Inpatient dietitians and outpatient nutrition counselors are, in many institutions, expected to form an effective team in the endeavor to improve the nutritional health of their shared clients through the use of "survival kits."

A "survival kit" may be a two-week menu to follow or a brief outline of the nutrition recommendations and a focus on one or two of the necessary dietary changes. The patient is then referred to the outpatient nutrition practice for further counseling and education. This system gives the patient time to recover and recognize his or her specific needs for dietary changes. Then the process of altering eating behaviors can be undertaken at a pace that will insure success. In this way, nutrition instruction prior to hospital discharge begins the counseling process. For this to occur successfully, the clinical nutrition staff must accept and support the idea of continued counseling. They must strongly promote outpatient counseling to the patient and physician, and stress the limitations of the survival kit.

The Bottom Line

Again, these facts suggest a strong need for reexamination of service offerings and service delivery methods, to determine the appropriateness of current service methods as they relate to the changing needs of clients, referring agents, and the institution. Challenge yourself to build new capabilities based on former competencies and the needs of those you serve.

Keep in mind that you may need to examine more than your service package and service delivery methods. To gain the attention of consumers and physicians, to draw business away from fraudulent and unqualified "nutrition" programs, and to sell administration on the need to establish the outpatient nutrition practice as its own entity requires nutrition care practitioners to use all of their marketing and business management capabilities. Most significantly, you must possess enthusiasm, an intrapreneurial spirit.

INTRAPRENEURSHIP AND BUSINESS MANAGEMENT SKILLS

Intrapreneur is defined as one who manages a business enterprise within a larger organization and has much of the same freedom and sense of accomplishment that entrepreneurs experience. The intrapreneur watches the marketplace for new needs, seizes opportunities, calculates risks, and monitors success. Intrapreneurs use creativity to provide superior quality services. Outpatient nutrition practitioners must possess an intrapreneurial spirit to achieve their goals.

During interviews with nutrition practitioners, certain characteristics became apparent that were common to the most successful practices. These intrapreneurs seemed intoxicated by the challenge of growing the practice, devoting boundless energy to this endeavor. They enthusiastically "owned" the responsibility to grow their practices. With vision, drive, and determination, these intrapreneurs sought ways to develop their own management skills to meet the needs of their practices. With sensitivity to the needs of their clients and the pulse of their institutional organizations, they were innovative, took risks, and had the ability to juggle a multitude of activities simultaneously. More over, they tied their personal success to the success of the practice.

The intrapreneurial spirit is a contagious condition. If you have it, your staff will too. Fortunately, these intrapreneurs, so eager to succeed, have more opportunity than ever to enhance their marketing and business management skills through formal training. Academic and professional organizations provide continuing education programs on such topics, and publications written specifically for outpatient nutrition practitioners are multiplying.

Note, however, the major factor that differentiates intrapreneurs from entrepreneurs. Whereas the entrepreneur is a "free agent," the intrapreneur is afforded the benefits of a larger organization. In most cases, this is a great advantage and should be recognized as such.

ADVANTAGES OF INSTITUTIONAL PRACTICES

Intrapreneurs seize the opportunities and resources available through the health care institution, to market their practices. They realize that the institution offers many advantages. Financial resources are one of the greatest advantages that an institution offers. While the entrepreneur must seek financial support in the form of investors, partners, and loans, the intrapreneur knows who the investors are and determines the appropriate approach and presentation for only one audience—the administrators of the institution. The institution provides assets in addition to finances. The facilities and equipment available may reduce capital expenditures to a minimum. Also, the wealth of expertise held by various departments is a tremendous advantage.

Reputation is another primary advantage. In focus groups, clients indicated strongly that they would choose a nutrition practice affiliated with a reputable health care institution over private practices. They indicated that the institution's reputation brought credibility to the practice, particularly in the start-up phase.

Institutional nutrition counselors also have the added support of marketing, public relations, media, and human resources departments to encourage them. The members of an institution's staff hold a vast amount of diverse knowledge. Seeking the expertise of colleagues will simplify the task of strategic planning and increase support. Time must be made to develop a team that can offer guidance. Establishing rapport with the dietary and food service departments is a good beginning, whether or not the outpatient practice is part of this department.

One of the most valuable assets to have in business planning may be the food service director. If the outpatient practice is part of the food and nutrition department, his or her support is imperative. Because his or her training usually requires a strong business curriculum, the food service director can guide strategic planning efforts. Due to the amount of financial planning involved in food service, the director may also provide valuable information on budgeting. He or she may have contacts and resources that meet specific needs.

The chief financial officer can outline the information required for a business plan in your institution. Financial officers can also answer questions related to taxation, depreciation, reimbursement, collection of fees, and accounting, or can provide other resource personnel who can. The chief financial officer is a strong ally for someone seeking administrative approval for a new endeavor.

Legal expertise may be required. All health care institutions have access to legal advisors. They offer guidance in meeting federal and state regulations that relate to the business. Assistance on such topics as contractual agreements, taxation, and liability should be sought from these advisors.

Marketing and public relations departments offer resources and expertise. The earlier they are contacted in the planning process, the better. In many cases, these departments have already accumulated important data and can provide the expertise for market research. The support of the clinical nutrition staff is imperative. With their help, a system of referral may be created, guaranteeing a steady flow of new clients to the outpatient nutrition practice. They can provide information on patient needs and develop links with physicians and staff who would be likely to use nutrition services. All of these individuals in the institution, along with the directors of patient education and human resources, provide a support network and a knowledge base.

SUMMARY

In order to succeed, your attitudes and perspectives must enable you to succeed. Misconceptions and an unwillingness to explore new approaches to nutrition care have handicapped many nutrition practitioners. The war stories are numerous.

Be willing to consider your practice a business. Recognize that profitability measures much more than financial status. It is also a direct measure of how well clients' needs are being met. As a consumer-oriented practitioner, expand upon your current capabilities, to better address the needs of your clients. Adapt your services and your skills and techniques. Recognize your competitive advantages as an institutional practitioner. Also, remember that a marketing mentality, which will lay the foundation of your success, means more than advertising products and services or promoting the dietitian as "the nutrition expert."

The remainder of this text deals specifically with the marketing and business management skills necessary to plan a new outpatient practice or to reevaluate and renovate an existing practice. Marketing is based on the ability to consistently identify, satisfy, and ensure the needs of customers, while making a profit (U.S. Small Business Association). Marketing aids nutrition practitioners in responding to opportunities and locating their niche in the health care marketplace. As you read through the following chapters, a stepwise approach to marketing and managing your practice will unfold.

Part 2

The Planning Process

Introduction

THE MARKETING PROCESS

What is marketing? As defined by Philip Kotler, the pioneer of service marketing, marketing is "the analysis, planning, implementation and control of carefully formulated programs designed to bring about voluntary exchanges of value with target markets for the purpose of achieving organizational objectives." (Kotler, 1982) In other words, marketing answers the what, to whom, where, when, and many hows of providing a service or product to the public. Marketing is not simply advertising and promoting products or services. It is a system for developing strategies to achieve goals, identifying groups of people who would be interested in services, determining the needs and wants of those groups, and actively competing for a share of the market (Dunlap, 1986).

Marketing skills are imperative to managing a successful nutrition practice. However, marketing is not an exact science. Human factors complicate the issues, and information on "what really works" is difficult to obtain (Kotler, 1971).

The marketing concept is based on the ability of marketers to consistently identify and satisfy customer needs, while making a profit (U.S. Small Business Association). Marketing allows nutrition practitioners to respond to opportunities and to locate their niche in the healthcare marketplace (Dunlap, 1986).

Fulfilling the marketing concept requires:

- Market research and analysis;
- Strategic planning;

- Gaining approval and funding;
- Fulfilling goals and objectives;
- Evaluating success; and
- Adapting to changing demands.

Each of these areas will be discussed thoroughly in the ensuing chapters of this book. Part 2 deals specifically with strategic planning, which includes market research and gaining approval and funding. However, you must first understand the concept of strategic planning.

STRATEGIC PLANNING

Some definitions are in order. *Strategic planning* is a process by which a group or organization defines its mission, assesses its current situation, determines a direction for the future, and maps out a plan to reach its goals (Policastro). Strategic planning is done for a period of three to five years, although programs are monitored and changes may be made during that period.

A *business plan* is a vehicle that aids in obtaining financing from the institution and directs the activities of the practice. Business plans usually define sales, service and administrative plans, the amount of cash needed, and the methods of financing the cash requirement (Rose, 1989). They also forecast expected results, probable risks, and reasonable timetables (Hysen, 1989).

Nutrition practitioners within healthcare facilities seldom understand the need for strategic planning. Aren't they already a part of the institution's business plan? Can't new programs and services simply be added to the existing document? Isn't planning the responsibility of the marketing and administrative experts? The answer to all of these questions is that, if you wish to establish a successful outpatient nutrition practice with the approval of your administration, the challenge of developing, writing, and presenting the business plan is yours.

In fact, as you begin to understand the purposes for strategic planning, you will realize that as the person responsible, you and your staff are the only ones in the institution qualified to prepare it.

The purposes of strategic and business planning are threefold:

1. Primarily, strategic planning is developing your services and strategies in a manner that will provide a reasonable return on your investment of time and capital. Even if your practice is already established, strategic planning can help you redirect your efforts toward a more profitable future.
2. Administrators will rely on the business plan in determining the value of your practice to the institution. With a business plan in their hands, they will be better prepared to decide how much they can and will invest in the practice. The business plan shows that you have done your homework and know the

institution's goals and objectives, thus creating a positive image in the minds of your superiors.

3. Finally, once approved and in place, the business plan directs your daily, monthly, and yearly activities. It not only provides a guide with which to run your business, but also a measuring stick for tracking your progress.

Strategic planning may require several months and depends on the information that is available to you, as well as the amount of expertise you can draw from other resources in the institution and the community. There are several ways to perform strategic planning, but basically they all require the same steps in varying order. The following outline profiles the steps as they are explained in this text.

OUTLINE STRATEGIC PLANNING PROCESS

I. Define your mission
II. Select services, products, and target markets
    A. Consider products/services that:
        1. You have resources for
        2. Fulfill organizational goals
        3. Serve selected groups of people
    B. Segment and select potential target markets
III. Analyze the market
    A. Use sources of information
        1. Learn from your history
        2. Tap available resources
        3. Network
        4. Survey potential targets
    B. Identify market forces
        1. Hospital usage changes
        2. Multi-health systems growth
        3. Increase/decrease in segments of the population
        4. Marketing emphasis of healthcare facility
        5. Changes in financial resources
    C. Identify key competitors
        1. Who?
        2. What services?
        3. What markets are they targeting?
        4. Market share?
    D. Analyze strengths and weaknesses
        1. Comparison to competitors
            a. Competitive advantages
            b. Competitive disadvantages

        2. Opportunities
        3. Threats

IV. Finalize selection of services/products for specific target markets
    A. Select target markets
    B. Select services/products

V. Determine goals
    A. Financial
    B. Nonfinancial

VI. Determine key action strategies
    A. Positioning and market mix
        1. Service offerings
        2. Place
        3. Price
        4. Promotion
    B. Staffing
    C. Scheduling

VII. Make financial projections
    A. Expense worksheet
    B. Cash flow statement
    C. Income statement
    D. Break-even analysis

VIII. Write strategic plan

IX. Prepare presentation
    A. Executive summary
    B. Presentation to administrators

X. Present to administrators

Chapter 2

Gathering Data for Strategic Planning

DEFINE YOUR MISSION

Before you can effectively begin market research, you must be able to state the mission of the business. A mission is the basis for existence (Parks and Moody, 1986). You will need to refine it as you become more aware of your plans and desired outcomes. Once formulated, your mission will become a more permanent statement of your intentions.

Be apprised of the mission statement of the organization in which you work and the mission statement of your own department. You must align your departments' goals, target markets, services, and marketing strategies with those of the larger organization. Once you have formulated or obtained a mission statement, you are ready to investigate the environment in which consumers and healthcare professionals interact.

Here are some examples of mission statements to consider:

- The American Dietetic Association stated that the mission of dietetics is "to promote and maintain health through encouragement of adequate nutritional status of individuals and groups." (Parks and Moody, 1986)
- A hospital mission statement might read: "To serve the community…and the surrounding region as a resource for high quality, cost effective primary, secondary and tertiary healthcare services.

  To meet the healthcare needs of the community in a comprehensive and coordinated manner by supporting the appropriate goals of area healthcare providers." (Akron City Hospital)

- In his book, *At America's Service* (Albrecht, 1988), Karl Albrecht suggests that support departments should create mission statements that define their service contributions. Thus, the outpatient nutrition department of the above hospital might read:

  "The outpatient nutrition services department is dedicated to providing personalized guidance to the community so that clients acquire the ability to self-manage their nutrition care. Our function is to support and facilitate the nutritional behavior changes of our clients through a variety of nutrition counseling activities and, thereby, provide the high-quality, cost effective healthcare in which the hospital prides itself."

SELECT SERVICES, PRODUCTS, AND MARKET SEGMENTS

The process of selecting services, products, and market segments requires four major steps:

1. Develop a list of potential service and product offerings.
2. Segment the market and list potential targets.
3. Conduct initial marketing research.
4. Select particular services and targets to pursue.

This section assumes that you are familiar with the community you will be serving and with the goals of the institution.

Throughout this chapter, the terms "marketing mix" and "positioning" will be used. Although these terms address more than services and products, their definitions are essential to understand what follows. Marketing mix encompasses the four key areas of marketing decision making (U.S. Small Business Administration), which are:

1. Product—What services/products will be offered?
2. Place—From what location will services be offered?
3. Price—What will be charged for each service/product?
4. Promotion—What techniques will be used in stimulating potential clients to purchase the services/products?

How the marketing mix is used to differentiate service offerings from those sold by the competition and to meet the needs of the target segment(s) is called positioning. Positioning and market mix go hand in hand. First, however, consider potential clients and services.

Determine Community Needs

Consider the following questions when listing potential services and products:

- What services does the community perceive to be desirable?
  Read the newspapers, check the news and special TV programs, and become aware of nutrition literature, services, and products currently on the market. Also, talk to potential clients and learn what they want.
- What are the services for which I have readily available resources (materials, staff, space, etc.)?
  Resources may be available through either an organization you are affiliated with or the inpatient practice. You or the nutrition department may have purchased or developed programs, visual aids, and materials in the past that could be of use. You may have a nutrition staff member who is well versed in a particular area of nutrition through continuing education or personal interest. Capitalize on such resources.
- What services would help the institution to meet its goals?
  Look closely at the institution's goals, specialties, and ambulatory healthcare programs. Know which physicians refer clients for outpatient services and what services they desire. Then, list the services you could offer to enhance these goals and desires.
- What products might I sell as accompaniments to these services?
  Services will be your primary concern; however, capitalizing on products that are associated with your service increases revenue. Having such products available may also enhance the image of the practice, in that you offer a complete package.

Possible Service Offerings

Basically, two classifications of nutrition services exist:

1. Direct influence—Those programs that offer education and counseling on an individual or group basis. Such programs include workshops, weight management programs, and support groups.
2. Environmental interventions—Those programs that influence awareness or increase opportunities for behavior change, without the personal attention. Such programs include printed nutrition information, provision of healthy food choices in the cafeteria, or scales in accessible locations.

The personal touch offered by direct influence services usually nets greater results in terms of behavior change and dietary compliance. However, services with direct influence are more expensive and require more time than indirect services. Therefore, they may be more difficult to sell to the healthcare institution, physicians, or worksite administrators. Indirect services may be a starting point for educating potential clients and enticing decision makers to offer more.

Six primary services, with dozens of variations, are commonly offered. You may be able to think of others not listed here, but these six are currently in greatest demand:

1. Individual education;
2. Individual counseling;
3. Group education;
4. Group counseling;
5. Nutrition information for the community (bulletin boards, table displays, nutrition fairs, etc.); and
6. Nutrition evaluations.

To understand these service offerings, you must understand the differences between "counseling" and "education" and the pros and cons of group versus individual programs (Chapter 1). A brief description of each primary service offering may help you develop some ideas.

Individual Education

Individual education can be given by a nutrition expert who offers information to a client and significant others. It includes such things as explaining a modified diet, meal patterns, and printed materials. Commonly, a client would see the nutrition practitioner once or twice. Such a service can be a precursor to individual counseling and/or group counseling or education.

Individual Counseling

Individual counseling includes some educating and is again primarily a one-on-one service. However, individual counseling is directed toward the client's self-sufficiency. Therefore, practices that offer individual counseling usually package several counseling sessions at one price. The service may even extend beyond the number of sessions in the package simply because the client needs further support from the counselor. As with individual education, individual counseling may also be prerequisite to a group program. This allows the counselor and client to assess individual needs and develop personal goals.

Group Education

Group education allows the nutrition practitioner to disseminate information to a large number of people at one time. The sessions are developed in advance and can easily be presented over and over again, with less preparation involved for each successive presentation. If limited discussion will be allowed, the group can be fairly large. However, a group of 6 to 12 is optimal for discussion and the formation of support networks (Raab and Tillotson, 1983; Shaw, 1971). Weight management programs, diabetes education programs, and programs on nutrition in cardiovascular disease are three examples of common group education programs.

Group Counseling

Group counseling may follow a group education program, or the two may be combined, with some education and some counseling being offered at each session. The elements that make group counseling successful are that it is:

- Client-directed (the participants determine the topics for discussion);
- Comprised of small groups that provide a supportive environment, continued until the clients feel their needs have been met; and
- Based on common goals, needs, and experiences of group members.

Group counseling sessions may also be packaged (several sessions for a combined price) to gain a commitment from participants in advance of the first session.

Public Displays

Public displays are most often sold to worksite programs. They include table displays, bulletin boards, short cooking demonstrations, and nutrition fairs. Nutrition fairs, the most popular form of public display, can be used in a variety of settings and in a variety of ways. Groups that might be interested in purchasing a nutrition fair or display include:

- Country clubs;
- Fitness centers;
- Gourmet food stores;
- Grocery stores;
- HMO/PPO;
- Medical centers;
- Schools, colleges, and universities;
- Retirement facilities; and
- Worksites.

Some of these groups would use a fair as a promotion for their own facility and services, others as a means to satisfy their clients, and still others to demonstrate the nutrition services that are provided in their facilities.

If the display is self-explanatory, the nutrition practitioner's presence may not be required at all times. However, experience indicates that the availability of a nutrition expert, for at least part of the time the display is present, improves the impact of the services and provides an opportunity to sell other services and products. The key to success in continued sales of public displays is the same as any other service: knowing the target market, their perceived needs, and what attracts them.

Nutrition Evaluations

Nutrition evaluations have, for the most part, taken the form of a computerized analysis. Clients record their food intake for one or more days, the data is entered into a computer, and the nutritional quality of the individual's dietary regimen is assessed. Such evaluations require time for explanation to the client, and are often done in combination with an education or counseling program. Nutrition evaluations are also quite popular at nutrition fairs and health fairs where other forms of screening are being provided. Computer programs available for such evaluations range from simple ones for quick, limited assessment that can easily be understood by the layman, to very complicated ones that must be interpreted by a nutrition expert. But both provide useful information for clients who want a thorough understanding of their dietary habits. Selection of software will depend on the intended use of the evaluation.

Possible Product Offerings

Although the outpatient nutrition practice is generally a service industry, nutrition practitioners can seize the opportunity to sell products related to their nutrition services, thereby increasing client education and raising additional revenue. Some of these products are developed by the practitioners, while others are purchased from wholesalers or retailers.

If you decide to sell products, be advised that legal, distribution, taxing, and promotion issues must be addressed. Keep in mind, also, that all products must carry your full endorsement and that of the institution. You may wish to have other experts (exercise specialists, physicians, etc.) evaluate products before you decide to offer them. Counsel from an accountant and a legal expert is imperative. Some of the more popular products that nutrition practitioners offer are mentioned below.

Printed Materials

Printed materials are more and more becoming a popular means of generating revenue. Nutrition practices sell informational brochures, newsletters, manuals, handout materials, cookbooks, and recipes. These materials may be developed by the practice or purchased from various publishers and agencies.

Food Products

Food products are often convenient to purchase where the program is held. The market for food products is rapidly expanding. Such products might include food supplements (mostly with rapid weight loss programs), convenience foods (frozen dinners, low calorie snacks, etc.), and seasonings.

Other Related Products

Some products that are popular accompaniments to nutrition services include food scales to weigh foods, videotapes, computer software, audiotapes, and exercise products.

Placing a Value on Free Services and Products

In the past, nutrition counselors willingly displayed at nutrition fairs, presented at meetings, and provided printed educational materials at no cost to consumers. Do not be afraid to charge for such products and services, particularly if they are not being used as promotional efforts. You must place a value on the time and knowledge of your professional staff.

Many practitioners have attempted and failed to build a practice by offering free or low-priced services with the intention of raising prices once the clientele was established. Experience shows that the clientele will leave the practice at this point and a new clientele must be sought. If you establish the value of a product or service as free, you will then have to overcome the client and physician perceptions of low value. Consider all products and services as potential revenue for the practice, even those you currently offer free.

When you choose to use services/products as promotions, evaluation is imperative. Strive to track the referrals you receive through such promotions. In this manner, you can place a value on staff time and determine how your promotion time will best be spent in the future.

At this point you have probably formulated some ideas about the types of services you might offer, changes or expansions in current service offerings, and people who might be interested in these services. The next step in the marketing process entails selecting target markets and understanding those markets.

Potential Target Markets

A market is all the people who could or would purchase a particular service or product. This is an overwhelming audience, and serving them all would mean generalizing the practice. Therefore, marketing experts suggest segmenting the market. As the word implies, segmenting entails breaking the market into smaller homogeneous groups. To be useful, members of a market segment should share characteristics that lead to similar buying practices. In planning a practice, intrapreneurial practitioners choose specific segments to serve. These groups are called target markets.

Segments may be based on such characteristics as client type, geographic, demographic, lifestyle, or behavioral differences. Each market segment will have different requirements and attitudes and will derive different benefits from nutrition services. For example, one target market might be adults with diabetes who live within a 30-mile radius of the hospital. By focusing your efforts on a segment of the market, you can better respond to consumer needs and market opportunities. You can more easily determine appropriate service/consumer match. Segmentation allows you to reduce costs and maximize the effectiveness of your marketing investment.

Look at the market segment of public service workers (police, fire fighters, and postal workers) as an example. These people want to know how to prevent chronic illness without drastic changes in their busy lifestyles and work schedules. Many of them are expected to be physically fit in order to perform their jobs effectively. Their needs are different from those of senior citizens or clerical workers. Therefore, programs should be tailored to the specific needs of public service workers in order to capture this market. Programs on nutrition and exercise, eating on the run, and cardiovascular risk reduction would be appropriate.

Finding the most attractive markets is challenging. Market segments must be:

- Measurable—Able to be designated by market size. (10 inpatient instructions with cardiac patients are done per week.)
- Accessible—Able to be reached through marketing efforts and served through programs, products, and services. (If the distance to travel is too far or you cannot offer the programs a group needs, the segment is not useful.)
- Identifiable—Able to be objectively grouped, based on common references and needs. (Referred from the same specialty group of physicians.)
- Substantial—Large enough to be profitable and warrant a special effort. (If the segment is limited to hypertensive fire fighters, it may not be a large enough group to consider.)
- Relevant—Based on objective criteria. (A group that has some reason to see a nutrition counselor.)

Table 2-1 provides some examples of market segmentation options. Once possible market segments are identified, the most promising should be selected as initial market segments. Expansion into additional market segments allows for planned growth as the practice matures.

Sometimes market segments can easily be defined. For instance, if you are setting up an outpatient practice in affiliation with a pediatric hospital, the market segments might be inpatients with chronic conditions, children with specific medical conditions, patients of the pediatricians who take an interest in nutrition, and so forth. From these segments, you will choose groups to direct marketing efforts toward. Your task is much greater if the institution is interested in expanding beyond its initial referral base.

TABLE 2-1 Market Segmentation for Nutrition Counseling Practices

Market	Segmented by
Individuals	Medical or dental condition Age Interests (exercise, nutrition, etc.) Occupation Sex Other demographic criteria Inpatient nutrition services required Previous involvement in nutrition counseling or education Home healthcare
Worksites	Size Location Number of employees Type of industry Interest in wellness education Money spent in educational programs Public vs. private sector
Community groups	Age Size Location Group interests
Health and fitness	Clinics HMO/PPO Health clubs
Organizations	Retirement centers Nursing homes Rehabilitation centers Hospitals (employees or patients) Athletic groups (schools, athletic teams, etc.)

A very common misconception among those starting outpatient practices is that they can be "all things to all people." In other words, they generalize their practices. Existing nutrition practices need to reevaluate their business, and new practices must begin by determining and understanding the markets they can best serve, to prevent generalization. Learn ways in which you can best affect specific populations, rather than react to situations that displease your clientele.

MARKET ANALYSIS

Marketing research is the process of analyzing the problems related to selling goods and services. Such analysis should answer the questions:

- Who are my potential customers?
- What are their common characteristics?
- Can and will they buy?
- How do I reach them?
- How do I compare with my competitors? (Laumer and Erffmeyer)

To make such decisions, marketing requires a research base.

The environmental forces that affect needs must be studied, as well as customers and their perceptions. Then, a practice must internalize its research to determine its ability to provide appropriate services (Parks and Moody, 1986). Once a business is established, marketing research can provide valuable information for growing and maintaining a healthy practice.

To determine specific service offerings and methods of attracting target groups, practitioners must base their decisions on consumers' perceived benefits—what people believe they want and need (Lewis, 1984). In addition, wise outpatient practitioners determine their strengths and weaknesses and become familiar with the competition—who they are and what they are offering (Parks and Moody, 1986). A thorough understanding of the market and how it affects your business is imperative when setting goals and developing strategies for marketing and operating the practice. Therefore, market analysis consists of four basic parts:

- Researching target markets;
- Examining market forces;
- Analyzing the competition; and
- Analyzing your strengths and weaknesses.

The market analysis provides descriptions of key factors that may affect the success of the business. A thorough investigation of target markets, market forces in your location, and the competition, along with an analysis of your strengths and weaknesses, enables you to determine marketing strategies that address the unique needs of target markets. These strategies set your nutrition practice apart from the rest. This section reviews the information you need and ways of obtaining it.

Researching Target Market

As you move into a consumer-oriented market, you must discover the consumers' economic, social, technological, and lifestyle needs and preferences. You must learn the perceived needs and desires of the market you target. Initial market research may help you to examine the markets you believe you have something to offer. Research provides you with specific information about each market segment as follows:

- Size;
- Growth potential;
- Economic status;
- Benefits the group is seeking;
- Features appealing to this group;
- The organizations serving this group;
- Locations where services would best be offered;
- Hours convenient to the target group;
- Forms of promotion that will help in acquiring clients;
- Stumbling blocks that might prevent you from reaching this group;
- Referring agents who could be instrumental in building clientele;
- Best ways to serve referring agents; and
- The share of the market that might realistically be captured.

Vehicles for Market Research

There are many ways to gather market information, depending on the time and/or financial resources you can afford. A corporate or institutional marketing department can be of service. However, hiring marketing specialists can be expensive.

The vehicles you use to research the market will depend on many things. The two largest dependents are whether the institution has marketing experts and whether you are beginning a new business, as opposed to having an existing practice. Your budget, potential target markets, potential services, and resources will all affect the research vehicles you use. Some methods of researching the market will prove more successful in your community than others will, as you may be able to determine from the marketing analysis efforts of others.

In this section we will examine what you can learn from:

- Your history and experiences;
- Your marketing department;
- Professional marketing groups;
- Networking;
- Available sources of information; and
- Surveys, interviews, and focus groups.

Your History and Experiences

If you and your staff have experience in providing outpatient nutrition services, you may be one of your own best resources. Use your own history and experiences as a starting point for market research. You can learn many things about people seeking nutrition services from the information you have in your head and in your files. And, the price is right. The following questions will lead you to critical information:

- What nutrition services are you presently providing?
- How many clients are using each service?
  — Inpatient by nutrition need (e.g., diabetic, cardiac); and
  — Outpatient by nutrition need.
- What are the demographic, geographic, and behavioral characteristics of these clients?
- Do you have an effective system for evaluating services and measuring effectiveness (follow-up interview, questionnaire, etc.)?
- Do you have an effective system for evaluating clients' and referring agents' perceptions of services?
- Which physicians regularly refer patients to your services?
- What are the specialties of these physicians?
- Why aren't you receiving referrals from other physicians?
- Have any physicians stopped referrals? Why?
- What is the sales/revenue from each of the services currently offered?
- What are current clients' reactions to pricing?
- What other nutrition practices or commercial nutrition programs have your clients used? What feedback have clients offered about these practices?
- Do your counselors encourage clients to return for multiple counseling sessions?
- What is the average number of sessions that clients return for?
- What percentage of clients return after an initial visit?
- Does a designated staff member contact those who do not return? If so, for what reasons do clients fail to return?
- Do you provide group programs?
- What is the dropout rate for group programs?
- For what reasons do group members drop out?
- How successful have clients been at getting reimbursement for your services?
- How much support have you received from the institution's administrators and/or other departments?
- Does your staff share a common vision and a high level of commitment to your goals?
- What is the relationship between other health facilities/community groups and your affiliated institution/practice?
- If you employed marketing/advertising strategies in the past, how successful were they?
- Do you or your staff communicate on a timely basis with referring physicians?
- Are clients satisfied with the times you offer services?
- Are you and your staff accessible to clients and physicians by phone?

- For what nutrition programs (and for which services) must you currently refer calls to other practices? How often?
- If you have offered programs at more than one location, which locations were the most successful?

Although you may feel you have a general understanding of the answers to these questions, the systematic compilation of the answers to these questions will provide valuable information for the experts who assist you. The data you collect will help direct decisions about markets to target, services to offer, and strategies to use.

Your Marketing Department

If the institution has a marketing department, you should first meet with them to determine how they can help and guide you and what research they have already done. Even healthcare organizations who do not have a marketing department usually have a staff member with marketing expertise. This person may be located in the public relations department.

The marketing specialists can usually direct you to data that is available within the institution. Such information includes community demographics, patient demographics, which insurance companies to contact, other departments in the institution who have gathered similar information, information on people who have participated in screening programs sponsored by the institution, and requests that have been made by individuals and groups for nutrition programs from the institution.

The marketing department may also be able to prepare and conduct surveys for you or to solicit the services of an outside agency. Their support to guide and refine marketing plans and/or to execute any part of them can be invaluable. This is, after all, their area of expertise, just as yours is nutrition.

If you have no support from a marketing department, you may gather information from other areas of the hospital. For instance, public relations can identify people who have done similar research. They can also track requests for nutrition information from media and community groups. Data processing will have demographic information about the patient population and number of patients receiving treatment for specific medical conditions. If the institution has an information and referral service or speakers bureau, they may be able to provide information on client interests.

Professional Marketing Groups

Professional resources may appear too expensive for your budget, but they may be well worth the money if the amount you risk losing is much greater than the cost of the research (ADA 1986). Marketing researchers can be located through local business schools, the yellow pages, health journals, and professional associations. Even if you cannot afford professionals to do all the research for you, you may be able to use their expertise for a portion of your research, such as providing mailing lists, developing surveys, and conducting focus groups. Many universities have a small business consulting program whereby students and educators analyze business and marketing plans and offer free advice. If you choose to perform surveys, interviews, or focus groups, professional marketing expertise is imperative.

Networking

You can learn many interesting and useful facts about your market from community activities and social contacts. An interview, whether casual or formal, with one physician can offer insight into the perceptions of a whole group of physicians. Peers can offer information on the competition by sharing their experience of participating in a program or the information they have gathered in pursuing a program. If you train students in a dietetic internship or coordinated program, chances are that they can give you information on other healthcare facilities in the area. The consumer affairs workers in grocery stores can provide ideas on nutrition information that the public is seeking.

As a member of one or many professional and/or community organizations, you may gather information about several aspects of the market. The local Dietetic Association is a good place to learn the focus and future plans of other outpatient nutrition practitioners. Volunteer work with health-related agencies, such as the American Heart Association and the American Cancer Society, increases your visibility, while offering you a chance to interact with influential people. Parent-teacher association, church group, and philanthropic organization meetings are great places to strike a conversation about nutrition and learn of people's interests and perceptions.

Available Sources of Information

Community resources offer a variety of information about the demographics, as well as health concerns, of your region. Highlighted below are a few of the most useful resources:

- Libraries—public, hospital, and university—are excellent resources. Before you approach a librarian, make a list of the kinds of information you are interested in so that he or she can lead you to the right information. For a nominal charge, many libraries can run computerized bibliographic searches. The computer databases Medline (healthcare issues) and PTS Mars or AMI (marketing information) may be particularly helpful (ADA, 1986). Larger libraries will offer many directories that can be of use in finding a consultant or in conducting market research (Laumer, Harris, Guffey, and Erffmeyer, 1988). Among the most helpful directories are:
  - *American Hospital Association Guide*—Provides census information by city.

- *Where to Find Business Information: A Worldwide Guide for Everyone Who Needs the Answers to Business Questions* (Brownstone, D.M. and Carruth, G. (2nd ed.) 1982)—A listing of over 500 publications indexed by subject areas, reference materials they contain, and publishers.
- *AUBER Bibliography of Publications of University Bureaus of Business and Economic Research* (Kloc, S., Ed. (Annually)—References business and economic research.
- *Rand McNally Commercial Atlas and Marketing Guide* (Annually)—Maps, census statistics, and information on marketing and retail sales.

- An organization that can be of service to anyone who needs guidance in establishing the business aspects of a practice is the U.S. Small Business Administration. The U.S. Small Business Administration offers a variety of publications at a nominal fee. A current publication listing can be obtained by writing: SBA, P.O. Box 15434, Fort Worth, TX 76119 (Laumer, Harris, Guffey, and Erffmeyer, 1988).

  Many communities have local associations, and retired business people often volunteer their expertise in guiding individuals who are developing small businesses.
- Table 2-2 outlines various sources of information and the types of information they may provide.

Surveys, Interviews, and Focus Groups

Surveys, interviews, and focus groups are the most common tools used by marketing experts for information on interest in certain products/services and intent to purchase products/services. In most cases, the size of the target and demographic information are gathered prior to surveying that market. Marketing experts strongly recommend that you seek professional guidance if you choose to conduct surveys. Experience shows that nutrition practitioners who have conducted surveys on their own have not been satisfied with the results. Table 2-3 provides a guide to various survey methods.

The value of each survey method cannot be judged on a pure cost basis. Instead, survey methods are chosen according to their cost effectiveness. In other words, how much useful information will you get for your dollar? Although mail surveys may appear to be the least expensive method of gathering this type of information, the low response rate can actually escalate the cost.

Mail surveys and telephone interviews tend to provide more quantitative information; they answer the question, "how many?" Personal interviews and focus groups, on the other hand, provide qualitative information; they offer insights on why consumers select services/products as they do. These two survey methods surface issues and problems that planners may have been unaware existed (Moosbrugger, 1986).

TABLE 2-2 Sources of Information

Source	Type of Information
Census Bureau	Demographics, including age, sex, marital status, family composition, income, and occupation
Libraries	Demographics
Chamber of Commerce	Demographics by county and city Community health organizations Competition Market forces
Health departments	Birth and death statistics Services needed
National organizations (local chapters) American Heart Association American Cancer Society Diabetes Association March of Dimes Red Cross Cooperative Extension Dairy Council AARP LaLeche League Visiting Nurse Association Home Health Agency YMCA/YWCA	Disease statistics with demographics Member interests Topic requests for speakers
Telephone directories	Local chapters of national organizations Competition
Media (local) Newspapers Radio Television	Competition Community health interests Local health concerns (water, soil contamination, etc.) Market forces
Health newsletters (local) HMO/PPO Healthcare facilities Fitness clubs	Competition Health interests of patrons
Insurance companies (annual reports)	Health statistics Coverage for various health services
Food purveyors and pharmaceutical companies (institution's affiliates)	Availability of special dietary products Regional market research

TABLE 2-3 Survey Methods

Type	Methodology	Pros	Cons
Personal interview	One to one conversation for the purpose of gathering specific information. Usually done in malls or the facility.	• Good response rate • High level of control • Useful for more in-depth probing than written or phone surveys • Verbal and non-verbal input	• Time comsuming • Involves travel time and expense • May be schedule difficulties
Telephone survey by practitioner or professional marketing group	Practitioner asks questions on telephone. The surveys must be short, and they may or may not be conducted by appointment.	• Requires less time than than personal interview • No travel time • Better response than mail survey • Possibility of probing • Begins the selling process	• Frequent use is irritationg to some people • Limited time/Limited information • Some reluctance to share information over the phone • Time consuming
Focus groups	Meeting with small groups representative of the target population, to gather information and reactions. A contracted interviewer is optimum, and incentives are usally offered to group members who participate.	• Smaller groups to gather for each group • Less time involved than interviewing • Begins the selling process • Allows for probing • Using a marketing expert allows coordinator to observe with a greater focus on interpreting the data	• Resistance of negative feedback or the appearance of defensiveness • Must assure a representative sample • Only hear from a small group unless multiple groups are formed • May be scheduling difficulties • Incentives may be costly
Mail survey	Questionnaires are sent to a representative sample of the target population with a pre-posted return envelope.	• Does not require scheduling or phone time • Can survey a large population in a small amount of time • Promotes the practice through visual image	• Printing and postage expense • Low response rate (about 10%) • Less control in collecting data • No opportunity for probing

TABLE 2-3 *(Continued)*

Type	Methodology	Pros	Cons
Telephone survey by support staff	Support personnel question a representative sample of the population by phone. The surveys must be short, and they may or may not be conducted by appointment.	• Requires less of coordinator time • Flexible scheduling • No travel time • Better response rate than mailing	• Expense of staff time • Staff is selling business and must be well trained • May not get specific feedback

Unfortunately, getting the information you require through surveys is not an easy process. In fact, full college courses are devoted to the subject. Therefore, many risks are involved when a nutrition practitioner decides to conduct any form of market survey without the assistance of professional marketing experts.

In conducting surveys without the aid of marketing experts, you may gather misleading information that may cause you to choose the wrong services and strategies. For instance, asking "What services are you interested in?" does not tell you what the person will purchase. By asking questions that people do not wish to answer, you may lose them as survey participants, as well as prospective clients. For example, when asked a question about income, 30 percent of the people will not answer the question and 15 to 25 percent will fail to respond to the survey entirely. Health practitioners conducting surveys on their own found that they failed to ask questions in a meaningful way. Thus, a physician might answer "no" to the question, "Would you refer clients to a dietitian-directed weight management program?" This data does not explain the physician's objections to the program or under what circumstances he or she might refer patients for the service.

Although you may be able to thoroughly describe the target market, locating them may be another problem. Obtaining a representative sample of the target market can be difficult. Large amounts of time and money can be wasted because:

- Such a small number of people respond to surveys.
- Mailings or phone calls are costly.
- Telephoning requires time.
- Compiling and analyzing the data collected is time consuming and requires specific expertise.

Offering incentives may increase the return on surveys, but providing a large enough incentive is also costly.

Although you must describe the new concepts you want reactions to, you cannot ethically sell products/services or look for leads in the survey process. For these reasons, you would be wise to involve a professional marketing service in conducting surveys. Even with the help of such a service, there are three tasks that will be required of you:

1. Write a survey proposal—Survey proposals organize your thoughts about the information you are interested in obtaining; provide a sense of direction to those preparing, distributing, and analyzing the survey; and provide a rationale to administrators, worksite decision makers, and yourself for conducting the survey.
2. Define terms—Neither the marketing experts or the survey participants will understand many of the terms used to describe nutritional conditions, nutrition services, or nutrition experts. In simple terms, clearly define any term (e.g., registered dietitian, nutrition counselor, group counseling) that you feel is necessary to use.
3. Explain to survey participants what you expect from them—Explain to the survey participants what you want them to do. Tell them what information you expect to obtain and why you need this information. Since this explanation will appear in the introduction to the survey, it is also important at that time to define the new concepts to which they will be reacting. Survey participants can hardly be expected to respond accurately if they don't know where, when, and how services will be offered.

When using a professional marketing service, one of the ways to reduce costs is by distributing and collecting the surveys yourself. There may also be some other steps in the survey process that you or your staff can address.

Two sample survey proposals and the accompanying surveys follow. The first sample survey (Figs. 2-1 and 2-2) is directed to potential clients within a specific target market. The second sample survey (Figs. 2-3 and 2-5) is directed to physicians who would refer clients. Most surveys are coded so that the data can be easily entered in a computer program. The codes (letters or numbers) are not included in these samples. Figure 2-4 provides a sample letter to the physicians. *These surveys are only samples.* You must develop surveys that are appropriate to your situation.

Examining Market Forces

Market forces are the financial, technical, and sociopolitical factors in the environment surrounding your practice that could affect the success of your business. Such factors might include:

- Changes in population or diversity of population;
- Changes in legislation;

PROPOSAL FOR SURVEY OF PROSPECTIVE CLIENTS OF ALWELL WOMEN'S HOSPITAL OUTPATIENT NUTRITION CENTER

Background

The Nutrition and Marketing Department of Alwell Women's Hospital have been discussing the marketing of a newly established outpatient nutrition practice. In order to have input from potential users, it was decided to conduct an interest survey. This study will focus on the kinds of nutrition services and the value of features of those services. This proposal discusses the ways to implement this survey.

Objectives

The principal objectives of this study are:

1. To determine the nutrition needs and desires of individuals; and
2. To discover the features that would encourage individuals to purchase such services.

Methodology

Questionnaires will be distributed through direct mail to a random sample of 1500 potential respondents gathered from the following organizations: local chapter American Cancer Society, local Diabetes Association, and local Association for Retired Persons. Surveys will also be distributed to patients of Alwell Women's Hospital.

All questionnaires will be distributed by (date).

The completed questionnaires will be returned in pre-posted envelopes to the Marketing Department of Alwell Women's Hospital for editing, coding, tabulation, and analysis. A return of 200 is anticipated.

Upon completion of the study, the Marketing Department will produce a written report containing findings, conclusions, and recommendations.

Expected Findings of the Study

This survey will offer information on the interests of individuals in:

- Purchasing various nutrition services;
- Various nutrition topics;
- Features that would encourage or discourage them from purchasing nutrition services; and
- Using nutrition services to meet specific needs.

Because of the groups we are surveying, these results will primarily tell us what people with either a current medical

FIGURE 2-1. Sample proposal for survey of prospective clients.

condition or a known threat of a medical condition would be interested in. These groups will form the nucleus of our market.

From these findings, the Nutrition Department and Administrators of Alwell Women's Hospital will have a better understanding of the interests of individuals in various nutrition services and what features will be necessary to market services successfully.

Responsibilities

The Marketing Department has developed a draft of a questionnaire as a part of this proposal.

The Nutrition Department will edit the draft and make any suggested changes by (date).

The Marketing Department will print and distribute questionnaires to the various organizations and the Nutrition Department by (date).

The sponsoring organizations and Nutrition Department will distribute the questionnaires, collect them, and forward them to the Marketing Department no later than (date).

If all of the above dates are met, the Marketing Department will be able to issue a report on the results of this study by (date).

FIGURE 2-1. *(Continued)*

NUTRITION SERVICES QUESTIONNAIRE

Alwell Women's Hospital is in the process of establishing an outpatient nutrition counseling center. This center would be designed to offer individual and group nutrition programs that meet the needs of our clients and referring physicians. We realize that nutrition is an important factor in improving health and that lifestyles affect the way we eat. Your input is critical. We hope that you will help us direct our efforts to serve you by answering the following survey questions, which probe your nutrition needs and interests.

Please complete the questions by placing an "X" in the appropriate response box. Feel free to add any comments that might help us better understand your needs.

This survey is completely anonymous. You will not be asked for your name or any identification that will associate you with your responses.

1. How interested are you in the following nutrition topics or concerns? Please check your answer on the grid below.

FIGURE 2-2. Sample questionnaire for surveying nutritional concerns of prospective clients.

	Very Interested	Somewhat Interested	Not too Interested	Not at all Interested
A. Weight management	[ ]	[ ]	[ ]	[ ]
B. Heart disease/high cholesterol	[ ]	[ ]	[ ]	[ ]
C. Diabetes	[ ]	[ ]	[ ]	[ ]
D. High blood pressure	[ ]	[ ]	[ ]	[ ]
E. Pregnancy	[ ]	[ ]	[ ]	[ ]
F. Eating disorders	[ ]	[ ]	[ ]	[ ]
G. Cancer	[ ]	[ ]	[ ]	[ ]
H. Osteoporosis	[ ]	[ ]	[ ]	[ ]
I. Premenstrual syndrome	[ ]	[ ]	[ ]	[ ]
J. Infant nutrition	[ ]	[ ]	[ ]	[ ]
K. Other (specify)	[ ]	[ ]	[ ]	[ ]
2. How interested would you be in working with a nutrition professional, individually, to help you change your eating behaviors to fit your needs and lifestyle?	[ ]	[ ]	[ ]	[ ]
3. How interested would you be in working with a group of people with similar nutrition problems, under the guidance of a nutrition counselor, to make desired changes in your eating habits?	[ ]	[ ]	[ ]	[ ]
4. How interested would you be in attending cooking classes to learn heal thier cooking methods?	[ ]	[ ]	[ ]	[ ]
5. How interested would you be in participating in supermarket tours designed to help you make healthier food choices?	[ ]	[ ]	[ ]	[ ]
6. How interested would you be in having a nutrition counselor visit your home to	[ ]	[ ]	[ ]	[ ]

FIGURE 2-2. *(Continued)*

inventory your food, make recommendations, and assist you in planning menus?				
7. How interested would you be in attending workshops that educate you regarding nutrition issues surrounding your specific nutrition needs?	[ ]	[ ]	[ ]	[ ]

8. Check the box that most reflects the degree of importance you would place on each item, if you were to choose a nutrition service:

	Very Important	Somewhat Important	Not too Important	Not at all Important
A. Physician referred you	[ ]	[ ]	[ ]	[ ]
B. Nutrition counselor is a registered dietitian	[ ]	[ ]	[ ]	[ ]
C. A friend or family member recommended the service	[ ]	[ ]	[ ]	[ ]
D. Personal working relationship with the nutrition counselor	[ ]	[ ]	[ ]	[ ]

9. How interested are you in using nutrition services to:

	Very Interested	Somewhat Interested	Not too Interested	Not at all Interested
A. Improve your health or reduce your risk of disease	[ ]	[ ]	[ ]	[ ]
B. Manage your weight	[ ]	[ ]	[ ]	[ ]
C. Feel better and look better	[ ]	[ ]	[ ]	[ ]
D. Support your current efforts to change eating habits	[ ]	[ ]	[ ]	[ ]
E. Obtain an eating plan that fits both your lifestyle and your special needs	[ ]	[ ]	[ ]	[ ]

FIGURE 2-2. *(Continued)*

10. If you were to use a nutrition service, during which time period would you most often schedule your appointments? (Check only one answer.)
    - ☐ Between 9:00 A.M. and 5:00 P.M.—Monday thru Friday
    - ☐ Evenings—Monday thru Friday
    - ☐ Weekends only
    - ☐ Combination of evenings and weekends

11. Which of the following locations would be convenient for you to receive nutrition services? (Check as many as apply.)
    - ☐ Community Medical Building (101 N. Main St.)
    - ☐ Health Maintenance Inc.
      - ☐ 505 N. Jefferson
      - ☐ 1500 E. Washington
      - ☐ 3555 Lincoln Lane
    - ☐ YMCA (Highway 3)
    - ☐ Elm Way Community Center (1200 Elm Way)

[Readers Note: Marketing experts have suggested a split survey. This means each half of your survey population would receive identical surveys, except for the prices indicated in the blanks of the following two questions. Test the range that you are considering.]

	Absolutely	Probably	No
12. Do you think most people who need nutrition services would be willing to pay $ ____ for a 1-hour individual session?	[ ]	[ ]	[ ]
13. Do you think most people who need nutrition services would be willing to pay $ ____ for each 1-hour group session? (This would include the cost of materials.)	[ ]	[ ]	[ ]
14. If 50% or more of the cost of nutrition services were reimbursed by medical insurance plans, would you be more apt to use nutrition services?	[ ]	[ ]	[ ]

15. Age: ☐ Under 30 ☐ 31-54 ☐ 55 or over

FIGURE 2-2. *(Continued)*

PROPOSAL FOR PHYSICIAN SURVEY

Background

The Ambulatory Care Center of Anywhere Community Hospital in coordination with the Nutrition Services Department have been discussing ways to establish an outpatient counseling practice. Realizing that the majority of referrals to outpatient nutrition programs are made by physicians, it was decided to conduct an opinion survey with physicians. This study will focus on the kinds of nutrition services to which physicians will refer patients. This proposal discusses ways to implement the survey.

Objectives

The principal objectives of the survey are to:

1. Discover how many patients each physician would refer to each service per month on average; and
2. Measure physicians' attitudes toward various topics and features of nutrition services.

Methodology

An announcement of the study will be made in the attached cover letter to physicians from the Medical Director of Anywhere Community Hospital.

Questionnaires will be mailed to 150 physicians on (date) and collected in the Physicians' Lounge and Dining Room or by return mail.

Complete questionnaires will be turned over to Anywhere Hospital's Marketing Department for editing, coding, tabulation, and analysis. A return of 75 questionnaires is expected because it will be requested by the Medical Director.

Upon completion of the study, the Marketing Department will produce a written report containing findings, conclusions, and recommendations to administration and all members of the medical staff.

Expected Findings of the Study

This survey will determine the attitude of physicians regarding:

1. Various nutrition services that could be offered;
2. How nutrition services should be provided;
3. Various features of nutrition services–price, location, number of sessions, and providers; and
4. Various nutrition topics.

From these findings, Anywhere Ambulatory Care Center would have a better understanding of the attitudes of physicians toward nutrition services and what programs they would most likely use for their patients.

Based on the number of physicians responding, we will be able to project the number of patient referrals that physicians will make to the center per month.

FIGURE 2-3. Sample proposal for survey of physicians.

Responsibilities

The Marketing and Nutrition departments have developed a draft of a questionnaire as part of this proposal.

The Medical Director and Ambulatory Care Center will edit these drafts and make any suggested changes by (date).

The Marketing Department will print and distribute these questionnaires on (date).

Physicians will be asked to return the completed questionnaire no later than (date), and they will be collected by the Marketing Department.

If all of the above dates are met, the Marketing Department will be able to issue a report on this study by (date).

FIGURE 2-3. *(Continued)*

Anywhere Community Hospital
123 Main Street
Nicetown, PA 19003

Jack Ormsby, M.D.
Cardiologist
Anywhere Community Hospital
123 Main Street
Nicetown, PA 19003

Dear Jack:

I want to share with you my enthusiasm over a new service center, The Anywhere Nutrition Center. This outpatient nutrition care center is being designed to meet the needs of physicians, like yourself, and their patients.

Most physicians are convinced that dietary changes do influence their patients' well-being. Hence, they continue to prescribe modified diets, even though they recognize that dietary compliance with modified diets is very low. Research on dietary compliance reveals several interesting facts for your consideration:

- FACT—Knowing how to change a diet and why dietary changes are important seldom results in lasting change. CONCLUSION—Patients need and want more than education.

FIGURE 2-4. Sample cover letter from administration that accompanies the physician survey.

- FACT—Nutrition counselors must tailor nutrition plans to individuals, taking into account needs, environmental and cultural influences, financial resources, personal preferences, expectations, motivation, and medical and allergic repercussions. CONCLUSION—A 1/2- to 1-hour session, either in or out of the hospital, isn't the answer. Understanding these influences and making lasting changes in eating behaviors requires time and a process with many steps.
- FACT—Changing behavior requires evaluation, practice, adjustment, and self-sufficiency. CONCLUSION—Most patients cannot make changes in their eating behaviors without consistent support throughout the process, support that enables patients to become self-sufficient.

Our dietitians and marketing staff have recognized that current approaches to nutrition care do not take these important considerations into account. Therefore, the time has come to employ new strategies for dealing with changing eating habits. With your support and input, our staff of registered dietitians is committed to designing a center that offers your patients ongoing counseling and support to modify their diets. And our expectation is that this center will help you:

- Provide more comprehensive medical care;
- Improve your track record of successful treatment;
- Promote a caring image; and
- Better utilize your time.

The enclosed survey will be the cornerstone in our decision-making process. This survey will identify specific services and features of those services that you feel would be most advantageous. Please take a few minutes to fill out the survey. Your comments and suggestions will be considered earnestly.

Thank you for your time and support of our newest endeavor, the Anywhere Nutrition Center.

Sincerely,

John Doe, M.D.
Medical Director

Enclosure

FIGURE 2-4. *(Continued)*

NUTRITION SERVICES QUESTIONNAIRE

The Anywhere Hospital is establishing an outpatient nutrition counseling center. The center will be located in the Professional Medical Building adjacent to the hospital. The center will be open during the following hours: Monday-Wednesday 9:00 A.M.-6:00 P.M., Thursday-Friday, Noon-9:00 P.M. and Saturday 9:00 A.M.-1:00 P.M. To serve physicians and their patients better, we are trying to determine the kinds of programs that would meet the needs of patients and physicians. The questionnaire will require only a few minutes of your time. We appreciate your time and assistance in completing the following survey.

Instructions:

If you are in a shared practice, indicate what you will do individually. Do not respond for your entire practice.

This survey is completely anonymous. You will not be asked for your name or any identification that will associate you or your practice with your responses.

Please return this questionnaire by (date) in the enclosed, self-addressed envelope or by dropping it in the box provided in the Physicians' Lounge.

1. How do you currently provide nutrition services? (Check as many as apply.)
   - ☐ Printed materials
   - ☐ You educate and counsel
   - ☐ Nurse educates and counsels
   - ☐ Internal nutrition counselor
   - ☐ Refer to hospital-affiliated nutrition counselor
   - ☐ Refer to private practice nutrition counselor
   - ☐ Refer to community programs
   - ☐ Other/specify ______________________________

   ____

2. Assume Anywhere Nutrition Center was to offer individualized nutrition education to patients and their families on an outpatient basis. The service would be provided by appointment at the center and would follow this format:

- Two sessions would be offered as a package, scheduled approximately a week apart.
- The first session (1 hour) would be used to complete a nutrition analysis of the current diet and review the prescribed diet.
- Follow-up sessions (½ hour) would address food preparation, food shopping tips, and label reading.
- The package of two sessions at 1 ½ hours would cost $90.

FIGURE 2-5. Sample questionnaire for surveying physician use of nutrition counseling center.

- With your referral, the fee would usually be at least partially reimbursed, depending on the insurance plan.

How likely would you be to refer patients to the program?

Very likely ☐ Somewhat likely ☐ Not too likely ☐

If likely, on average, how many per month?________

If not likely, why wouldn't you refer patients to this service? (Check as many as apply.)

☐ Cost
☐ Prefer another provider
☐ Can address these needs in my own practice
☐ Location
☐ Patients won't be interested
☐ Don't need that many sessions
☐ Other/specify ____________________

____

3. Assume Anywhere Nutrition Center were to offer a series of four individual nutrition counseling sessions to patients and their families. In addition to the educational component mentioned above, these counseling sessions are designed to influence difficult behavior changes, while encouraging self-sufficiency, taking into account needs, influences, financial resources, lifestyle, and motivation. It would follow this format:

- The service would be provided at the center, by appointment.
- Participants meet once a week for four weeks.
- The first session is 1 hour and the three follow-up sessions would be 1/2 hour.
- The total cost is $150.
- With your referral, the fee would usually be at least partially reimbursed, depending on the insurance plan.

How likely would you be to refer patients to this program?

Very likely ☐ Somewhat likely ☐ Not too likely ☐

If likely, on average, how many per month?________

If not likely, why wouldn't you refer patients to this service? (Check as many as apply.)

☐ Cost
☐ Prefer another provider
☐ Can address these needs in my own practice
☐ Location
☐ Patients won't be interested
☐ Don't need four sessions
☐ Feel that group counseling is more effective than individual

FIGURE 2-5. *(Continued)*

☐ Not a priority
☐ Other/specify ______________________________

____

4. Assume that Anywhere Nutrition Center were to offer group education workshops on the nutrition topics listed below, with the following conditions:

- Services would be offered at the center.
- Workshops would be offered once a month, except where demand is greater.
- Both evening and weekday programs would be offered.
- The size of the groups—7–35 people.
- Each 1-hour program would cost $25 per participant.

Would you refer patients to these programs? Yes ☐ No ☐

If yes, indicate how many patients you would refer each month on average by placing a number in the blank next to each workshop topic:

☐ Heart-healthy eating
☐ Nutrition and cancer
☐ Low-sodium diets
☐ Guided supermarket tours
☐ Cooking classes for special diets
☐ Nutrition and osteoporosis
☐ Stress management through nutrition
☐ Other/specify ______________________________

____

If no, why wouldn't you refer patients to this service? (Check as many as apply.)

☐ Cost
☐ Prefer another provider
☐ Can address these needs in my own practice
☐ Location
☐ Patients won't be interested
☐ Feel that individual education is more effective than group
☐ Not a priority
☐ Other/specify ______________________________

____

5. Assume Anywhere Nutrition Center were to offer a series of eight group counseling sessions on each of the topics listed below. Like individual counseling, these sessions are designed to help patients make difficult changes in their eating habits. The idea exchange, group problem-solving methods, and group support benefit all members of the group. It would contain:

FIGURE 2-5. *(Continued)*

- A 1-hour individual counseling session as a prerequisite for the program, during which individual needs will be assessed and a specific diet recommended.
- A group of—7-18 members.
- Group meetings for one hour each week for 8 consecutive weeks.
- Both weekday and evening sessions offered at the center.
- All nine sessions would cost $295.
- With your referral, the fee would usually be at least partially reimbursed, depending on the insurance plan.

Would you refer patients to these programs? Yes ☐ No ☐

If yes, indicate how many patients you would refer each month on average by placing a number in the blank next to each program topic:

☐ Weight management
☐ Heart-healthy nutrition
☐ Nutrition and diabetes
☐ Nutrition and pregnancy (4 weeks only)
☐ Other/specify ______________________________

____

If no, why wouldn't you refer patients to this service? (Check as many as apply.)

☐ Cost
☐ Prefer another provider
☐ Can address these needs in my own practice
☐ Location
☐ Patients won't be interested
☐ Don't need eight sessions
☐ Feel that individual counseling is more effective than group
☐ Not a priority
☐ Other/specify ______________________________

____

6. Please rate the following factors according to the importance you place on them in choosing a nutrition services provider:

	Very Important	Somewhat Important	Not too Important	Not at all Important
Your relationship with provider	[ ]	[ ]	[ ]	[ ]
Nutrition counselor is a registered dietitian	[ ]	[ ]	[ ]	[ ]
Patient satisfaction	[ ]	[ ]	[ ]	[ ]
Evidence of compliance	[ ]	[ ]	[ ]	[ ]
Feedback to the physician	[ ]	[ ]	[ ]	[ ]

FIGURE 2-5. *(Continued)*

Direct physician involvement	[ ]	[ ]	[ ]	[ ]
Flexibility of scheduling	[ ]	[ ]	[ ]	[ ]
Practice offers computerized nutrition analysis	[ ]	[ ]	[ ]	[ ]
Ongoing support of a nutrition expert	[ ]	[ ]	[ ]	[ ]
Periodic review and updating of your nutrition materials	[ ]	[ ]	[ ]	[ ]
Tailoring nutrition plans to individual lifestyles	[ ]	[ ]	[ ]	[ ]
Reimbursability of payment	[ ]	[ ]	[ ]	[ ]

Other/specify ____

____

Comments: (Indicate the letter your comment(s) refer to.)

7. How interested do you think physicians would be in using outpatient nutrition services to:

	Very Interested	Somewhat Interested	Not too Interested	Not at all Interested
Promote a caring image?	[ ]	[ ]	[ ]	[ ]
Provide more comprehensive medical care?	[ ]	[ ]	[ ]	[ ]
Increase accuracy in your nutrition instruction?	[ ]	[ ]	[ ]	[ ]
Conserve your time?	[ ]	[ ]	[ ]	[ ]
Increase your credibility?	[ ]	[ ]	[ ]	[ ]
Improve your track record of successful treatment?	[ ]	[ ]	[ ]	[ ]

8. Check the type of practice you are in:

☐ General
☐ Family
☐ OB/GYN
☐ Cardiology
☐ Orthopedics
☐ Pediatrics
☐ Osteopathy
☐ Oncology
☐ Other

FIGURE 2-5. *(Continued)*

- New technology;
- New information that impacts healthcare;
- Economics of the community;
- Social attitudes and trends;
- New businesses that may compete; and
- Changes in healthcare institutions (mergers, specialization, expansion, etc.).

An examination of market forces allows you to take advantage of opportunities that present themselves. This can be illustrated with the following example.

> An outpatient nutrition practice is providing services to senior citizens, highlighting the role of nutrition in minimizing complications to chronic disease and/or preventing them. Just the prior week an article appeared in the *New England Journal of Medicine* that stated that nutrition is the number one factor in reducing recurrence of heart attacks in older Americans. The article spurs a nationwide media blitz. This is a market force that creates an opportunity. The practice may now consider starting a group program on nutrition and heart disease sooner than anticipated in order to take advantage of the publicity and build promotions around the current fanfare.

On the other hand, some market forces threaten the success of your practice, and knowing of them permits you to protect the practice against them. An illustration of such a market force might be a new drug on the market that allows diabetics to eat as they please without fluctuations in their blood sugar. If a nutrition practice was intending to offer group and individual counseling to diabetics, this might alter their approach, promotion, and projected start-up. The market forces that will most likely have the greatest impact on your strategies are created by the competition. Therefore, competition will be given more in-depth consideration.

Analyzing the Competition

The competition includes anyone who offers a service or product that might be purchased instead of your service/product. Your competition can sometimes be an elusive nemesis: it could be a business very similar to yours; it could be a different means of achieving the same need satisfaction; or it could be ignorance on the part of the potential clients/customers. Finding similar businesses in direct competition with your own is a fairly simple process. You can obtain information about the competition through personal contact, information from clients, and other professionals or personal experience. The more you can learn about your competitors, the easier it will be to distinguish your practice as unique. You should learn their:

- Service/product offerings;
- Target markets;

- Qualifications as service providers;
- Image in the community;
- Marketing strategies; and
- Pricing structures/fees.

Indirect competition is competition from businesses that offer other ways of satisfying the same need. These competitors may be harder to determine, but are best sought through a survey or focus group from the target market. Your marketing strategy must emphasize the weaknesses of such opponents and clearly show the superiority of your services. Health food stores, printed information, media programs, mail order products, health clubs, and those who promote misinterpreted information are all forms of indirect competition.

Finally, your ultimate competitor may be lack of knowledge. Potential clients may not understand the benefits they stand to gain from your services. Your strategies may need to aim at educating prospective clients on the need for a service by emphasizing its benefits. Not only are clients unaware of the services that you provide, but referring physicians also often lack knowledge of your service offerings. Even after clients and referring agents are aware of your services and the benefits to them, they still may not understand how your practice differs from other providers.

Surveying the competition is not as complex as surveying target markets. In fact, you can probably conduct these surveys on your own. Personal interviews with the provider are the most direct method of gathering information about the competition. However, some businesses are reluctant to reveal their strategies. Therefore, you may be forced to complete your surveys with the help of other people who have knowledge of the competitor.

A competitive analysis should be conducted on each of your major competitors. The sample competitive analysis form (shown in Fig. 2-6) can be adapted for your use. Gathering information on each point on the form may not be possible, but the more you know about the competition, the easier it will be to plan strategies.

Analyzing Your Strengths and Weaknesses

Up to this point you have gathered much information on the target markets, the market forces surrounding the practice, and the competition. Before you can actually plan the strategies that will set the practice apart, you must organize the information in a usable form—the strengths and weaknesses analysis.

The strengths and weaknesses analysis consists of four parts:

- Competitive advantages;
- Competitive disadvantages;
- Opportunities; and
- Threats.

COMPETITIVE ANALYSIS FORM

Business Name: Anywhere Hospital Date: 1/90

Address: 1000 Anyplace Avenue

Program Reference: Clinical Nutrition Manager

Director or
Nutrition Counselor: Angie Bodine

Service Program: Weight Management—a physician-monitored quick weight loss program.

Target Market: All overweight persons.

Reputation/Image: Hospital is well recognized in the community, although weight loss program has not drawn the clientele they hoped.

Location/Schedule: On hospital premises (9-5 weekdays). Screening; two 1-hour meetings per week for 4 months; maintenance—one 1-hour meeting per week for 1 month.

Price: Total program $4,000/year.

Service Provider: Physician, nurse, psychologist, dietitian.

Support Materials: Materials provided by Mint Labs, the program purveyor.

Promotion Strategies: Newspaper ads, word-of-mouth.

Payment Policy: Cash at the time of service.
Reimbursement Available: All participants have received reimbursement at a rate of 50-80%.

Competitor's Strengths: Established program; has made enough money to advertise heavily; hospital is easily accessible by public transit.

Competitor's Weaknesses: No specified target market; name not tied to institution; inflexible schedule.

FIGURE 2-6. Sample competitive analysis form.

The information gathered from the market analysis and historical data will help you compile this analysis. This analysis will lay the groundwork for marketing strategies. First, examine your competitive advantages.

Competitive Advantages

Competitive advantages range from the very specific features of your services to the availability of funds to develop and run your services. Until marketing of outpatient nutrition practices becomes more universal, one of your greatest advantages will probably be to target specific segments and tailor your services to those segments. The expertise and experience of your professional staff is also an advantage. If you are offering nutrition counseling as well as education (see Chapter 1 for differences), you may be the only outpatient nutrition facility providing this service. This is a definite strength.

Make use of the competitive analyses you have completed, as well as your knowledge about your community and institution. Then, use the following questions to guide you in determining your competitive advantages:

- What will you offer that will be perceived by the referring agent and the users as superior?
- What are your competitors' weaknesses?
- What services will you be first in the community to offer?
- What support does the community or institution offer you in contrast to other nutrition services in the area?
- What special equipment or services does the institution offer that will draw people to your services (e.g., screening equipment, shuttle service, home healthcare)?
- What special expertise or experience does your staff offer that others do not?

Competitive Disadvantages

Determining competitive advantages aids you in determining which features and benefits you should highlight in your promotional efforts. Combating competitive disadvantages may require more than promotional efforts. You may need to make changes in the ways that you will offer services or operate the business. In fact, minimizing competitive disadvantages can be a greater challenge than capitalizing on advantages is.

To embrace the extent of your competitive disadvantages, answer the following questions:

- What do the competitors offer that will be perceived by the referring agent and the users as superior?
- What services have they been the first to offer to the community?
- What support does the community and their affiliates offer the competition, in contrast to what they offer your nutrition practice?
- What special equipment or services do the competitors have access to that will draw people to their services?
- What special expertise or experience does the competition have that you and your staff do not have?

Opportunities

What factors in the market analysis can you capitalize on? Are there changes in the community that affect the business in a positive way? For example, if in a particular community the senior citizens centers have just expanded their programming to include a health topic twice a month, the outpatient nutrition counselor may see this as a key opportunity to market a new senior nutrition program. Other opportunities might include:

- Media stories that strengthen or promote your services;
- Sophisticated equipment in the practice or institution;
- Improved specialty services in the institution or affiliate;
- Support from influential people or groups; and
- A community award that might strengthen your advertising campaign.

Any factors that could enhance your service, improve your promotional efforts, or increase your business are opportunities. Look carefully at market forces and competitive advantages. The possible ways that you can use these factors to your benefit are your opportunities.

Threats

Any factor that might jeopardize your success presents a threat. Such factors include:

- Media stories that challenge your service or philosophy or the credibility of the nutrition profession;
- Strengths of the competition;
- Changes in the local healthcare market;
- Lack of support from staff, institution, or community;
- Changing reputation of the institution from good to bad; and
- Changes in medical plans of local business.

A specific example may help.

> An outpatient nutrition practice decided to develop a program to educate postmenopausal women on osteoporosis. An orthopedic group in the city recently purchased state-of-the-art equipment for bone density screening. The private practice nutrition counselor who works for this particular group is now in a perfect position to market both treatment and prevention programs through the new screening process. Therefore, the new equipment poses a threat to the outpatient nutrition practice.

Strategies must aim at minimizing threats while maximizing opportunities. You are now in a position to select services, products, and target markets and to determine the specific goals of the practice.

Chapter 3

Key Action Strategies

FINALIZE SELECTION OF SERVICES AND PRODUCTS FOR SPECIFIC TARGET MARKETS

You now have enough information to select the particular services you will market and the target markets you will pursue. Use your market research to develop services tailored to the needs and desires of the target market.

Selecting Market Segments to Target

With the data you have acquired on specific segments, you can make intelligent decisions about the groups you will target. Select those that will offer the greatest return on your investment. The determining factors in selecting market segments includes:

- Size;
- Ability to pay for nutrition services;
- Interest in nutrition services; and
- Ease with which they can be reached.

Hopefully, marketing research has confirmed your initial feelings about which markets to target. If not, some adjustments must be made. Consider the following questions:

- Is the target market interested in the services you wish to provide?
- Is the target market large enough to be lucrative?
- Are you willing to develop the services desired by the target?

- If a targeted segment is too small to prove lucrative, can you expand the target so that enough business can be generated?

Once you select specific target markets, your strategies should be focused toward those groups only. Your primary goal in selecting services then becomes meeting the needs and desires of the specific market groups.

Selecting Services and Products to Pursue

As you design nutrition services and products for your targeted segments, continue to focus on the consumers' needs and desired benefits (Ward, 1984). You may choose any combination of the seven primary services, or you may find that offering just one particular service is most profitable. This will be determined by the demand, competition, marketing methods, and the capabilities of your practice.

Besides the needs and desires of the target markets, you must consider revenue potential of the service, goals of the institution, time necessary to provide and promote each service, and your budget. For example, one nutrition practice's target segment was upper- and middle-class postpartum women who had chosen not to return to work after delivering their babies. During the surveying process, they found that this group was interested in learning to feed their babies at various ages, losing the weight gained during pregnancy, social interaction, support from other mothers, and time management. Surveys of the competition showed that this need was being addressed only through individual counseling. Based on this information, the practice decided to offer a group approach that provided education and counseling combined with a minimal number of individual sessions to tailor eating plans. This program should meet the needs of the target segment. In addition, surveys indicated that the service would draw enough business for the revenue to cover costs. The program would draw women to the hospital because the institution would then be offering complete prenatal and postnatal care.

Once you have determined primary service offerings, you may be able to identify collateral products that would interest the target segment or additional segments into which you could expand your programs (ADA, 1986). Using the example above, the postpartum women might be interested in exercise videotapes, prepackaged gourmet foods, measuring devices for portion control, and so forth. As their children get older, the nutrition practice might expand services to include a nutrition-for-toddlers program.

Products and services have life cycles. At some point, the need for nutrition education on osteoporosis may become obsolete. On the other hand, weight management programs will most likely continue to be popular for decades. Projecting the life cycle of a service or product is difficult. However, in doing so, you can introduce new services as old ones are phased out. In this manner, you allow for periods of development and marketing for each service. Also, as one service declines in profitability, another will be reaching its peak and generating a relatively constant income. Remember, the strategic plan is a living document that changes in response to clients and the environment. Once you have chosen services and target markets, you are ready to refine the goals you established at the onset.

SET GOALS

Unlike your mission statement, which was broad and all encompassing, goals provide specific direction to the practice. Both financial and nonfinancial goals should be defined. Initially goals may be fairly general. Ultimately, each goal will specify a time frame, dollar amounts, and/or numbers where applicable. Consider the primary and secondary reasons for the business to exist, profit objectives, service objectives, and the reasons you would contemplate terminating the business (ADA, 1986). You will have both financial and nonfinancial goals.

Financial Goals

Financial goals relate directly to the monetary needs and expectations of the practice. The following questions will help you define them:

- How much income does the practice need to generate to provide for future needs?
- What does the institution expect from the practice?
- At what point in time must the practice break even (income = expenses)?
- What financial factors will be considered grounds for changing or terminating the business?
- When and for how long will various services be expected to earn a profit?
- Will major investments in equipment be necessary over time (computers, screening devices, etc.)?
- How much profit would make it worthwhile to make the commitment?

Nonfinancial Goals

Although non-financial goals may have an indirect relationship to financial goals, they are not defined in monetary terms. Some such goals can be addressed by answering the following questions:

- How does the practice expect to serve the institution and/or community?
- What image does the practice hope to gain from the market?
- What share of the market does the practice expect to obtain?
- What expansions or improvements does the practice expect over time?

- How many new clients per a specified time period will be required to maintain the business?

The case study (Chapter 4) provides an example of the goals set by an outpatient nutrition practice.

DETERMINE KEY STRATEGIES

With all of your data in hand, you are prepared to develop strategies that will form the cornerstone of your success. Your plan should answer the following questions:

- How will you ensure that goals will be met?
- How will you capitalize on opportunities?
- How will you reduce risks and threats?
- How will you position the practice in the market?
- What time frame will you use for evaluation?

As you develop the specifics of your services, you will begin to project needs for staff, equipment, materials, and, ultimately, finances. Although the section on financial projections follows this one, you will quickly learn that you must work with strategies and finances simultaneously, making adjustments in both as you progress. An example follows.

> Suppose you decide to offer group education programs for senior citizens. You realize that transportation to your current location is not readily available. Therefore, your strategy includes working out of locations in several neighborhood centers. As you calculate the costs of renting space, traveling, and equipment, you realize that the program will be very costly. You then adjust the strategy by deciding on the two locations that provide for your equipment needs and are accessible and affordable.

Positioning and Marketing Mix

Positioning is the strategy of differentiating your services from those sold by the competition, by determining or creating what your client or referring agent wants or needs and then managing your practice accordingly. The process is complex and requires a good knowledge of the target market and an appropriate selection of services. Providing service in a desirable location and pricing so that you deliver value at reasonable rates are also positioning strategies. Positioning to attract clients requires that you promote your services in a manner that will reach your audience and evaluate the outcome of your efforts regularly.

An example may help.

> During their initial marketing research, an outpatient nutrition practice that offers nutrition services to the healthy community was limited to an educational

program in the local hospital. They decided to target community members who were involved in fitness programs, and surveyed this population in two area health clubs and the YMCA. They found that the greatest perceived needs of this group were weight management, nutrition for peak performance in athletic competitions, and good nutrition for busy people.

The practice decided that they would begin by offering group programs for weight management and peak performance and expand over time. As the survey population noted that convenience of location and timing would be key in their decision to join such programs, the practice developed agreements with one of the health clubs and the YMCA to provide services on site during the times when the most adults were present in the sites. An office was provided for individual consultations, and classrooms were available. As a further measure of convenience, clients could sign up for programs at the facility, as well as by calling the nutrition office for appointments.

A competitive price was established that reflected the value of nutrition programs as comparable to other programs offered within the facilities. Promotion was accomplished through the member newsletters, posters within the facilities, and personal selling through instructors at the sites and physical therapists and dietitians at the hospital. The message of all advertisements were composed to appeal directly to this group.

Six months after implementing the program, an evaluation was conducted. The practice found that competitive athletes were not interested in group programs and responded better in one-on-one counseling. Therefore, the practice shifted their services to meet that need. The weight management program was progressing nicely, but the need to develop support groups arose and a plan was developed to implement such a program. The practice also decided to expand their services by marketing to a third facility.

As you can see, the practice mentioned above positioned themselves by selecting appropriate services, localities, prices, marketing media, and conveniences to a very select group of people. They paid careful attention to market research and reevaluated their services regularly. Throughout the following section, you will be able to gather positioning ideas related to each facet of the market mix.

Service Offerings

Often, the most effective strategy for establishing a position in the market is *be there first*. Being the first to offer a product or service provides an advantage over those who may later enter the market and will force your competition to work around your practice. However, being first may cost you more in time and resources to educate the public on the service and to promote it. If you select services offered by the competition, try a new twist or approach. For instance, computerized nutrition analysis programs are becoming a popular means of generating revenue. To separate your practice from the competition, you might offer a service package that includes the computerized nutrition analysis and four brown bag lunch seminars.

The key is to apply creative and innovative approaches in providing products and services that will place the practice in a leadership position in this competitive marketplace. Remember that what works today may not work tomorrow. Therefore, continuous appraisal of your product mix is vital to long-term success. Personal feedback, current customer flow, waiting lists, program evaluations, and satisfaction surveys are all ways to continuously evaluate your services.

Location of the Services

Issues in determining a location include accessibility, environment, and appearance of the facility. Level or quality of services being offered also have a bearing on choosing a location.

You may choose a central location for services or several branches, depending on the geographic and demographic information you have gathered and what your positioning strategy is. If you are dealing with a population that is not particularly mobile (e.g., senior citizens or handicapped), you will want to locate your services at a common meeting place or a place close to their homes. Accessibility also encompasses the ease with which your outlet can be reached. One particular outpatient practice was located so deeply within the hospital that clients literally needed a guide to find it. An outside entrance directly into the point of service and in close proximity to the parking lot is ideal.

The level and quality of services affect all aspects of location in regard to the position you wish to hold in the marketplace. If you are serving an upper-class market, the accessibility, environment, and appearance must all be optimum. If you are serving an outpatient clinic where half of your clients are handicapped, you may be more concerned about accessibility and a comfortable environment than about the aesthetics of the surroundings. Some points that will enhance the quality of your services are:

- Parking accessibility and security;
- Privacy of counseling facilities;
- Adequate space for group programs; and
- Availability of proper equipment.

Healthy clients may be resistant to visiting the hospital or clinic for nutrition services. They may associate such places with illness or past painful experiences. Therefore, other points of service might be explored. Although outpatient services have been administered in the hospital kitchen, cafeteria, or nutrition office, these are not adequate environments for counseling. These settings are unprofessional.

The environment should be comfortable for both the client and counselor and free from interruptions (Ward, 1984).

The appearance of the facility used in delivering services creates an image that affects client attitude and behavior. When considering location, factors such as color, neatness, cleanliness, condition of the rooms, furnishings, and space should be considered. Ask yourself:

- Will this setting have a positive affect on my clients?
- Is it large enough for the services I am offering?
- Is it a pleasant atmosphere?
- Is it comfortable?
- Does it compare favorably with offices of other health care professionals?

Institutions offer credibility and a broad referral base. You may choose to offer services at various other locations even though you are sponsored by the institution. Use the institution's name in the name of your practice. Focus group interviews conducted with physicians and business people indicated that association with an institution significantly increases credibility. Although 95 percent of referrals currently being made to institutional outpatient practices are from physicians, you are not limited to this referral base. Nurses, physical therapists, and social workers are all good sources of referrals.

A very difficult barrier to overcome is the perception of the value of nutrition services. This perception will not only affect the location where services are provided, but also the price and promotion of services. Often, these perceptions are formulated on the basis of the quality of inpatient services and the rapport built with physicians and nursing staff. Therefore, you may find that changing the institution's perception is the largest stumbling block you will encounter.

If you provide services within the institution, be sensitive to the accessibility to your area of service. Every effort should be made to avoid traipsing your clients through areas of the institution where patients are treated. Negotiate for an office that is yours alone, or a conference room specifically for nutrition counseling, so that you will be able to provide confidentiality to your clients. When sharing facilities for group programs, establish permanent times that you will be using that space, and try to eliminate interruptions before they occur.

Several alternatives to hospital locations exist, including worksites, private offices, the client's home, or shopping malls. Two options that merit further discussion are physician's offices or clinics and community facilities (public or private).

Physician's offices and clinics offer a referral base, physician satisfaction, a built-in administrative staff, and a preexisting location that is conducive to medical services. However, when questioned, counselors affiliated with institutions who had provided services in a physician's office or clinic stated that the cons far outweighed the pros. Generally, these dietitians were paid a fee per hour for an agreed upon time each week or month, and the physician charged his or her patients so that he or she would make a profit for the nutrition services offered. For example, the physician paid the nutrition counselor $40.00 per hour. He or she charged $60.00 for the first visit (1 hour) and $30.00 for follow-up visits (15–20 minutes). The nutrition practice would hardly break even once salary, fringe benefits, and loss of time traveling to and from the physician's office were calculated into costs.

Another disadvantage of providing services in the physician's offices is that physicians maintain control over the quality and type of service provided by the dietitian. Also, if you market services through one physician at a low rate in order to get your practice started, others will expect the same low rate. Although a physician may guarantee payment for the specified time period whether or not the counselor sees clients, more revenue might be gained by seeing clients in a group or by charging the physician's rate in another location.

Experience shows that physicians who are interested in establishing nutrition services within their practices are those with large referral bases. Once nutrition services are established within the physician's office and these physicians are making a profit, institutional nutrition practices seldom survive because the referral base becomes limited. These physicians will view the institutional services as competition.

Avoid allowing the physician or clinic to control your activities and fee schedules. Establish an agreement to keep the physician from hiring the institutional nutrition counselor himself or herself. Agreement to prevent the physician from terminating services at a moment's notice are also important so that a conflict of interest does not result. If you do decide to base your services in a physician's office or clinic, some physicians may be enticed by a fee for renting space or support staff time. *Contractual agreements are imperative to such situations.*

You should also be aware of the federal and various state fraud and abuse statutes relating to patients receiving government medical payment assistance. The fraud and abuse statutes prohibit, among other things, a medical service provider from soliciting, receiving, offering to pay, or paying any remuneration (including any kickback, bribe, or rebate) in return for referring an individual to another for the furnishing of any service.

Subletting may be an option in clinics and physicians offices. In this case, they are leasing the building/offices and you rent space from them. In many cases, practitioners find it more practical to share space for group programs at the onset and consider renting added space as the program grows. However, a large practice (three or more counselors) may find the space for group programs useful for meetings and promotional activities, allowing them to use the space to its full potential.

Community facilities can be prime locations for nutrition services and may be available for nominal rent. Some possible contacts would be community centers, YMCA/YWCAs, senior citizen centers, schools, colleges and universities, park departments, public libraries, and churches.

Price

Valuing and pricing products and services properly may be the most important set of decisions you will make. Selling price is cost and market sensitive. The price you place on any service or product will also be directly related to your mission statement. What are the objectives of your pricing strategy?

A nutrition counseling practice is likely to be a combination of products and services catering to different markets. The pricing approach would, therefore, be a combination of pricing objectives and strategies. Setting specific prices considers four factors:

1. Cost;
2. Demand;
3. Competition; and
4. Desired return.

Each of these considerations deserves further review.

Cost Cost considerations are important no matter what your objectives. Beyond salary and benefits are developmental costs, operating expenses, equipment and materials, and overhead. When calculating costs, you must be sure to include these "hidden costs" or else suffer from a reduced profit margin. Pricing is often based on "billable" hours. Billable hours are the hours it takes to perform a specific service. For worksite clients, what is billable is usually agreed upon at the onset of the project or contract. Keep in mind that there is a dramatic difference between the amount of time necessary to provide a service and the time spent with a client (Rose 1986). Therefore, projects must be estimated at full cost and priced accordingly. Before you can understand the formula for pricing services in this manner, you must first be exposed to the following terms and their definitions:

- Salary—Annual rate of pay.
- Fringe benefits—The dollar value of employee insurance, vacation time, and benefits of employment upon which a value can be placed. Benefits range from 25 percent to 40 percent of salary.
- Productive hours—The time spent generating revenues such as counseling, presenting programs, and screening. (Productive hours average about 1600 per year or 32 per week.)
- Overhead—All costs involved in maintaining and operating the business, usually calculated as 150 percent of salary and benefits (office, phone, housekeeping, etc.).
- Profit—The amount you intend to make after all costs are covered. A fair profit in the service industry would be 20 to 30 percent of total costs.

The following is the pricing formula, based on cost, that is most often suggested by large accounting firms.

Formula:

(SALARY % PRODUCTIVE HOURS) + FRINGE BENEFITS + OVERHEAD + PROFIT = HOURLY RATE

WHERE: FRINGE BENEFITS = SALARY × BENEFIT (AS A PERCENTAGE)
OVERHEAD = (SALARY + BENEFITS) × 1.5

PROFITS = (SALARY + BENEFITS + OVERHEAD) × DESIRED PROFIT %

Example:

Salary	=	\$20,000	
Productive Hours	=	1,600 =	
		20,000 ÷ 1,600 =	\$12.50
Fringe Benefits	=	12.50 ×.25 =	3.13
Overhead	=	(12.50 + 3.13) × 1.5 =	23.43
Profit	=	(12.50 + 3.13 + 23.43) ×.30 =	11.71
		Total	50.77
		or	\$50.00/Hr.

Demand Demand for your services depends upon your marketing ability and the image you create. Prices create a perception or expectation about the level of service and its benefits in the minds of clients. Prices set too low or services or products given away diminish perceived value. It will become increasingly important to stop "giving away" products and services. Rather, find a fair value and confidently promote the level of service, quality, and benefits associated with the product. Success and profitability are not determined strictly by the number of clients in a program. Therefore, if prices are too low, higher volume can increase losses.

Prices are influenced by the socioeconomic character of the community. If your services are offered primarily to persons of lower economic status, you should consider:

- Tailoring services to reduce costs. (Be careful not to limit necessary services. Xeroxing materials, eliminating promotional costs, and eliminating computer analysis would all be acceptable options.)
- Marketing services to a different clientele.
- Using more group programs and less individual counseling and education.
- Not going into this particular business.

Wise nutrition counselors will look at reimbursement during their marketing efforts, but they will not allow reimbursement to dictate pricing. Presently, very few outpatient nutrition services are being paid for by insurance, medicaid, or medicare. As more outpatient practitioners and their clients pursue reimbursement, more nutrition services may be covered by these plans. If you promote your programs and products as valuable health care commodities, people will be willing to pay the fair price. Then, reimbursement will only increase the satisfaction of an already satisfied client.

Competition Competition is an extremely important variable in determining price of services. You cannot legally discuss price with others offering similar nutrition services in your area and agree upon rates to charge. However, you can look at various rates for particular services to determine where you want to position yourself among the competition. You might also check the rates of other health professionals (e.g., psychologists, physical therapist).

The independent practitioner often has little overhead and purchases limited amounts of fringe benefits. Therefore, the independent practitioner may be able to offer services at a lower price and gain the same amount of profit as the institutional practice. On the other hand, the institutional practice will be able to market the benefits of additional resources as the rationale for a higher price.

For instance, the institutional practice might offer a quick weight loss program with medical monitoring for the obese client, plus a weight management program for those who have smaller amounts of weight to lose, whereas the private practitioner without physician or some financial support would have difficulty managing and financing both programs.

If you price the service at the low end of the market, your services may be perceived as lower quality (or lower value) than the competition. However, you will need to consider whether your reputation will bring in clients if you price yourself at the upper end of the market (Helm, 1987).

Desired Return Desired return implies that you expect financial reward in return for services beyond coverage for expenses. In some instances, you and/or your institution may decide that a break-even price is adequate because you expect other benefits for offering the service. For instance, a nutrition fair may provide exposure and the opportunity to promote another program. You may sell frozen entrees at a low cost to clients who are members of your weight loss program as an enticement to join the class.

In other cases, your goal may be profit. You may actually determine the desired amount of profit as a first step in formulating the price.

Formula:

(DESIRED SALARY + EXPENSES) ÷ BILLABLE HOURS = HOURLY RATE

Let's look at a price formula based on the desired return of a practice with one counselor whose expenses are fairly low.

Desired salary + expenses: $60,000
Billable hours:

(Based on a 40-hour week)	
Hours per year	2080 hours
2 weeks vacation	-80 hours
1 week sick leave	-40 hours
1 week paid time off	-40 hours
Marketing (10%)	-200 hours
Administration (12%)	-220 hours
Billable hours	1500 hours

Therefore: $60,000/1500 hours = $40.00/hour

Fee Structure

A discussion of pricing would not be complete without some basic information on fee structures. The most common fee structures now in use by outpatient nutrition practices are time factor pricing, unit of service, and package pricing. However, other fee arrangements can be very satisfying to both the practice and the client. Let's explore all the options.

Time Factor Pricing Time factor pricing sets a price on the amount of time required to provide a service. A situation where time factor pricing might be effective is in the worksite setting. A charge of $70.00/hour might be charged for time spent at the worksite. If a physician contracts your services, an hourly rate prevents loss of income due to cancellations and "slow" days. The general public is resistant to this method of pricing (Rose, 1986). When time factor pricing is used, caution must be taken to give a consistent amount of service in a specific amount of time. If one counselor spends an hour during the initial session and another spends an hour and a half, clients will begin to compare notes and realize the difference in price.

Many pioneer practitioners have offered a word of caution. Using a per-hour rate rather than a half- or full-day rate can be a significant profit drain unless this price is high enough to cover all costs. Preparation, administration, and travel time should be included in the cost.

Unit of Service Pricing Unit of service pricing is more familiar to the general public because the majority of physicians use this method of pricing. In unit of service pricing, each service is given a set price (e.g., $40.00 for an initial counseling session and $25.00 for each follow-up session). Cost accounting is more difficult when unit of service pricing is used because services to individual clients may take varying amounts of time and nonproductive time must somehow be accounted for (Rose, 1986). One way to deal with the time issue is to set limits on the time that counselors will spend with the client. You may want to explore the unit prices of other professionals, such as psychologists.

Package Pricing Package pricing has proven to be very effective in outpatient practices. In package pricing, a set of services is priced as a whole. A group weight management program with eight group sessions and two individual sessions would be package priced, and even individual counseling sessions can be packaged (three sessions for $75). One of the great advantages to packaging programs is that the nutrition counselors can gain a greater commitment to continue services from clients who have already paid for them. You are also guaranteed payment for services whether or not the client returns. This arrangement is quite pleasing to the client who wants to know what the total cost for services will be (ADA, 1986). As for accounting, all costs can be built into the package price.

Per-head Pricing Per-head pricing is a method often used in workshops, educational programs, or speaking engagements where a larger organization is paying for the services (worksite group, HMO, community organization, etc.). When charging a per-head rate, you must protect the practice by requesting payment for the minimum number of participants estimated, no matter how many attend. Or you can charge a flat fee for the program and a per-head fee for any participants in excess of an agreed upon number (ADA, 1986). If the practice is being paid a per-head rate for multiple sessions, guard against dropouts by basing the price on the first session's attendance.

Retainers Retainers are fees paid for agreed upon services that are normally based on time and expertise. Retainers are appropriate if an organization (health club or clinic) wishes to utilize a nutrition counselor's services, but cannot offer steady income from fee-for-service arrangements. Under a retainer, the practice is paid to have a nutrition counselor available a certain number of hours per month. The practice would be paid for that time whether or not services were used. Your contract or written agreement should state that the practice would receive an additional fee in those months when counselors work more than the agreed upon hours.

Project Pricing Project pricing is less common in outpatient practices, but might be feasible in worksite programs. You would propose a fee for an entire project (possibly a nutrition fair, a series of activities for nutrition month, or a consultation service to improve the healthy food choices in a food service). In quoting a project price, you risk underestimating the cost of the project. Worksite clients, however, like project pricing because they can compare with competitors more easily (ADA, 1986).

Price Adjustments

No matter what your pricing strategies are, you will need to evaluate them on a regular basis and adjust prices accordingly. Clients may expect incremental increases in fees, but they often feel betrayed and become angry when price increases are significant. When setting prices, anticipate increasing costs and market trends so as not to require frequent price adjustments.

When making adjustments, anticipate how the affected parties will react and be prepared to discuss the reasons. Consider these approaches to price adjustments:

- Change prices across the board—Add 10 percent to all services offered.
- Adjust individual programs—Increase the price of the Risk Reduction Program, and market improved services or add a new section.
- Add a higher priced program—Rather than raising the price of the Risk Reduction program, change it somewhat, rename it, and market it at a higher price.
- Sell products and services previously given away—Place a value on professionally printed materials.

Many practices made the decision to build a clientele without charging for services. Then, once the client base was established, they began to charge a fee. This approach is strongly discouraged. Clients angered by fees charged for services they perceive should be free do not return, and a whole new client base must be established. When you provide services for little or no fee, you create the perception of low value with your clients and the community.

Worksite Pricing

Pricing telegraphs the most significant difference between worksite and other types of nutrition services. Specifically, the message is:

Pricing—stop—Reconsider your current approach—stop—Pricing for worksite nutrition services are not tied in any way to reimbursement—stop—If by "low cost benefit" you mean low pricing, Stop—stop.

For most nutrition practitioners, a reference point for pricing is reimbursement. *This is not so for worksite services.* Businesses understand profitability and expect to pay a market price for the services. Usually, your fees will be compared to the cost of other health care benefits and, if applicable, your competitors' fees. The Employee Benefit Research Institute recently indicated that the average cost of all health care benefits is 16 percent of total compensation (*Benefits Today*, 1989). A recent study of manufacturing organizations indicated that "the cost of providing health insurance represented an average of 37% of profit." (*Wall Street Journal*, 1989) Comparatively speaking, nutrition services are a "low-cost benefit."

Another pricing advantage associated with the worksite is the opportunity to use guarantees. If your fees are based on a certain number of participants, be sure to ask the organization to guarantee the participation level. If the level of participation is lower than expected, the organization would pay for the difference between the participants attending and those guaranteed to attend.

Be sure to consider the following costs associated specifically with the worksite when determining fees:

- Expenses—Phone calls, proposal assembly and materials, administrative costs, and travel costs.

- Cost of time may include:
  - Time to sell the account;
  - Proposal development time;
  - Time to administer surveys;
  - Time tabulating and summarizing surveys;
  - Preview sessions;
  - Service delivery time;
  - Downtime between appointments or activities;
  - Setup/dismantle time;
  - Meeting time;
  - Record-keeping time;
  - Phone time;
  - Travel time; and
  - Time dedicated to nurturing the client relationship.

Some experienced worksite practitioners have suggested that it is wise to inflate the cost of time by an additional 25 to 30 percent to account for unanticipated time needs.

- If surveys are administered and/or results are tabulated and summarized by an outside agency, their fees must be considered.
- Program materials.
- Promotions—Buy-one-get-one-free coupons, giveaways, gift certificates, discounts, and so forth.)
- Competitions and associated materials.
- Incentives built into fees. (For example, if weight groups are offered partial reimbursement for achieving their goal-weight and the organization is not subsidizing this, fees should be inflated to account for the incentive.)

Since there are many alternative ways to provide services, knowing the client's budget before you propose services and fees is helpful. Some prospective clients will be cryptic about the amount of money they are willing to spend for your services. Usually, they are concerned that their budget may be more lucrative than the services warrant. They don't want to influence you to increase your fee. If appropriate, directly ask clients what they are willing to spend, then tailor your services to that amount. You will lose credibility if you state a price and then you lower it based on their reaction.

Not every organization can afford or is willing to pay your standard fee, nor do you want every opportunity you consider. The most financially successful practices seek out business that is the most profitable use of their time rather than compromise pricing. When you finish estimating the fees for each worksite opportunity, ask:

"Could I spend this time more profitably somewhere else?"

If your answer is "no," you probably want to proceed. If the answer is "yes," you have three viable options:

- Increase your price to make it worth the time investment.
- Decline the opportunity to provide services, and spend time either finding or performing more profitable work.
- Make a conscious choice to reduce profit potential because there is a payoff that makes it worthwhile for you (e.g., opportunity for additional community visibility, more profitable referral business, experience).

Don't make a habit of exercising the third option. You may not be in business in the long run if you can't pay your bills in the short term.

When a price is submitted to your prospective clients, it is best not to itemize costs or show the profit margin. This invites them to scrutinize your fee calculation or to bargain on a partial package that won't cover all costs. Instead, if you suspect that a client is going to haggle or reject your services based on costs, you might present a flat fee with some potential ways to reduce costs. Copayment by employers and employees will reduce the burden of the employer. Copayment also increases the value of the service to the employee, while sending a message of commitment from the employer. Some prospective clients may prefer to assume more of the administrative responsibilities (administering surveys, tabulating surveys, coordinating activities, room set-up, appointment scheduling, etc.). Obviously, providing facilities and equipment could reduce costs, or you could suggest that the client print handout materials internally.

You can make decisions to reduce costs, too. As you analyze the options, be careful not to compromise professionalism, rapport building, quality, or the perception of quality. Some common methods to reduce costs include altering the services or performing the contract in fewer hours. Reduce break periods, administrative time, and downtime used as a cushion between service periods. Control the use of time in performing services. Find ways to make fewer trips to the worksite.

Review materials. Are they all necessary? Could some be available by purchase only? Could the same message be sent effectively with less expensive audiovisual aids? Ask yourself and your staff: "Are there cheaper ways to deliver the same message in an interesting way to groups without compromising quality?"

Local universities or colleges may be helpful in reducing costs. Professors are always open to special projects that students might complete for hands-on experience. Consolidated job responsibilities and reduced staff are also possibilities for curtailing costs. Food demonstrations and audiovisuals may also be eliminated.

While flexibility is the name of the game, consistency is important too! Consistency here means that you may have several approaches to pricing—flat rate, per-hour rate, and so on—but you establish a pricing policy that is applied to all worksites. If there are good reasons to make exceptions, build the exceptions into the pricing policy. You don't want two clients chatting over an Elks Dinner to be comparing prices if you haven't been consistent. A carefully considered pricing policy is an excellent tool for you as well.

It is wise to build annual rate increases into the schedule in advance. The amount of increase may vary from year to year, based on market rates, inflation, or increased costs. This enables you to use the proposed rate schedule in estimating fees in the worksite sales process.

Promotion

Promotion refers to marketing efforts designed to;

- Increase awareness of the services or products;
- Persuade current clients to use more of the services or products;
- Persuade users of competitive services to use your services; and
- Remind past and potential clients that your services are still available.

Promotion can be seen as a series of communication activities that influence attitudes, knowledge, and consumer behavior (Ward, 1984). The medium for communication, message content, and the format of the message are all based on consumer needs (Parks and Moody, 1986).

Perhaps the most complex strategy in positioning the practice is that of promotion. You must be able to show the target market why your services fit their particular needs better than the competition can. Your promotional strategies should reach out and grab potential clients and leave no doubt as to whom your target audience is. Ask yourself the following questions:

- What services or products do we provide to address a perceived need that the competition does not?
- What expertise, experience, or skills can we offer to address a perceived need that the competition cannot?
- What unique resources or conveniences can we offer that would cause a client to choose our services over others? In other words, what sets our practice apart?
- How can we ensure that our target audience will understand the benefits of the product or service offerings?

While overall promotional strategies must be developed at this point, the promotional planning and development are detailed closer to start-up. Consequently, you will find more extensive information on promotion provided in the section entitled "Promoting Your Practice" in Chapter 7.

Staffing

Determining the kind and number of staff you will need is very important in planning strategies. If you have planned to start new services over the three-year time frame, be sure to forecast the need for more staff as these services grow.

As you develop strategies, your main concerns with staffing are:

- What kinds of personnel (managers, nutrition counselors, support staff) does the practice require?
- How many positions are needed to run the business successfully?
- What level of expertise and experience will be required?
- What salary level will be required to attract and maintain such personnel?

Take a closer look at the types of staff you may need.

Administrative Support Staff (Receptionists/Secretaries)

In deciding on the type and amount of administrative support you will need, you must look carefully at:

- How much time will you require from an assistant?
- How many hours per day must someone else cover the phone(s)?
- What duties will you expect this person to carry out?
- Will there be much public exposure involved?
- How much paper work is involved?

Once you have answered these questions, look at the options. Many practitioners begin with an answering machine or service and some contract clerical services. On the other hand, you may realize that you need a part- or full-time employee to handle the office so that you and your staff's time is spent counseling, developing, or marketing.

Practices in the institution often locate offices in the dietary department or affiliated outpatient clinic. Phone calls may filter through diet clerks, other dietitians, and clinic staff. These people are very busy and may not be attuned to your services and schedule. Many times messages are lost, forgotten, or difficult to decipher. Prospective clients who cannot obtain information from those answering your phone will not be impressed and may look elsewhere for nutrition services. Staff your practice to prevent such unpleasant effects.

Nutrition Counselors

Although the nutrition counselor is the most critical factor in delivering service and maintaining the business, past experience reveals many mistakes in staffing. Commonly, outpatient programs were an extension of the inpatient department. Clinical dietitians were asked to share the responsibility of outpatient counseling, or one particular dietitian was to split her time between inpatient and outpatient services. The outpatient programs suffered due to excessive clinical hours.

Rotating nutrition counselors through the outpatient practice is also detrimental to the business. Once a client establishes rapport with a counselor, his or her success in changing behavior often hinges on the continuation of that relationship. Clients are reluctant to "spill their guts" to more than one counselor, and counselors must often start from the beginning to fully understand the client's progress. Therefore, the counseling process never progresses when more than one counselor is involved.

Such historical information indicates that nutrition counselors chosen for outpatient nutrition practices should be educated and experienced in the field of nutrition in wellness, as well as in nutrition and disease, and dedicated to the provision of outpatient nutrition services. More information on hiring nutrition counselors along with job dimensions and descriptions can be found in Chapters 6 and 7.

Outpatient Nutrition Managers

If you are in practice alone, you are the manager, counselor, and possibly your own receptionist. As the practice grows or if you begin with a larger practice, someone must take the responsibility of managing the practice. In many institutions, the clinical nutrition manager manages both the outpatient and the inpatient practice. This was not a difficult task when outpatient services were offered relatively free of charge. Now the duties of the outpatient nutrition manager are much greater.

These duties include:

- Managing financial resources;
- Promoting services and products;
- Public relations with clients, physicians, and purveyors;
- Monitoring the practice;
- Updating policies and procedures to meet regulations;
- Orienting new staff; and
- Supervising staff.

In small practices, the nutrition counselor can divide his or her time between managing and counseling. But over time, these responsibilities will eat into counseling hours and more staff will be necessary. Programs such as quick weight loss require a full-time nutrition manager very early in the program.

Scheduling

Providing service at convenient hours is essential. Since many of your clients will be working people, some evening and Saturday hours will be necessary. Often, practices find it necessary to staff the phones during regular work hours for convenience of physicians making referrals and clients scheduling appointments. However, the nutrition counselor need not be present during all of those hours.

If the practice includes more than one counselor, you might consider staggering the hours the counselor works. This sample schedule may help explain:

Sample Schedule

	Counselor I	Counselor II
Monday	12:00 P.M.–8:00 P.M.	8:00 A.M.–4:00 P.M.
Tuesday	12:00 P.M.–8:00 P.M.	8:00 A.M.–4:00 P.M.
Wednesday	8:00 A.M.–4:00 P.M.	12:00 P.M.–8:00 P.M.
Thursday	8:00 A.M.–4:00 P.M.	12:00 P.M.–8:00 P.M.
Friday	8:00 A.M.–4:00 P.M.	8:00 A.M.–4:00 P.M.
Saturday	10:00 A.M.–2:00 P.M. (every 1st Saturday)	10:00 A.M.–2:00 P.M. (every 3rd Saturday)

The more regular the schedule, the easier it will be for clients to schedule follow-up appointments.

TRANSLATE YOUR PLANS INTO DOLLARS AND CENTS

The majority of health care providers see their primary work responsibilities as tending to the physical and emotional well-being of their clients. Much further down their list of priorities come the financial aspects of providing this care. That responsibility has been left to the health care administrators. However, these traditional roles are changing. Department heads are finding it necessary to justify the care and the resulting cost it incurs. This justification must be based not only on the benefit to the patient's health, but also on the financial benefit it brings the institution.

Attention to the financial realities of health care is very important to emerging services, for these services will never gain the support of the institution if they are seen as still another drain on financial resources. Institutions are offering optional patient services only if they will generate revenue.

This section focuses on the financial planning necessary for your strategic plan. However, be prepared to continue extensive financial analysis of the nutrition practice. This analysis will guide your practice toward those services that meet the needs of your clients, because the better the financial viability of your practice, the better chance it will survive. The institution's accountants can help you prepare the necessary financial analyses for your business plan. They may also be able to suggest computer software that will simplify the ongoing financial analysis of your practice.

At a minimum, four basic forms of financial analysis must be presented as a part of your plan for an outpatient nutrition practice. Each one will be discussed at length. They are:

1. Profit and loss projections;
2. Cash flow;
3. Balance sheet; and
4. Break-even analysis.

The first three forms of analyses will become financial statements that you will use to report and monitor the financial success of the business. These statements will be prepared on a regular basis. Break-even analysis is usually performed at the onset of a business, service, or product, as well as when any changes occur in price, costs, or distribution.

All four types of analyses require that you know what revenue and expenses you expect over the period for which the projections are being made. Therefore, you should develop an estimate of revenue and an expense worksheet for your own use, detailing the costs of everything from setting up the office to performing the various services. As you will see in the following descriptions, the expenses fit into each form of analyses in very different ways. Before describing each form of financial analysis, the most common expenses a nutrition practice has require definition.

Start-up Cash Outlays and Expenses

Before the practice begins to function, many expenses will be incurred. Some of these expenses are one time at the onset. Others occur at start-up and then again as the business grows and more staff, supplies, and equipment are needed. Still others are incurred on a regular basis. The following list attempts to describe the basic categories of expenses for an outpatient nutrition practice.

Rent or Overhead Rent or overhead is dependent upon where you choose to offer your services and operate your business. Often, practices are established within the institution and later move to a location that better serves their market. Therefore, you may want to plan the expense of renting space into your initial budget. If utilities are paid separately from rent, they must also be considered.

Overhead includes much more than rent. Whereas rent is the price of space and possibly utilities, overhead includes all the services that are part of maintaining and operating the institution. If you had to pay the full cost of these services, you would never start into business. However, these costs are spread over all the departments within the institution. Institutional nutrition practitioners may not be charged directly for the space they use within the institution. Your finance department will be able to explain how overhead is dealt with in your facility.

At the onset, consider sharing space with other departments in the institution. Administrators in health care facilities are now forced to compare health care services and select those that will generate the greatest revenue per square foot of space used. Following is an example:

> The Food and Nutrition Services Department submits a proposal for an outpatient nutrition service that will utilize a section of a vacant medical wing. At the same time, hospital administrators are looking at opening a fertility clinic and/or a sports medicine center. The proposal for the fertility clinic forecasts the

greatest income in the smallest amount of space and is approved. The department resubmits their proposal, offering to share space with the Prenatal Clinic, which only runs three days per week. The practice will now generate revenue in space where the hospital was previously losing money.

Equipment Equipment is purchased at the start-up of the business and when new services are added or the clientele grows to a certain point. Large equipment includes:

- Furniture;
- Electronic equipment (computers, answering machines, etc.);
- Audiovisual equipment; and
- Medical equipment (medical scales, sphygmomanometer, etc.).

Many nutrition professionals have found that they can cut the cost of furniture and equipment by using what is available in the institution. A scavenger hunt through the facility may uncover unused desks, tables, and chairs. Select those that are in good repair and be sure the furniture matches to some degree. The cost of servicing old audiovisual and medical equipment may be cheaper than purchasing something new.

If you purchase new equipment, you may be offered service contracts once the warranty ends. A separate expense line will be required to express these costs. Small items must be included in your expense budget under direct expenses or office supplies. Calculators, clocks, and computer disc storage are examples of such equipment.

Program Licensure Fees Program licensure fees tend to be quite high, but offer some features that can be of great benefit. Usually, a commercial program that expects a licensure fee offers training, supportive data for your marketing presentation, and continued monitoring of the program. Often, computer software is available through the commercial organization for ease of record keeping and accounting.

Labor Costs Labor costs must be considered for counselors, managers, and administrative support personnel. You must work with your human resources department to learn the cost of benefits and the salaries that would be offered. A separate expense line may be needed to address the cost of recruiting nutrition professionals. Be sure that the institution has malpractice coverage; otherwise, you may need to purchase it for yourself and your professional staff.

Supplies Supplies can be divided into several categories. Paper goods, pens, staples, and so on, are all considered office supplies. You may include printed educational materials, business cards, and brochures as supplies. However, be aware that there will be separate charges for the initial development of these items that must be included in your expenses.

Medical or lab supply costs will be incurred if the program requires medical screening and/or monitoring. If you choose to do demonstrations in your educational programs, they will necessitate cooking supplies. Program supplies encompass such items as audiovisuals, printed materials, and manuals that support the program, as well as any food supplements that are used.

Promotional Costs Promotional costs are comprised of advertising expenses, mailing charges, and money spent for publicity purposes. If expenses are incurred in preparing press kits, they should be listed as promotion costs. In soliciting business from worksite clients, a great amount of salesmanship is involved. Traditionally, the public relations department covers all promotion costs of the institution. However, they also have control over the promotional efforts. In many cases this arrangement is no problem, but some outpatient nutrition practitioners have learned that paying for promotion out of their own budgets allows them the freedom to choose the promotional vehicles and mediums they wish.

Professional Fees Professional fees include the cost of contracting other health professionals and certification fees. The lab may charge a fee to read test results, as will the cardiologist who runs an EKG. The professionals who administer quick weight loss programs are often contracted rather than hired as part-time employees. Institutions seldom reimburse employees for registration in a professional organization; however, a certification that would inevitably increase business might be covered. Certification for a diabetes education center is an example.

Training and Education Training and Education covers expenses for continuing education and seminars and workshops that enhance the programs you offer. For instance, you may wish to begin an adolescent weight management program, but you have not been able to find a dietitian with expertise and experience in this area. Paying to send a dietitian through some training may be the best option. Training can be very costly and should be chosen carefully. Some institutions may pay for education that leads to a higher degree if it benefits the practice and the institution. Reference materials and publication subscriptions are also a part of professional fees.

Travel Travel expenses are the costs of getting to and from job-related, off-site activities, such as promotional activities, program sites, physicians' offices, meetings, and continuing education programs. Most businesses determine a rate per mile for car travel. On longer trips, such expenses as food and lodging, along with air transportation, will be included.

Bad Debt Bad debt is revenue that is not collected for services or products. For instance, a client joins an eight-week nutrition counseling program at a cost of $300. The outpatient nutrition practice that offers the program does not require full payment for the program in advance. The participant is billed for the program, but the bill is never paid. This is bad debt and should be forecasted as a percentage of income.

Bad debt can be practically eliminated by requiring payment at the time or before the service is rendered. Establishing payment plans that allow for bad debt may sink the practice. In some instances, bad debt cannot be helped. Checks do bounce on occasion, and the bill may then be difficult to collect.

Community or Indigent Expense Community or indigent expense may be a line item in many practices. A particular outpatient nutrition practice established their programs by targeting people with middle to high incomes. However, they were informed by the institution that an endowment agreement would force them to accept indigent clients at no charge. The practice did not advertise this fact, but occasionally an indigent client enrolled in their program, requiring them to write off the cost, which translates to an expense. If you expect such an expense in your practice, your prices should cover it, or you may wish to look for funding for indigent service.

Profit and Loss Projections

Profit and loss projections (P&L) provide you with the ammunition you need to prove the financial benefit of your practice to your institution. Also known as an income statement, the P&L is the basic tool a business uses to determine whether the business is taking in more money than it spends or spending more money than it takes in during a given period of time. Generally speaking, when you take in more money than you spend you have a profit, and when you spend more than you take in you have a loss. If you can project a profit in the business plan for your nutrition services, you have a much better chance of receiving approval from your administration. In fact, the chief financial officer may be able to tell you what percent of the profit the institution expects.

Profit and loss statements are not forgotten after the original business plan, however. Once your nutrition practice is up and running, you will be preparing monthly and annual P&L statements. Therefore, you want to project realistically, since your actual results will be compared to projected results. This is the primary method of evaluating the performance of the practice.

The actual profit and loss statement is a summary of all the revenues and expenses you have during a specific period of time. For the business plan, you will make projections on the revenues and expenses you expect. This is similar to the budgeting process, with which you may already be familiar. However, you must consider the revenue you will generate, as well as the expenses.

P&L statements follow a second basic accounting equation:

$$\text{Profit} = \text{Revenues} - \text{Expenses}$$

Note two important factors about the above statement:

1. If expenses are greater than revenues, a loss will occur, rather than a profit.
2. The words revenue and expense have very specific definitions in accounting.

Revenue Revenue is the money or the right to receive money, exchanged for a product or service you provide. For example, a client pays you $40 in cash after a consultation. You would have $40 in revenue. If instead you bill the client for the $40, you still have $40 in revenue because you have a right to receive the $40. In both of these cases, you have earned the revenue by providing the service or product to a client.

Generally, it is reasonably easy to determine when revenue is earned and is, therefore, easily recorded in your P&L. The determination of expenses is not so apparent. Expenditure, or the spending of money, is not the same as expense.

Expense Expense is an accounting term used to describe the using up of an asset or the creation of liability that is a direct result of receiving revenue. For example, if a client pays, comes in for a consultation with a staff member, and buys a three-week supply of nutritional supplements, you have created two expenses. One, you have an obligation or liability to pay the staff member for counseling time. In addition, you have used part of an asset—part of the supply of nutritional supplements.

Accountants generally divide expenditures, or spending of money, into several categories:

- *Period expenses* are expenditures that will provide no future benefit. They will be used immediately or at least by the end of the accounting period.

  Example: If you pay a staff worker today for work done today, you will have to pay him or her again to work tomorrow. Today's wages will not prevent you from needing to pay wages tomorrow.

  Another example might be rent paid for the month. You still have to pay next month's rent. Any costs that are in this category will be considered a cost for the period in which they occur.
- *Inventory expense* is the expense incurred upon the use of supplies or sale of products. At the purchase of supplies or products, they are considered assets. Once they are used or sold, they become expenses.

  Example: You buy 10 scales for $10 each to resell to your clients. When you buy the scales, you trade $100 cash for $100 worth of scales, but you still have $100 worth of assets. If a customer buys a scale, you have only $90 worth of scales left. You have used up $10 worth of your assets, so you would have $10 of expense. Obviously, you will also have a cash revenue of $10 or more from the sale.
- *Capital expenditures* are expenditures that will provide future benefit by preventing you from making an expenditure in the future. The accountants say that you are simply exchanging one asset (cash) for a different asset. Only when the new asset is exchanged for payment or used completely should you consider it an expense.

  Example: You purchase a computer for $2,000. You still have $2,000 worth of assets in the form of a computer. The computer only becomes an expense when its $2,000 worth of use is exhausted or it is sold.

Generally, larger, more expensive tangible items are capitalized so that their costs can be expended over the time periods that they benefit. For a nutritional services center, these might include:

— Office furniture;
— Computers;
— Audiovisual equipment;
— Medical equipment; and
— Building and/or lease improvements.

- *Depreciation* is the name given to the process that estimates the economic life of an asset and divides the cost of that asset among the years of its expected use. How do you know when you have used the total cost of the computer or a building? Many assets are used gradually, over a long period of time; and it is difficult to say how and when they are being used. These assets that will be used for more than one year are known as capital assets, and the process of recording them in the accounting records is called capitalization.

  For example, if you buy a body fat analyzer, it might last for 5 years. You need to divide up the cost of the analyzer among the years. If an analyzer was purchased for $5,000 and was to be used for 5 years, figuratively speaking, each year you would use $1,000 worth of the analyzer. The $1,000 would be considered depreciation and treated as a yearly expense.

  Your institution's accountants are probably good sources for guidance on determining what items should be capitalized and the appropriate method to depreciate them. Note that many assets continue to be used after the depreciation period (e.g., buildings).

  The distinction between items that are expenses and those that are capitalized is particularly important to a start-up business. Remember the P&L equation—Revenue - Expenses = Profit (Loss). If all the expenditures of a start-up business were treated as expenses, even those that were going to be used for several years, start-up businesses would seldom be able to show a profit. And businesses that had been in business several years would show large profits because many items they use would have been deducted from profits in previous years.

Matching Expenses to Revenue

A primary tenant of accounting when creating P&L statements is that you must match expenses in a particular time period to revenues during that same time period. The premise suggests that there is no reason to have expenses if not to bring in revenue. Sometimes it is easy to see the relationship between the revenue that a client provides and the expenses that should be matched to it. It is fairly simple to match the cost of nutritional supplements to the money the client paid for them.

The relationship between revenue and other expenses may be more difficult to see. How much of the value of the scale do you use up each time a client steps on it? What about the cost of the building in which you locate your practice? How do you allocate these costs to match the revenue you will receive over a number of years? These are not simple questions to answer and require the advice of your institution's accountants.

In many cases, the institution's accountants can prepare your P&L projections for you if you have determined your needs (expenses) and desired returns (prices and projected number of clients) in advance. However, you should have some understanding of how profit and loss statements are prepared.

Preparing Profit and Loss Statements

Profit and loss statements can be prepared for each service and/or product you intend to offer or for the entire outpatient nutrition practice. The level of aggregation in your final profit and loss to be included in your business plan is up to you, but, for your planning purposes, you probably need to prepare statements that are as detailed as you are able to make them.

The basic profit and loss statement (which doesn't provide much information) takes on the following form:

Revenue	$ 107,000
less expenses	81,000
Profit	$ 26,000

This can and should be expanded to provide more information to your reader. This brief P&L does not tell the reader how well you have planned the financial aspects of your proposed nutrition practice. He or she may have reason to doubt the extent of your planning and the validity of your projections. The P&L (Figure 3-1), while still simple, provides more information to your reader.

The reader has far more information on which to judge your predictions than if all he or she had was the original P&L statement. Ultimately, you too will be far better off, because your projected P&L can be used to evaluate your performance once your outpatient nutrition center is operating.

Cash Flow

Cash flow is used to describe the flow of monies into and out of a business enterprise, as well as the timing of these inflows. Cash flow projections include not only the plan of expenditures, but also the sources of funds to pay for these expenditures. Cash flow projections are extremely important for a start-up business, because money will inevitably flow out of the practice faster than it will come in. You will need to prove to your administrators that you can identify the sources

Proposed Outpatient Nutrition Practice
Statement of Profit and Loss
For the Year Ending 12/31/XX

	Counseling Services	Nutritional Supplements	Total
Revenue	$ 100,000	$ 7,000	$107,000
Less inventory expense		(2,000)	(2,000)
Gross profit	100,000	5,000	105,000
Less operating expenses:			
Rent	(12,000)		(12,000)
Salaries	(50,000)		(50,000)
Depreciation on:			
Equipment	(1,000)	(100)	(12,100)
Advertising	(15,000)	(900)	(15,900)
Profit	$ 22,000	$ 4,000	$ 26,000

FIGURE 3-1. Sample profit and loss statement.

and uses of money in your practice and that the outflow will be more than offset by inflow.

At least two steps are required to prepare a cash flow for your business plan:

1. Detail the cash outflow necessary to set up the practice.
2. Illustrate the ongoing intake and outflow of cash from an operating nutrition practice once the P&L projections have been made.

Before the first clients walk in the door, bringing their checkbooks along, a large amount of money may need to be spent setting up the practice. These expenditures are commonly called start-up costs and include a wide variety of items. The following list is not intended to be inclusive, rather to explore the breadth of items that may be needed before your outpatient nutrition practice can open:

- Rent (if the institution does not provide rent-free space);
- Telephone installation;
- Program licensure fees;
- Office equipment;
- Legal and accounting fees;
- Medical equipment;
- Staff training;

- Promotional costs; and
- Supplies (office, medical, etc.).

All of these items are necessary to begin an outpatient nutrition practice, and most must be paid for before you receive any payment from your clients. Your cash flow projections should include the amount and timing of payments for these items.

In the second part of your cash flow projection, you will need to detail the expected outflow of cash and, in addition, project the inflow. For a start-up business, the best way to do this is often with a month-by-month projection, usually done by adapting monthly profit and loss statements.

Adapting Profit and Loss Statements to Cash Flow Statements

Profit and loss statements are the basis of cash flow statements for most enterprises, but they must be adapted for this use. Cash inflow for the new practice is fairly simple to determine. You chart the revenue you expect to collect, just as it appears on the P&L statement, to provide most of your cash inflow. The first year you are in operation, you must also include the start-up capital you receive from the institution or funding agencies as part of your cash inflow. These monies are recorded in the month they are received.

The cash flow statement records expenditures rather than expenses. Whereas capital expenses (furniture, equipment, etc.) were depreciated over several years on the P&L statement, they must be completely accounted for in the month they are purchased on the cash flow statement. You must therefore examine your capital expenditures and your expenditures for day-to-day items, and make a detailed analysis of when the cash actually goes out. For the most part, period expenses will be recorded as they are on the P&L. Again, the institution's accountants will be of great help.

If you adapt the preceding P&L statement to a cash flow statement, you would need to know when revenues were earned and in what months equipment, supplements inventory, and advertisements were purchased. For the sake of simplicity, say that revenues were divided equally over 10 months, beginning in March. Equipment and supplements were purchased in January. Also, $5000 of advertising was paid for in January, May, and August. The first five months of the cash flow statement are shown in Figure 3-2.

Balance Sheet

A balance sheet is defined as a summary of the economic resources of an enterprise, the economic obligations of the enterprise to others, and the equity in the enterprise. This summary can be compared to a snapshot of the financial situation

Proposed Outpatient Nutrition Practice
Statement of Cash Flow
For the Year Ending 12/31/XX

	January	February	March	April	May
Revenue					
Counsel	$8,333	$8,333	$8,333	$8,333	$8,333
Supplement	583	583	583	583	583
Expenses					
Rent	1,000	1,000	1,000	1,000	1,000
Salaries	4,166	4,166	4,166	4,166	4,166
Equipment	5,500				
Ads	5,000				5,000
Supplement	2,000				
Total	$(8,750)	$3,750	$3,750	$3,750	$1,750

FIGURE 3-2. Sample cash flow statement.

of the enterprise on one date in time. The balance sheet you prepare for the business plan shows what you expect your balance sheet to look like the day you open for business. Administrators use the balance sheet to determine the amount of financial support they are expected to provide. To understand the balance sheet, you must be apprised of some accounting terminology.

Assets Assets are the economic resources of an enterprise and include not only cash, but items that could be turned into cash. For example, an inventory of office supplies could be sold for cash. Therefore, the inventory is an asset. Accounts receivable represent the cash you will receive from clients who do not pay cash at the time a service is performed. Again, accounts receivable is an asset. Buildings, equipment, and furniture are all examples of assets.

Liabilities Liabilities are the economic obligations an enterprise owes to others. For example, when you buy supplies on credit, you create the obligation, or liability, to pay for those supplies. If you borrow money to finance the start-up of your nutrition practice, you create the obligation or liability to repay the loan. Other examples of liabilities would include wages owed to workers that have not been paid and taxes owed.

Equity Equity or residual interest are terms that label the excess of assets over liabilities. This is the amount that would be left over if all of the assets were turned into cash and used to pay off all of the liabilities of the enterprise.

The "Accounting Equation" is an important concept to remember if you want to understand the financial workings of a business enterprise. It follows:

Assets = Liabilities + Equity

This equation is the basis for the balance in the term balance sheet. The terms on either side of the equal sign must balance. A simple example is a good starting point. Say that a hospital invests $10,000 in an outpatient nutrition practice, Nutrabiz. For Nutrabiz, the accounting equation looks like this:

Assets = Liabilities + Equity
$10,000 = 0 + $10,000

Trading one asset for another does not change the equation. For example, when the manager of Nutrabiz buys a $2,000 computer to use in the practice, Nutrabiz has an asset called cash and an asset called computer instead of only an asset called cash. Your equation still balances:

Assets = Liabilities + Equity
Cash ($8,000) + Computer ($2,000) = Liabilities ($0) + Equity ($10,000)

Another possible transaction is that Nutrabiz buys supplies on account for $2,000. Now, even though the assets increase by $2,000, the equation still balances because there is also a $2,000 liability. The equation now reads:

Assets = Liabilities + Equity
Cash ($8,000) + Supplies ($2,000) + Computer ($2,000) = Liabilities ($2,000) + Equity ($10,000)

Each year, you will prepare a new balance sheet showing your assets, liabilities, and equity because they will change. Assets and liabilities will increase or decrease as a result of each transaction you enter. Equity will increase or decrease as your business produces profits or losses.

Break-Even Analysis

Profit and loss statements are based on your projections of revenues and expenses. However, if projections of revenues and expenses are inaccurate, so are projections of profit or loss. The problem is in determining how inaccurate they are. Break-even analysis allows you to project the magnitude of your profit or loss at varying levels of activity.

The break-even point is the point at which the revenue produced exactly equals the fixed expenses plus variable expenses. The break-even point is the point at which you neither make a profit or suffer a loss. To perform break-even analysis, you must be able to separate your expenses into expenses that are fixed and those that are variable.

Fixed expenses are those that remain the same, regardless of changes (increases or decreases) in revenue. An example of a fixed cost would be rent. You will pay the same amount of rent every month whether you see one client or many. The manager's salary is also a fixed expense.

Variable expenses are costs that increase or decrease with changes in revenue. Variable expenses may or may not vary in direct proportion to sales. An example of a variable expense is the cost of nutritional supplements and printed handout materials. The cost will vary directly with the number of packages you sell. Another example might be a fee paid to a commercial weight loss program for every client you put through the program.

To illustrate these fixed and variable cost concepts, assume you have one product, "Clo-low"—a commercial cholesterol reduction program for which you pay the owner a fee of $100 for each client who begins the program. This cost covers training, promotion and all client materials. Your only other cost is payment of $2,000 per month in wages to the nutrition counselor who you hire to conduct the "Clo-low" program. Table 3-1 illustrates the monthly costs for the program with different numbers of clients. Notice that the total wage expense is the same no matter how many clients you have (a fixed expense), while the expense associated with the fee changes with every additional client (a variable expense).

Revenue is almost always dependent on the level of activity at which you are operating. If you have no clients, you have no revenue. As you acquire paying clients, your revenue increases.

Profit is also activity dependent, for the most part. The more activity you have, the more profit you will most likely have. To illustrate this, let's expand on our previous example and assume that for each client on the "Clo-low" program, you charge $300 (revenue). Table 3-2 now includes the revenue you will receive and the profit to be made with different numbers of clients. Remember, Revenue - Expenses = Profit (Loss).

An important level of activity to note on the table is the 10-customer level. When the service has 10 customers, the revenue that they bring in is exactly equal

TABLE 3-1 Fixed and Variable Costs of "Clo-Low"

Number of clients	Fixed cost (wages)	Variable cost (fee expense)
0	2,000	0
1	2,000	100
2	2,000	200
10	2,000	1,000
100	2,000	10,000

TABLE 3-2 Break-Even Table for "Clo-low"

Number of clients	Total revenue	Total wage expense	Total fee expense	Total profit (loss)
0	0	2,000	0	(2,000)
1	300	2,000	100	(1,800)
2	600	2,000	200	(1,600)
9	2,700	2,000	900	(200)
10	3,000	2,000	1,000	0
11	3,300	2,000	1,100	200
50	15,000	2,000	5,500	7,800
100	30,000	2,000	10,000	18,000

to the expenses of serving the customers. This is known as the *break-even point.* If the service has fewer than 10 customers, there is a loss. If more than 10 customers enter the program, the practice makes a profit. Break-even analysis thus illustrates how much profit can be made at a given level of activity.

In this example, calculating the revenue and expenses generated at each level of clients would have been relatively easy. But, many times this is not the case. Mathematical formulas can be used to calculate the break-even point for you. The break-even point is the point at which the revenue produced exactly equals the fixed expenses plus variable expenses.

$$R * C = (V.E. * C) + F.E.$$

where:

R = Revenue per client
C = The number of clients
V.E. = Variable expenses per client
F.E. = Total fixed expenses

By solving the equation for C, you know the number of clients it will take to break even.

Using the Clo-low example, the equation reads:

$$300 * C = (100 * C) + 2{,}000$$

the solution, $C = 10$.

You can see that the equation produces the same answer; 10 clients are needed for the "Clo-low" program to break even. Once you know your break-even point and project the number of clients you expect to attract, the comparison will give a basis for making decisions. The comparisons indicate whether your program provides the opportunity to meet your financial objectives.

Break-even analysis can also be done graphically, and, for many people, graphical break-even presents the range of financial projections in a very understandable fashion. To perform graphical break-even, create a graph where the X-axis represents the number of clients served and the Y-axis represents dollars.

Calculate the revenue and the total expenses at two levels of activity. (Hint: Use no activity (0) as one of your levels—it is the easiest calculation.) Locate the two revenue levels and draw a line between them. Locate the two levels of total expense and draw a line between them. The intersection of the two lines you have drawn is the break-even point.

Continuing with the "Clo-low" example, Figure 3-3 would be produced.

The break-even graph not only presents a picture of the break-even point, but also some additional information. The difference between the revenue line and the expense line represents the profit or loss that is expected at any given level of activity. If the activity level is to the left of break-even, it represents loss; if it's to the right, it represents profit. You can indicate an expected range of activity levels

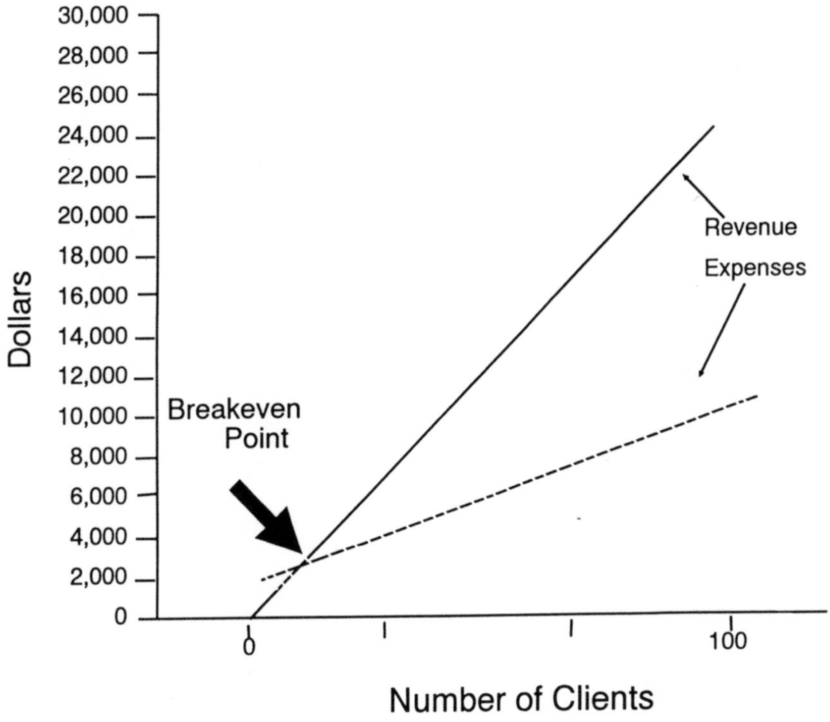

FIGURE 3-3.

on your graph, indicating your projected profit and many levels of activity. Again, the marketing and financial experts in your institution can be of service.

No matter how carefully you prepare your financial spread sheets, develop your strategies, and prepare your business plans, you can only put them into action on the acceptance of administration. How you develop rapport with key decision makers, express your enthusiasm for the practice, and present an effective plan will set the direction for the future of the practice.

Chapter 4

Case Study—Strategic Plan

ABOUT THE CASE STUDY

This case study was developed using the steps outlined in this book. The outline can be found on page 21.

The purposes of this case study are twofold:

1. To provide an example of the information presented in this book; and
2. To validate the earnings potential of outpatient nutrition practices.

Bear in mind that this example shows a brand new outpatient practice. As with most businesses, the earnings potential increases each year. Research for this publication indicated that many outpatient practices that have been established for 6 to 10 years are seeing profit margins between 15 and 17 percent. Some basic assumptions are necessary to develop a scenario for this sample.

BACKGROUND OF THE INSTITUTION

Alwell Community Hospital, a hospital in a community of 250,000 people, was in the process of becoming a women's hospital. The hospital was a 404-bed acute care facility that had been operating at about one-half of its capacity for 3 years. Because the hospital realized their strength in the area of high risk pregnancies and maternity care, they had expanded these services 1 year ago and increased their marketing to OB/GYN specialists and women in their childbearing years. At that time, they changed their name to Alwell Women's Health Center.

Alwell's administrators were encouraging efforts of all departments to develop ideas for revenue production and/or support of the new goals of the institution. The goals of the institution that might affect the nutrition staff follow. Note that market share is the percentage of people who currently purchase that particular service and *not* a percentage of the entire target market. The "projected" share is what the hospital hopes to gain over the next 3 years.

- Increase occupancy to 70 percent (283 beds);
- Gain a market share of each of the following services:

Inpatient service	*Current share*	*Projected*
Medical/surgical unit specializing in surgery for females	20%	50%
High-risk pregnancy	20%	40%
Maternity	50%	75%
Perinatal unit	50%	75%
Oncology	10%	30%
Endocrinology	20%	40%
Outpatient service		
Outpatient surgery	20%	40%
Genetic and fertility counseling	0%	50%
Prenatal care and education	50%	75%
PMS clinic	0%	100%
Screening programs for osteoporosis and cancer	0%	50%
Osteoporosis treatment, prevention, and education	20%	60%

- Reduce bad debt to 5 percent; and
- Attract specialists who are female.

In summary, the goals suggest the hospital's desire to grow by 200 to 300 percent in the areas of high-risk pregnancy, oncology, and endocrinology. By increasing these services, along with an expansion of their maternity and perinatal services, they expect a growth in both inpatient and outpatient surgery by 150 percent and 200 percent, respectively. The institution intends to dramatically increase outpatient services to entice a greater share of the female population, as well as female specialists (Note: Research indicates that women prefer female medical specialists over males). Therefore, they will be renovating a portion of the hospital for outpatient services and offices for specialists.

Community Demographics

Industry in the community is mixed, with a large number of people employed at three major factories. Unemployment is 5 percent, and the working population is about half blue collar, half white collar. Five hospitals are located within a 15-mile radius of Alwell, all of which are traditional and conservative in their treatment approaches. Due to the university and college of medicine in the area, most of the health care facilities offer career training in a variety of health care fields.

The Nutrition Services Department

The professional nutrition staff at Alwell consists of a clinical nutrition manager and three clinical dietitians. Inpatient nutrition services have not been directly charged to the patients in the past. Outpatient nutrition services, which were provided by one of the inpatient dietitians, were limited to a weight management program, one prenatal nutrition session as part of the hospital's prenatal education program, and individual counseling for modified diets.

The clinical nutrition manager realized that this was an excellent opportunity to create an outpatient nutrition practice that would support the hospital's new endeavor. She gathered her staff, the director of the patient education department, and a representative from the marketing department together to discuss the possibilities. Below are the steps that led to the business plan.

DEFINING THE MISSION

A mission statement was drafted, stating that the outpatient nutrition practice would support the goals of the hospital.

SELECTING SERVICES AND PRODUCTS AND TARGET MARKETS

Possible Services and Products

The committee first produced a list of "possible services," in relationship to the resources they had readily available, the goals of the institution, and their perception of market needs and desires. The following list was generated:

- *Services for which some resources are readily available*
  Prenatal nutrition
  Individual counseling for modified diets
  Education for prevention of:
  — Heart disease
  — Cancer
  — Osteoporosis (materials developed for nutrition month)
  — Weight management

- *Services that relate to the hospital's goals*
  Individual counseling for:
  — High-risk pregnancy
  — Osteoporosis (diagnosed or high-risk)
  — Referred modified diets
  Group counseling and education for:
  — Osteoporosis treatment and prevention
  — Prenatal nutrition
  — Well baby nutrition
  — PMS
  — Cancer prevention
  — Migraine headaches
  — Diabetes education
  — Weight management
  Home care
  WIC grant program
- *Services perceived to be desirable to the hospital's target market*
  Weight management
  Eating disorders
  Osteoporosis prevention
  Cancer prevention
  Heart healthy cooking
  PMS programs
  Migraine headache programs
  Computerized nutrition analysis
  Grocery tours
  Worksite programs
  Nutrition in fitness

Possible Targets

Although the committee knew that their larger target market would be women in general, they segmented the female population into groups that might be interested in the services they might offer. These segments were:

- Females over age 55;
- Females in their childbearing years;
- Pregnant women;
- Working women;
- Female adolescents; and
- Women actively participating in fitness programs.

ANALYZING THE MARKET

The committee then explored the various segments of the market to determine their perceived needs and desires and to determine the potential of various services. Most of the information they gathered came from three sources and revealed some very helpful information:

1. Information was gathered from national statistics and research data. Statistics from the American Heart Association and the American Cancer Society provided information on at-risk groups for heart disease and breast cancer.
2. Journal articles provided statistics on PMS, eating disorders, and health conscious shoppers.
3. Census Bureau data was needed to extrapolate actual numbers in specific age ranges.

The marketing department had already researched the interest in osteoporosis diagnosis, treatment, and prevention. They also had some statistics on various disease entities, the demographics on those who would use a women's center, and overall interest in nutrition services.

One of the dietitians contacted a friend who worked at a women's hospital in a similar community that had been functioning for about three years. She had some data on the types of women actually using the services. Generally, the information gathered indicated that women who are educated are more likely to pursue nutrition services than those with no post-high school training or education. This factor influenced the committee's decision not to pursue welfare recipients. Also, because there would be a charge for education/counseling, targeting those in mid- to high income ranges was indicated. According to census data for this community, 60 percent of the females over 20 are educated with an income of $25,000 or more. Table 4-1 indicates the data by medical condition that was collected.

Target Market Data

Table 4-1 shows health conditions that might aid in segmenting the female population. Column two explains the factors that predispose women to the health condition. These factors identify the segments of the female population who are educated and have mid- to high incomes with the greatest chance of having or getting the condition. For instance, many unmarried women have babies, but the greatest number of educated mid- to high income level females having their first child are married. Using the best data sources where actual numbers or percentages could be found, a total number in the target market was extrapolated (column

TABLE 4-1 Target Market Data

Health Condition	Predisposing Factors	Target Market	Source of Data
Heart disease	Over 45, family history, smokers, working away from home	39,000	Am. Heart Assoc. Am. Hosp. Assoc.
Breast cancer	Over 40, family history, never pregnant	4,290 (diagnosed)	Am. Cancer Society
Osteoporosis Treatment	Postmenstrual, Caucasian/ Oriental	11,700	Research/National (hospital stats)
Prevention	Over 45, Caucasian/Oriental, family history	5,850	Research/National
High-risk pregnancy	Over 35 or teenage, Diabetic, Other medical cond., African-American/Caucasian	667/year	Hospital stats
First pregnancy	15–40 years, married	1,110/year	Hospital stats
Diabetes	Over 40, family history, gestational	1,300/year	Hospital stats
PMS	20–50 years	10,608	Journal article and census data
Overweight	All ages, African-American/ Caucasian	37,500	Journal article and census data
	Age 45–54 largest group	60/year	Current program
Modified diets	All ages, hospitalized	3,686/year*	Dietary stats
Eating Disorders	Age 15–25	780	Journal article and census data
Interest in nutrition/ fitness services	Age 25–54, married	22,620	Hospital stats
Health conscious grocery shoppers			
Weight conscious	Age 15–44	21,840	Marketing, journal article and census data
Prevention conscious	Age 30–60	26,202	
Medical problem	Age 45+	21,840	

*The dietitian from the women's hospital contacted indicated that the changes in specialization cause insignificant changes in the number of inpatients instructed on modified diets.

labeled Target Market). Unless noted as a per year figure, this number represents an estimate of the present population. The last column notes the sources of data.

Survey of Potential Targets

Using this information, the committee decided to conduct focus groups and surveys on target markets and services that looked to be most advantageous. Some populations that were readily available to the institution—prenatal class members, maternity and high-risk pregnancy patients, and female medical and surgical patients—were surveyed on the premises either in a direct conversation with a committee member or in writing. A list of physicians to survey was obtained from the hospital. The local chapter of the American Association of Retired Persons sent surveys along with their regular mailing. With the help of the university and a community college, focus groups were done with women who had a wide range of age and interests.

The surveys provided the committee with information regarding not only the best target markets and services to offer, but also on convenient times to offer services, the desired features of nutrition services, and projections of the number that would purchase the services. The survey results pertinent to choosing services and target markets indicated:

- A strong interest among pregnant women in expanded nutrition counseling during pregnancy with follow-up education on feeding infants and group programs on weight management.
- A desire for greater compliance among physician's patients and a need for more follow-up and feedback from nutrition counselors. If such features were part of the nutrition services, physicians would refer patients mostly for modified diets and weight management. Of the physicians surveyed, 75 percent felt that offering inpatients a survival kit to be followed by outpatient counseling would be very appealing.
- A great concern about cancer, heart disease, and osteoporosis among women over 55. Of the women surveyed, 50 percent were concerned about weight, 10 percent were interested in physician-monitored quick weight loss, and 15 percent were interested in group weight management as explained in the survey. About 10 percent would participate in workshops or seminars, and 20 percent were interested in grocery tours.
- The most positive responses to the use of nutrition services was from health conscious women between the ages of 30 and 45. As a whole, they were interested in nutrition programs associated with screening, weight reduction, and PMS education. This population was mostly working women who preferred group counseling and wanted convenience and time-saving ideas.
- All patients surveyed who were experiencing a medical condition for the first

time were interested in more nutrition counseling following discharge, while only 20 percent of those who had been hospitalized for the condition in the past were interested in such counseling. Of those who were interested, 70 percent felt that individual counseling would be most beneficial.

- The services that appeared to be in greatest demand were:
  - — Weight management;
  - — Physician monitored quick weight loss;
  - — Comprehensive group education and counseling;
  - — Workshops and seminars on:
    - Osteoporosis treatment and prevention,
    - Prenatal nutrition,
    - Infant nutrition,
    - Heart-healthy eating, and
    - Cancer prevention, and
- Group counseling and support for:
  - — PMS,
  - — Diabetes,
  - — Cancer, and
  - — Weight management.

Market Forces

The market forces that may affect the outpatient nutrition practice follow:

- The Surgeon General's Report cites nutrition as a key factor in preventing chronic disease.
  Impact anticipated: A greater interest in nutrition counseling in the general population.
- The population over age 60 who can continue to care for themselves is rising.
  Impact anticipated: More interest in nutrition to alleviate symptoms of and prevent chronic disease among senior citizens.
- As of 1990, Medicare will pay for osteoporosis screening every other year for women over 65.
  Impact anticipated: Increased number of women participating in screening and treatment for osteoporosis.
- Hospitals in the area are becoming more marketing-oriented.
  Impact anticipated: More hospitals will be competing vigorously for health care revenues.
- Two hospitals in the area plan to merge within the next year.
  Impact anticipated: Increased credibility and marketing of programs in these institutions.
- A Quickie Weight Management franchise will open in the city in one month.

Impact anticipated: More competition for clients interested in quick weight loss.

- Registered dietitians are readily available in the community due to the fact that many of the graduates from the Coordinated Undergraduate Dietetics program available at the university have remained in the area over the years.
  Impact anticipated: Although recruitment of competent nutrition professionals will be easier, more nutrition counselors are likely to develop private practices, which would increase competition.

Competition

Competition for health and nutrition markets includes:

- The two major HMOs to which area businesses subscribe. They contract with area health care providers for services with no centralized location in the community.
- Only one private practice nutrition counselor consults for physicians, and she has aligned herself with one physician's group.
- A competitive analysis was done on each competitor. From those analyses, the committee determined the following descriptions, competitive advantages, and disadvantages.

Five hospitals are located within a 15-mile radius of the Women's Hospital as follows:

1. Hospital A—618-bed acute care facility with specialized services for renal care, cardiac care, and rehabilitation. This hospital will merge with Hospital B in 1 year. A variety of inpatient, fee-for-service nutrition programs are offered. The outpatient nutrition counselors work exclusively in the outpatient programs but report to the clinical nutrition manager. Services include the following.
   Private counseling:
   a. Eight PPO (preferred provider organizations) locations;
   b. Internal medicine center;
   c. Family practice center; and
   d. Renal/dialysis center.
   Weight management programs:
   a. Dietitian directed; and
   b. Comprehensive weight management ($300 for eight 1-hour group sessions, one 1-hour individual session, and six 1/2-hour group follow-up sessions); Childbirth education (no money credited to nutrition practice).
   Wellness programs (prices dependent upon services):
   a. Internal program for employees; and
   b. Worksite programs at three locations.

Cardiac rehabilitation (included in cardiac program package price, no money credited to nutrition practice):

a. Phase II nutrition classes; and

b. Phase III nutrition classes.

Individual counseling ($52/1-hour initial, $38/1/2-hour follow-up).

2. Hospital B—A 230-bed osteopathic hospital that will specialize in orthopedic surgery and rehabilitation after the merger with Hospital A. Currently, the inpatient nutrition services are offered, with revenue going to the general fund and no credit to the food and nutrition services department. Outpatient, individual counseling is done occasionally by the clinical dietitian.
   The service includes an occasional individual counseling session ($25/initial visit, $10/hour follow-up).
3. Hospital C—A 430-bed acute care facility with strong programs in oncology, cardiac care, and eating disorders. Prenatal and maternity services are provided. Some inpatient programs are fee-for-service. The dietitians report to the specialty area they work with and are responsible for both inpatient and outpatient services in that area, including individual counseling and any group programs. Services include the following.
   Weight management:
   a. Dietitian-directed, on the hospital premises ($200/ten 1-hour group sessions); and
   b. Physician-monitored quick loss ($4000/year, two 1-hour meetings/week, 2 months plus individual and support group sessions over one year).

   Cardiac rehabilitation program (no money credited to nutrition practice)—Phase II nutrition education.
   Eating disorders clinic:
   a. Physician-directed; and
   b. Individual and group counseling ($30/1/2-hour, $100/four 1-hour group).
4. Hospital D—A 250-bed hospital that is generalized in its services. Prenatal and maternity services are provided. One clinical dietitian covers all inpatient nutrition services, with no reimbursement to the food and nutrition services department. No outpatient services are offered at this time.
5. Hospital E—A 215-bed children's hospital with two clinical dietitians who handle all inpatient nutrition services and individual counseling on the outpatient basis specifically for children and infants. Services include:
   Outpatient individual counseling (no charge)—Infant and adolescent.
   Weight management ($150/ 12 1-hour group sessions)
   a. Adolescent; and
   b. Dietitian-directed.
6. Facility F—One rehabilitation facility, located 25 miles from the Women's

Hospital. A clinical dietitian provides group and individual education to inpatients for a competitive fee. The following services are offered.
Alcohol and chemical dependency rehabilitation.
Physical medicine and rehabilitation.
Long-term care for chronic illness.

Competitive Advantages

The competitive advantages of providing the nutrition services that were selected include:

- Alwell would be the first outpatient practice to offer women's nutrition seminar series and grocery tours.
- Presently, other outpatient practices in the area do not seem to be targeting specific segments of the market.
- An evening and Saturday schedule, currently unavailable at other institutions, will attract a greater proportion of the working women.
- The combination of quick weight loss, weight management, and weight management counseling and support will provide a more comprehensive program than any other facility.
- More group programs will be offered than any other facility.
- The use of "nutrition counselors" who are actually trained to counsel, as well as to educate, will promote greater compliance, achievement of desired results, and more satisfied clients, increasing both referrals and word-of-mouth advertising over time.
- A certified diabetes educator will enhance the program for those who have diabetes.
- Parking is free, and security is excellent at this hospital location.

Competitive Disadvantages

The features of other nutrition programs that place Alwell's practice at a disadvantage include:

- Location of services limited to the hospital, whereas Hospital A provides services in a variety of locations and the private practitioner provides services in the physician's office.
- Weight management programs are well established at Hospital A and C, and physician-monitored quick weight loss programs are provided by Hospital C, giving them a competitive advantage.
- Hospital C has an aggressive marketing campaign for their weight management program.
- Hospitals C and E often provide community nutrition programs on timely topics free of charge.

- The private practitioner has promoted herself to the media, limiting publicity of other nutrition professionals in the area.

Key Opportunities

Alwell's outpatient nutrition practice could capitalize on the following opportunities:

- First outpatient nutrition practice in the community to offer services specifically for women.
- First to offer group nutrition counseling for high-risk pregnancy and grocery tours.
- Hospital has recently acquired state-of-the-art equipment for osteoporosis screening.
- The recent Surgeon General's Report has increased the awareness of nutrition's role in preventing and treating chronic diseases. The media is ripe for nutrition news.

Threats and Risks

Problems that Alwell's nutrition practice must overcome to succeed follow:

- The merger of Hospitals A and B will heighten their reputation in the community. The specialization of Hospital B in orthopedics will increase their market share in osteoporosis screening and treatment.
- The opening of the Quickie Weight Management franchise will increase the competition in the weight loss market.

FINALIZING SELECTION OF SERVICES AND TARGET MARKETS

Considering the data collected and the goals of the institution, the committee discussed the services that would most likely generate revenue and those that would support the hospital's goals. The services that seemed to have the greatest possibilities were:

- Individual counseling for physician-referred patients on modified diets. (Although the committee realized that group counseling would be more effective, physicians and potential clients were more interested in individual counseling. Therefore, the committee decided to offer individual counseling at the onset and then work toward greater acceptance of group programs.)
- Weight management, including:
  - Physician monitored quick weight loss;
  - Comprehensive group education and counseling; and
  - Ongoing support groups.

- Educational workshops and seminars on:
  - Prenatal nutrition through childbirth education; and
  - Timely women's nutrition issues.
- Counseling and support groups for:
  - Diabetes; and
  - High-risk pregnancy.
- Grocery tours.
- Computerized nutrition analysis.

Services and products that were considered ideas to look at in the future were:

- Certified diabetes education;
- Heart-healthy cooking classes;
- Recipes/cookbooks;
- Home care; and
- Infant nutrition education programs.

Target markets were also specified at this time to include women who were educated with mid- to high incomes in the following groups:

- Over age 55;
- Working, age 30–45; or
- Pregnant for the first time.

Although the hospital would most likely draw many of its prenatal/maternity/postnatal clients from the welfare population, the committee decided against programs that draw this target market. They reasoned that, at best, the services would break even and would require large amounts of time and capital to start. Therefore, the outpatient nutrition practice would hope to draw more middle and upper income clients to the hospital, in support of its goals.

DETERMINING GOALS

Both financial and nonfinancial goals that coordinated with the goals of the hospital were established. Goals were set for a time frame of 3 years. The goals follow:

Nonfinancial	*Financial*
Provide two referrals/month to other programs in the facility	Recover all direct costs by first year end
Coordinate the efforts of the inpatient and outpatient nutrition staff to create a team approach	Break even by month 13 Payback the initial investment by month 19
Continue to offer the following services: • Individualized counseling • Prenatal nutrition education	Produce a profit of: $60,000 by second year end $180,000 by third year end

Nonfinancial	*Financial*
• Weight management program	Acquire 100 new clients/month by first year end

Expand services to include:
- Weight management support groups by month 3
- Quick weight loss by month 4

Counseling and support groups for:
- Diabetes by month 6
- High-risk pregnancy by month 13
- Grocery tours by month 13
- Certified diabetes education center by month 15
- Box lunch seminar series by month 17

Offer computerized nutrition analysis as part of any counseling program

DETERMINING KEY ACTION STRATEGIES

Positioning

The Alwell Women's Nutrition Center will position itself as the community resource for women's nutritional concerns. This position will be established through location, service offerings, and promotion. The center will target women who are educated (high school diploma or above) in mid- to high income levels. Through pricing and promotion, this position will be developed. More specifically, three groups of women will be targeted, including those:

1. Over age 55;
2. Working, age 30 to 45; and
3. Who are pregnant for the first time.

Service

Assumptions

1. The outpatient nutrition programs that are already established (individual counseling, comprehensive weight management, and prenatal nutrition education) will continue with some modifications.
2. A weight management program that meets the needs of the morbidly obese to the moderately overweight is necessary to establish credibility and serve the proposed target market.
3. Research shows that counseling and support are key factors in establishing new dietary patterns with individuals.
4. Prenatal nutrition education will be offered to support the hospital's prenatal and maternity services.

Strategies

Year One

1. Individual counseling—One-on-one counseling tailored to the individual's nutritional and lifestyle needs. The 1-hour initial counseling session includes nutritional assessment through diet history and 24-hour recall until computerized analysis is available. Follow-up sessions of 30 minutes can be purchased separately or as part of a package.
2. Prenatal nutrition education—As part of the seven-session prenatal program, group programs would be offered on nutrition during pregnancy for 1-hour of sessions 1 and 3.
3. Weight management—A dietitian-supervised weight management program, including:
   a. Eight 1 ⅓-hour group sessions with nutrition education, behavior modification, and activity;
   b. Two 1-hour individual counseling sessions; and
   c. One computerized nutrition analysis.

   This program will differ from the current program in the use of computerized nutrition analysis, incorporation of a 20-minute walk with every group session, and use of professionally prepared audiovisuals.
4. Weight management counseling and support—Six 1-hour group sessions to follow the more structured, education-oriented weight management program. This program would be client-directed, focusing on the specific needs and problems of the small group. This program begins in month 3.
5. Quick weight loss—A physician-monitored weight loss program combining the expertise and counseling of dietitian, psychologist, nurse, and physician with a liquid protein supplement for controlled weight loss.

   For those who are more than 40 lb. overweight. The three components of the program are:
   a. *Screening phase*—Blood work, physical examination, and psychological and nutritional evaluation.
   b. *Program phase*—Five months of 1-hour, weekly meetings with physician monitoring, nutrition education, and behavior modification. Diet consists of liquid protein supplements.
   c. *Adaptive phase*—Four weekly 1-hour meetings limiting the supplement and adding food to the diet.

   A pre-developed program that includes training, consultation, and all necessary support materials will be purchased. This program begins in month 4.
6. Diabetes management counseling—One individualized counseling session with computer analysis and four, 1-hour group counseling sessions to aid diabetics in adapting their new eating patterns to daily living.
   This program begins in month 6.

Year Two

1. High-risk pregnancy counseling—A package of two individualized counseling sessions with computer analysis and three group sessions. The purpose of this program is to address the specific nutritional needs and problems of those who have diabetes, hypertension, or some other high risk during pregnancy. This program will begin in month 13.
2. Grocery tours—A 1 1/2-hour tour through the grocery store to educate people on healthy food selection, economics, and label reading. Aimed primarily at the senior population. This program begins in month 13.
3. Certified diabetes education center—A comprehensive education program approved by the American Diabetes Association.
4. Box lunch seminar series—A series of group educational programs on timely nutrition topics. Topics include Osteoporosis, PMS and Nutrition, Cancer and Nutrition, Eating Heart-Healthy, and Nutrition for Children. This series will be targeted toward working women. The series begins in month 15.

Year Three

1. Development of services that meet the needs of worksite nutrition programs.

Staffing

Assumptions

1. Physicians, psychologists, nurses, and dietitians can be contracted to provide services for the quick weight loss program.
2. Registered dietitians will be hired for the manager and counselor positions.
3. Starting salaries will be established at a level that would attract experienced professionals.

Strategies

1. Implementing these programs over a period of 15 months would require the following staff:

Outpatient nutrition manager/counselor	
Full-time	Day 1
Secretary/receptionist	
Full-time	Day 1
Nutrition counselor	
Part-time	At month 6
Full-time	At year 2
Quick weight loss manager	
Full-time	Day 1

2. Either a certified diabetes educator will be hired; or one counselor will become certified, with the cost of training paid by the practice.

Scheduling

Assumptions

1. Since most of the target market consists of working women, they will not be able to schedule appointments during regular business hours.
2. Most contact with physicians and allied health professionals will be made during regular business hours on weekdays.
3. Grocery stores are less crowded during the early afternoon weekdays, with the exception of the first Tuesday of the month. Senior discounts are offered on Thursdays.

Strategies

1. A receptionist/secretary will be available Monday-Friday, 8:00 A.M. to 4:30 P.M. Calls will be taken by the ambulatory care switchboard during lunch hours.
2. The nutrition center will be staffed by one of the nutrition professionals from 9:00 A.M.-5:00 P.M. weekdays.
3. Evening programs will be held Tuesday, Wednesday, and Thursday.
4. Individual counseling will be available every other Saturday morning and one evening per week until more Saturday and evening hours are deemed necessary.

Location

Assumptions

1. The price of renting space is much higher than using hospital space.
2. Clients are willing to come to the hospital for nutrition services.
3. The hospital offers free parking, security, and housekeeping services as part of office overhead.
4. The number of group programs being offered does not warrant the cost of a classroom.

Strategies

1. The practice will be located in the newly renovated ambulatory care wing, easily accessible from the parking lot.
2. The space will include a reception area, two offices, a meeting room that seats 20, and a small conference room.
3. Adjacent to the Nutrition Center is a fertility clinic that is staffed by the physician only during morning hours. The examining room is accessible from

the Nutrition Center. Therefore, when the quick weight loss program begins, the practice will use the fertility clinic examining room for medical screening.
4. As the quick weight loss program grows, a third office will be necessary. Two possibilities are the office across the hall, currently housing an occupational therapist, or a large storeroom next to the Nutrition Center, currently used for office supplies.

Pricing

Assumptions

1. Less revenue is made from individual counseling than from group counseling.
2. The major intent of the prenatal nutrition program is to aid in acquiring clients for the hospital and for other outpatient nutrition programs.
3. Computerized nutrition analysis will be offered as part of packaged services.
4. The center intends to become a certified diabetes education center.
5. Collection of fees will be the responsibility of the ambulatory care cashier. Collecting fees at the first session will limit bad debt.
6. Asking for payment at the onset of a program increases the commitment of the client.

Strategies

1. Table 4-2 explains the pricing strategy and the number of clients necessary in each service to meet financial goals.
2. The following price increase will occur during the second year:
   Weight management $330/package
   Weight management counseling and support$100/package
3. When the practice becomes a certified diabetes education center, the charge for education and counseling will rise.
4. All fees will be collected prior to the first session of any program.

Promotion

Assumptions

1. The institution is reluctant to pay large sums of money for advertising before the practice can show its ability to generate revenue.
2. Promotion to referring agents is likely to generate more business than promotion to prospective clients.
3. So that inexpensive yet enticing giveaways can be offered, the hospital food service will prepare food baskets to be taken to physicians' offices.
4. People with osteoporosis will be interested in weight management, seminars, grocery tours, and individual counseling.

TABLE 4-2 Pricing Services

Service/ Start Month	Package Description	Price	New Clients Needed to Meet Goals Year 1	Year 2
Individual counseling (month 1)	Initial (1 hr.)	$60.00	2/wk.	3/wk.
	Follow-up (30 min.)	30.00		
	Initial + 2 follow-ups	100.00		
Prenatal nutrition education (month 1)	2 ½-hour sessions (part of prenatal classes)	5.00/2 sessions	10/wk.	10/wk.
Weight management (month1)	2 Individual + 8 1⅓-hr. group sessions (8–14 participants/group)	300.00	130/yr.	150/yr.
Weight management counseling and support (month 3)	6 1-hr./wk. group sessions	75.00 w/pkg. 15.00 per session	65/yr.	85/yr.
Quick weight loss (month 4)				
Screening	1 hr.	350.00	120/yr.	200/yr.
Program	1 hr./wk. group	450.00 monthly	120/yr.	200/yr.
Adaptive phase	1 hr./wk. group	360.00 monthly	45/yr.	180/yr.
Diabetes counseling (month 6)	4 1-hr. group sessions	100.00	16/mo.	20/mo.
Nutrition counseling for high-risk pregnancy (month 13)	2 1-hr. individual 3 1-hr. group sessions	115.00		16/mo.
Grocery tours (month 13)	1 ½-hour group	30.00		16/wk.
Box lunch seminars (month 15)	2 1-hour group	15.00/session		40/mo.

5. Referring agents who would potentially refer clients include physicians who are affiliated with the hospital, especially family practitioners, obstetricians, gynecologists, endocrinologists, inpatient dietitians, social workers, physical therapists, occupational therapists, and nurses.

Strategies

1. Publicity will include:
   a. Public speaking at community organization meetings such as the American Cancer Society, AARP, women's church organizations, and local women's professional organizations. Notification of all community events will be sent to local newspaper and radio stations.
   b. Brief presentations at meetings of hospital physicians, interns, and residents, as each new service begins.
   c. Staff training programs to teach nurses and inpatient dietitians how to promote the outpatient nutrition services to inpatients and physicians.

   d. A referral procedure with the inpatient dietitians that recommends to the physician that the inpatient be given a "survival kit" while in the hospital and be scheduled for the appropriate outpatient nutrition services within two weeks of discharge.
   e. A referral system with other outpatient services in the ambulatory care wing, to promote a team approach to women's health care.
   f. Involvement in teen pregnancy programs and local cancer and diabetes organizations, as well as other organizations where networking could be established.
   g. News releases sent to local newspapers, TV, and radio stations, along with a list of topics on which the outpatient nutrition practitioners could offer expert information and advice.
   h. Newspaper article with client's success story.
   i. A nutrition display to be set up and brochures to be provided at every osteoporosis screening the hospital offers, with a nutrition counselor available to answer questions during peak hours.
2. Promotion to physicians and their support staff will include:
   a. A scope of services brochure.
   b. A brochure explaining weight management offerings.
   c. Letters mailed to the home.
   d. Personal visit to physicians' offices with giveaways and materials.
   e. Thank you note for each referral.
   f. Invitation to physician staff for free nutrition analysis.
3. Promotion of each service is shown in Table 4-3.

FINANCIAL PROJECTIONS

As the strategies were being developed, the committee compiled a list of supplies, equipment, and other expenses and placed dollar figures on each, as shown in the Expense Worksheet (Table 4-4). Expenses were estimated fairly high to allow for unexpected price changes.

Note that labor appears on the expense worksheet in two places. The cost of each employee is calculated, and the fixed cost of labor for each service is calculated. The second calculation is for the purpose of preparing break-even analysis on individual services.

Some assumptions had to be made regarding expenses, as follows:

1. Direct labor will include benefits at a rate of 25 percent of salary. A pay increase of 5 percent is estimated for year 2.
2. All handouts are purchased or have been developed in the past.

TABLE 4-3 Program Promotion

Program	Promotional Vehicles	Rationale
Individual counseling	None	Not profitable
Prenatal nutrition	None	Promoted by staff
Weight management	Yellow pages Brochure Word of mouth Preview session	Already in place; Little promotion needed
Weight management counseling and support	Through weight management program Brochure	Follow-up program to weight management
Quick weight loss	Newspaper ads Yellow pages Word of mouth Brochure Preview session	Largest revenue producer; Demands largest promotional effort
Diabetes counseling	Discharge packet brochure Automatic referral from physician inpatient services of newly diagnosed diabetics	Target market readily available through inpatient services
High-risk pregnancy	Same as diabetes counseling	Same as diabetes counseling
Grocery tours	Grocery bag stuffers Posters in grocery Announcement in the grocery ads Food demonstrations	High revenue producer; Some help from the store with ads and demos
Box lunch seminars	Mailers to worksite Human resource directors (HRD) and organization presidents Luncheon/preview for HRDs and industrial nurses	First marketing effort to worksites

3. Because all fees will be collected prior to rendering services, the only bad debt will be associated with overdrawn checks.
4. Overhead includes the services of maintenance, housekeeping, security, distribution, the library, marketing, and public relations, as well as utilities and mail service.
5. Professional assistance will be required for the development of the brochures.
6. The grocery store would be willing to include announcements of the tours in its ads and donate the cost of food used in demonstrations for the promotion of the tour and the tour itself.

The income figures were calculated using Table 4-2. Again, some assumptions were made.

TABLE 4-4 Expense Worksheet

	Year 1	Year 2
Direct labor*		
(Beginning Jan.)		
Manager	$37,500	$39,375
Clerk	18,938	19,885
Quick weight loss manager	35,350	37,118
(Beginning July)		
Nutrition counselor		
Part-time	8,333	
Full-time		36,750
Overhead	12,000	14,400
Reception area		
3 offices		
Meeting room, seats 20		
Conference room, seats 4		
Equipment		
Medical scale	500	500
Typewriter	300	
Slide projector	250	
Television	500	
VCR	500	
Computer w/printer and software	3,500	
Copier		1,000
Furniture		
2 computer tables	400	
3 desks	750	
5 chairs	300	
3 file cabinets	250	
3 waiting room chairs	150	
Brochure rack	50	
Bookcase	150	
Blackboard	50	
Conference room table	250	
4 chairs	200	
Typing table	50	
20 folding chairs	600	
Telephone		
Monthly service charge	600	600
Installation	150	
Phones—4 (multiple line) 1 w/answering machine	350	
Supplies		
Office supplies	700	800
Small equipment	600	100
Demonstration supplies	200	

TABLE 4-4 Expense Worksheet *(continued)*

	Year 1	Year 2
Dues and subscriptions		
Books	$ 500	
Subscriptions	200	$ 250
Travel and education		
Off-site training	1,000	1,500
Travel	1,500	1,000
Miscellaneous expenses	1,000	1,000
Promotion		
Brochures (2 different)		
Development	3,050	
Printing	750	
Yellow pages listing	600	600
Physician campaign	2,000	
Display for public presentations	150	
Maintenance contracts		300
Expenses by Service		
Individual Counseling		
Variable (per person)		
Labor	16	17
Handouts	2	2
Prenatal Nutrition		
Expenses will be covered by the Prenatal Education Department		
Weight Management		
Variable (per person)		
Labor	45	48
Materials	70	70
Computer analysis	35	40
Food supplies	2	2
Fixed		
Promotion supplies	150	
Audiovisuals	260	
Quick Weight Loss		
Screening—Variable (per person)		
Medical history	7	10
Lab fees	115	130
EKG	15	20
Psychological screening	30	32
Professional services	10	13
One Month Participation—Variable (per person)		
Physical exam	28	30
Lab fees	112	127
Professional services	50	65

TABLE 4-4 Expense Worksheet *(continued)*

	Year 1	Year 2
Dietary supplement	$ 160	$ 180
EKG	15	20
Fixed		
Program licensure	5,000	
Computer and software	3,000	
Training	10,000	
Manuals	500	
Promotion	1,500	
Lab supplies	800	800
Scale	500	500
Counter weights	84	
BP cuffs	66	
Recruiting	200	
Manager salary	36,400	38,220
Secretary salary	9,750	10,238
Diabetes Counseling		
Variable (per person)		
Labor	24	26
Materials	5	5
Food supplies	2	2
Computer analysis	35	40
Fixed		
Audiovisuals	200	
Promotion	200	50
Weight Management Counseling and Support		
Variable (per person)		
Labor	20	21
Materials	5	5
Food supplies	2	2
High-Risk Pregnancy Counseling		
Variable (per person)		
Labor		39
Materials		1
Computer analysis		40
Food supplies		2
Fixed		
Audiovisuals		100
Promotion		200
Grocery Tours		
Variable (per person)		
Labor		5
Materials		2
Fixed		
Training and visuals		360

TABLE 4-4 Expense Worksheet *(continued)*

	Year 1	Year 2
Promotion		$ 100
Travel		40
Box Lunch Seminar Series		
Variable (per person)		
Labor		2
Materials		2
Box lunch		5
Fixed		
Audiovisuals		200
Promotion		800
Travel		100

*Note: For the purpose of profit/loss and cash flow, labor must be combined. However, it must be broken down into variable expense for break-even analysis on each service.

1. For accounting purposes in this case study, the assumption is made that a steady flow of clients will be maintained. Therefore, income was divided by the number of months from the start-up month to month 12. (Note: This does not generally happen in outpatient practices. Enrollment rates change monthly.)
2. A 50-week per year schedule allows for holidays and vacations.
3. Where a package program is offered, the assumption is made that all clients purchase the package as opposed to individual sessions.
4. Only half of those who participate in weight management will purchase the weight management counseling package. The first month of this service will only be offered to one class that has finished weight management. In month 4, two classes per month will be eligible, and in month 6, three classes per month.
5. Table 4-5 shows the flow of clients through the quick weight loss program. Because each phase is priced differently and incurs different expenses, the chart is broken down by phases.

The rest of the year shows the same number of clients as month 18.

The committee found it useful to develop a table (Table 4-6) matching each service's revenues to its expenses.

P & L Statement

The profit and loss statement was developed using the expense worksheet, services chart, and revenue/expense per service chart. To understand how the P&L statement was developed, some basic calculations and explanations may be helpful.

TABLE 4-5 Proposed Number of Clients

Month	Screening	Program	Adaptive
4	13	13	
5	13	26	
6	13	39	
7	13	52	
8	13	65	
9	13	65	13
10	13	65	13
11	13	65	13
12	13	65	13
13	17	69	13
14	17	73	13
15	17	77	13
16	17	81	13
17	17	85	13
18	17	85	17

1. Revenue was calculated using the formula:
   Cost/Client * Projected Number of Clients/Month = Revenue
2. Clients in the quick weight loss program pay for the program monthly for five months. Therefore, during the first five months of the program, the number of new clients will be added to the number of clients seen in the previous month, to determine the total number of clients per month.
3. Capital expenditures are detailed in Table 4-7.
4. All capital expenditures were depreciated over 4 years for simplicity. Therefore, the P&L statement shows the monthly expense for capital expenditures as:
   9500 ÷ 4 ÷ 12
   (Total expenditures ÷ Years of depreciation ÷ Months/year)
5. Table 4-8 shows expenses spread over two years.
6. Phone expenses include $600 per month for phone bills and $50 per month for yellow pages advertising.

The profit and loss statement used by the committee can be found in Figure 4-1. This statement was condensed for the presentation to the administration.

Cash Flow Statement

The committee used the profit and loss statement, and the revenue/expenses by service chart to develop the cash flow statement (Figure 4-2). Remember that these are projections and do not represent the actual statement of cash flow that accoun-

TABLE 4-6 Revenue and Expenses by Service

	Income	Year 1 Expenses	Year 2 Expenses
Individual Counseling			
Income (per client/package)	$100		
Variable (per person)			
Labor		$16	$17
Handouts		2	2
Prenatal Nutrition Education			
Income (per person)	5		
Costs incurred by the prenatal program other than the 1-hour of counselor's time			
Weight Management			
Income (per client/package)	300		
Variable (per person)			
Labor		45	48
Materials		70	70
Computer analysis		35	40
Food supplies		2	2
Fixed			
Promotion supplies		150	
Audiovisuals		260	
Quick Weight Loss			
Screening			
Income per person		350	
Variable (per person)			
Medical history		7	10
Lab fees		115	130
EKG		15	20
Psychological screening		30	32
Professional services		10	13
Program phase—one month participation			
Income (per person)	450		
Variable (per person)			
Physical exam		28	30
Lab fees		112	127
Professional services		50	65
Dietary supplement		160	180
EKG		15	20
Fixed costs			
Program licensure		5,000	
Computer and software		3,000	
Training		10,000	
Manuals		500	
Promotion		1,500	
Lab supplies		800	800
Scale		500	500

TABLE 4-6 Revenue and Expenses by Service *(continued)*

	Income	Year 1 Expenses	Year 2 Expenses
Counter weights		$84	
BP cuffs		66	
Recruiting		200	
Manager salary		36,400	$38,220
Secretary salary		9,750	10,238
Adaptive Phase			
Income per person	360		
Costs are limited to labor, which has been included in the program phase.			
Diabetes Counseling			
Income per person/package	100		
Variable (per person)			
Labor		24	26
Materials		5	5
Food supplies		2	2
Computer analysis		35	40
Fixed			
Audiovisuals		200	
Promotion		200	50
Weight Management Counseling and Support			
Income per person/package	75		
Variable (per person)			
Labor		20	21
Materials		5	5
Food supplies		2	2
High-Risk Pregnancy Counseling			
Income (per person/package)	115		
Variable (per person)			
Labor			39
Materials			1
Computer analysis			40
Food Supplies			2
Fixed			
Audiovisuals			100
Promotion			200
Grocery Tours			
Income (per person)	30		
Variable (per person)			
Labor			5
Materials			2
Fixed			
Training and visuals			360
Promotion			100
Travel			40

TABLE 4-6 Revenue and Expenses by Service *(continued)*

	Income	Year 1 Expenses	Year 2 Expenses
Box Lunch Seminar Series			
Income (per person/package)		$15	
Variable (per person)			
Labor			2
Materials			2
Box lunch			5
Fixed			
Audiovisuals			200
Promotion			800
Travel			100

TABLE 4-7 Capital Expenditures

	Year 1	Year 2
Scale	$500	
Typewriter	300	
Slide projector	250	
Television	500	
VCR	500	
Computer	3,500	
Copier		$1,000
Furniture	2,950	
Books	500	
Phones/installation	500	
Total capital expenditures	9,500	1,000

TABLE 4-8 Two-year Expenses

	Year 1	Year 2
Physician campaign	$2,000	
displays	150	
Weight management	260	
Quick weight loss		
Licensure	5,000	
Computer	3,000	
Training	10,000	
Manuals	500	
Scale	500	$500
Diabetic counseling	400	50
High-risk pregnancy		300
Grocery tours		500
Box lunch seminars		1,100
	$21,876	$2,450

ALWELL OUTPATIENT NUTRITION SERVICE CENTER

PROFIT AND LOSS PROJECTIONS FOR THE FIRST TWO YEARS OF OPERATION

	Year 1												
	Jan	Feb	Mar	Apr	May	Jun	Jul	Aug	Sep	Oct	Nov	Dec	Total
Revenue													
Individual counseling	800	800	800	800	800	800	800	800	800	800	800	800	9,600
Prenatal nutrition	50	50	50	50	50	50	50	50	50	50	50	50	600
Weight management	3,300	3,300	3,300	3,300	3,300	3,300	3,300	3,300	3,300	3,300	3,300	3,300	39,600
Weight management													
Counseling and support			450	450	450	450	450	525	525	525	525	525	4,875
Quick weight loss													
Screening				4,500	4,500	4,500	4,500	4,500	4,500	4,500	4,500	4,500	40,950
Program				5,850	9,100	13,650	18,200	29,250	29,250	29,250	29,250	29,250	193,050
Adaptive phase									4,680	4,680	4,680	4,680	18,720
Diabetic counseling						1,600	1,600	1,600	1,600	1,600	1,600	1,600	11,200
Nutrition counseling													
for high-risk pregnancy													
Grocery tours													
Box lunch seminars													
Total revenue	4,150	4,150	4,600	15,000	18,250	24,400	28,950	40,075	44,755	44,755	44,755	44,755	318,595
Expenses													
Salaries and wages	7,649	7,649	7,649	7,649	7,649	7,649	8,333	8,333	8,333	8,333	8,333	8,333	95,892
Office rental	1,000	1,000	1,000	1,000	1,000	1,000	1,000	1,000	1,000	1,000	1,000	1,000	12,000
Depreciation expense	198	198	198	198	198	198	198	198	198	198	198	198	2,376
Phone (note 1)	650	650	650	650	650	650	650	650	650	650	650	650	7,800
Promotion—Brochures	158	158	158	158	158	158	158	158	158	158	158	158	1,896
Travel and education	208	208	208	208	208	208	208	208	208	208	208	208	2,496
Miscellaneous expense	642	442	442	442	442	442	442	442	442	422	442	442	5,504
Expenses for specific programs													
Individual counseling handouts	16	16	16	16	16	16	16	16	16	16	16	16	192
Weight management													
materials and supplies	792	792	792	792	792	792	792	792	792	792	792	792	9,504
Computer analysis	385	385	385	385	385	385	385	385	385	385	385	385	4,620
Weight management													
counseling and support													
materials and supplies			42	42	42	42	42	49	49	49	49	49	455
Quick weight loss													
Amoritization of startup costs				908	908	908	908	908	908	908	908	908	8,172
Lab supplies				67	67	67	67	67	67	67	67	67	603
Screening													
Lab fees				1,495	1,495	1,495	1,495	1,495	1,495	1,496	1,495	1,495	13,455
EKG				195	195	195	195	195	195	195	195	195	1,755
Professional services				130	130	130	130	130	130	130	130	130	1,170
Program													
Physical				364	728	1,092	1,456	1,820	1,820	1,820	1,820	1,820	12,740
Lab fees				1,040	2,080	3,120	4,160	5,200	5,200	5,200	5,200	5,200	36,400
Professional services				520	1,040	1,560	2,080	2,600	2,600	2,600	2,600	2,600	18,200
EKG				195	780	585	780	975	1,125	1,125	1,125	1,125	7,815
Supplement				2,080	4,160	6,240	8,320	10,400	10,400	10,400	10,400	10,400	72,800
Adaptive phase													
None listed													
Diabetic counseling						1,600	1,600	1,600	1,600	1,600	1,600	1,600	11,200
Supplies						112	112	122	112	112	112	112	784
Computer analysis						640	640	640	640	640	640	640	4,480
Nutrition counseling													
for high-risk pregnancy													
Material and supplies													
Computer analysis													
Grocery tours													
Box lunch seminars													
Total expenses	11,698	11,498	11,540	18,534	23,123	29,284	34,167	38,373	38,523	38,523	38,523	38,523	332,309
Profit (Loss)	(7,548)	(7,348)	(6,940)	(3,534)	(4,873)	(4,884)	(5,217)	1,702	6,232	6,232	6,232	6,232	(13,714)

Note 1 - Phone expenses include $600 per month for phone bills and $50 per month for yellow page advertising.

FIGURE 4.1. Detailed Profit and loss statement.

					Year 2							
Jan	Feb	Mar	Apr	May	Jun	Jul	Aug	Sep	Oct	Nov	Dec	Total
1,200	1,200	1,200	1,200	1,200	1,200	1,200	1,200	1,200	1,200	1,200	1,200	14,400
50	50	50	50	50	50	50	50	50	50	50	50	600
3,960	3,960	3,960	3,960	3,960	3,960	4,290	4,290	4,290	4,290	4,290	4,290	49,500
700	700	700	700	700	700	700	700	700	700	700	800	8,500
5,950	5,950	5,950	5,950	5,950	5,950	5,950	5,950	5,950	5,950	5,950	5,950	71,400
31,050	32,850	34,650	36,450	38,250	38,250	38,250	38,250	38,250	38,250	38,250	38,250	441,000
4,680	4,680	4,680	4,680	4,680	6,120	6,120	6,120	6,120	6,120	6,120	6,120	66,240
2,000	2,000	2,000	2,000	2,000	2,000	2,000	2,000	2,000	2,000	2,000	2,000	24,000
1,840	1,840	1,840	1,840	1,840	1,840	1,840	1,840	1,840	1,840	1,840	1,840	22,080
1,920	1,920	1,920	1,920	1,920	1,920	1,920	1,920	1,920	1,920	1,920	1,920	23,040
		600	600	600	600	600	600	600	600	600	600	6,000
53,350	55,150	57,550	59,350	61,150	62,590	62,920	62,920	62,920	62,920	62,920	62,920	726,760
10,904	10,904	10,904	10,904	10,904	10,904	10,904	10,904	10,904	10,904	10,904	10,904	130,848
1,200	1,200	1,200	1,200	1,200	1,200	1,200	1,200	1,200	1,200	1,200	1,200	14,400
219	219	219	219	219	219	219	219	219	219	219	219	2,628
650	650	650	650	650	650	650	650	650	650	650	650	7,800
158	158	158	158	158	158	158	158	158	158	158	158	1,896
208	208	208	208	208	208	208	208	208	208	208	208	2,496
408	158	158	158	158	158	158	158	158	158	158	158	2,146
24	24	24	24	24	24	24	24	24	24	24	24	288
864	864	864	864	864	864	864	864	864	864	864	864	10,368
480	480	480	480	480	480	480	480	480	480	480	480	5,760
49	49	49	49	49	49	49	49	49	49	49	56	595
950	950	950	950	950	950	950	950	950	950	950	950	11,400
67	67	67	67	67	67	67	67	67	67	67	67	804
2,080	2,080	2,080	2,080	2,080	2,080	2,080	2,080	2,080	2,080	2,080	2,080	24,960
320	320	320	320	320	320	320	320	320	320	320	320	3,840
208	208	208	208	208	208	208	208	208	208	208	208	2,496
2,070	2,190	2,310	2,430	2,550	2,550	2,550	2,550	2,550	2,550	2,550	2,550	29,400
6,900	7,300	7,700	8,100	8,500	8,500	8,500	8,500	8,500	8,500	8,500	8,500	98,000
3,450	3,650	3,850	4,050	4,250	4,250	4,250	4,250	4,250	4,250	4,250	4,250	49,000
1,380	1,460	1,540	1,620	1,700	1,700	1,700	1,700	1,700	1,700	1,700	1,700	19,600
12,420	13,140	13,860	14,580	15,300	15,300	15,300	15,300	15,300	15,300	15,300	15,300	176,400
2,000	2,000	2,000	2,000	2,000	2,000	2,000	2,000	2,000	2,000	2,000	2,000	24,000
140	140	140	140	140	140	140	140	140	140	140	140	1,680
800	800	800	800	800	800	800	800	800	800	800	800	9,600
1,840	1,840	1,840	1,840	1,840	1,840	1,840	1,840	1,840	1,840	1,840	1,840	22,080
48	48	48	48	48	48	48	48	48	48	48	48	576
640	640	640	640	640	640	640	640	640	640	640	640	7,680
128	128	128	128	128	128	128	128	128	128	128	128	1,536
		280	280	280	280	280	280	280	280	280	280	2,800
50,605	51,875	53,675	55,195	56,715	56,715	56,715	56,715	56,715	56,715	56,715	56,722	665,077
2,745	3,275	3,875	4,155	4,435	5,875	6,205	6,205	6,205	6,205	6,205	6,298	61,683

ALWELL OUTPATIENT NUTRITION SERVICE CENTER
SCHEDULE OF CASH INFLOW AND OUTFLOW

Note: This not the same as a statement of cash flows. This projection assumes that expenditures that may benefit several months are made at the beginning of the month in which the program will begin.

	Year 1											
	Jan	Feb	Mar	Apr	May	Jun	Jul	Aug	Sep	Oct	Nov	Dec
Revenue from operations												
(Rounded to lower $1,000)	4,100	4,100	4,600	15,000	18,000	24,000	28,000	40,000	44,000	44,000	44,000	44,000
Cash outflow												
Salaries and wages	7,649	7,649	7,649	7,649	7,649	7,649	8,333	8,333	8,333	8,333	8,333	8,333
Office rental	1,000	1,000	1,000	1,000	1,000	1,000	1,000	1,000	1,000	1,000	1,000	1,000
Phone												
Monthly bill	600	600	600	600	600	600	600	600	600	600	600	600
Yellow pages	600											
Promotion												
Brochures	3,800											
Doctor promotion	2,000											
Display	150											
Travel and education	2,500											
Miscellaneous supplies and equip												
Supplies (note a)	1,900											
Books	500											
Subscriptions	200											
Small equip	600											
Furniture and equipment	9,500											
Expenses for specific programs												
Quick weight loss												
Startup	19,066											
Lab supplies				800								
Expenses from program												
Screening				1,820	1,820	1,820	1,820	1,820	1,820	1,820	1,820	1,820
Program phase				4,199	8,788	12,597	16,796	20,995	21,245	21,145	21,145	21,145
Adaptive phase												
Individual counseling												
Handouts	500											
Weight management												
Materials and supplies	9,900											
Computer analysis	385	385	385	385	385	385	385	385	385	385	385	385
Weight management counseling and support materials and supplies			450									
Diabetic counseling												
Supplies						1,200						
Computer analysis						640	640	640	640	640	640	640
Nutrition counseling for high-risk pregnancy material and supplies												
Computer analysis												
Grocery tours												
Box lunch seminars												
Total cash outflow	60,850	9,634	10,084	16,453	20,242	25,891	29,574	33,773	33,923	33,923	33,923	33,923
Excess of inflow over outflow	(56,750)	(5,534)	(5,484)	(1,453)	(2,242)	(1,891)	(1,574)	6,227	10,077	10,077	10,077	10,077

Note a: Supplies, misc. expense, demo supplies

FIGURE 4.2. Detailed cash flow statement.

Year 2

Jan	Feb	Mar	Apr	May	Jun	Jul	Aug	Sep	Oct	Nov	Dec
53,000	55,000	57,000	59,000	61,000	62,000	62,000	62,000	62,000	62,000	62,000	63,000
10,904	10,904	10,904	10,904	10,904	10,904	10,904	10,904	10,904	10,904	10,904	10,904
1,200	1,200	1,200	1,200	1,200	1,200	1,200	1,200	1,200	1,200	1,200	1,200
600	600	600	600	600	600	600	600	600	600	600	600
600											
2,500											
1,800											
250											
100											
1,500											
1,300											
2,608	2,608	2,608	2,608	2,608	2,608	2,608	2,608	2,608	2,608	2,608	2,608
26,220	27,740	29,260	30,780	32,300	32,300	32,300	32,300	32,300	32,300	32,300	32,300
9,500											
480	480	480	480	480	480	480	480	480	480	480	480
600											
1,700											
800	800	800	800	800	800	800	800	800	800	800	800
1,840	1,840	1,840	1,840	1,840	1,840	1,840	1,840	1,840	1,840	1,840	1,840
900											
640	640	640	640	640	640	640	640	640	640	640	640
2,000											
		2,800									
68,042	46,812	51,132	49,852	51,372	51,372	51,372	51,372	51,372	51,372	51,372	51,372
(15,042)	8,188	5,868	9,148	9,628	10,628	10,628	10,628	10,628	10,628	10,628	11,628

tants develop prior to the start of the services. Also remember that cash flow does not represent profit or loss. Again, some explanations of calculations are in order:

1. Revenue was determined by adding the revenues for each month on the profit and loss statement and rounding to the lower $1,000.
2. The assumption was made that expenditures that may benefit several months are incurred in the month that the service begins.
3. Under miscellaneous supplies and equipment, "Supplies" includes supplies, miscellaneous expenses, and demonstration supplies.
4. All capital expenses are represented in the month of purchase.

As with the profit and loss statement, the cash flow statement was condensed for presentation to administration. Refer to the sample "Executive Summary," Chapter 5.

From the cash flow statement, the committee learned that the practice would require an initial investment of $60,000 (the "Excess of inflow over outflow" for January, Year 1, plus the expected revenue for that month). They also realized that $5,000 of support money would be necessary to operate the practice each month through July (an approximation). Realistically, the cash inflow from August through December, Year 1, would cover the outflow in January of Year 2, and the practice could begin to pay back some of the investment. By the end of Year 2, the initial investment and support money would be completely paid back.

Break-Even Analysis

Break-even analysis was conducted for Year 1 and the combined Years 1 and 2. Rather than solving the break-even equation for the number of clients, as is done for individual services, the committee used dollar sales as the unknown variable. The formula for this equation is:

where:

$$DS = FE + (VE \div TR)\,DS$$

DS = Dollar Sales (Revenue)
FE = Total Fixed Expenses
VE = Variable Expenses (determined by subtracting fixed expenses from total expenses)
TR = Total Revenue (in this case, for the period of 12 and 24 months)

Thus, the calculations were as follows:

Year 1

FE = $158,212 (the sum of all expenses with the exception of specific program expenses)

VE = \$174,097 (total expenses for Year 1 - fixed expenses)
TR = \$318,595 (total revenue for Year 1 on P&L statement)
DS = \$158,212 + (\$174,097 ÷ \$318,595) DS
DS = \$699,791

Year 2

FE = \$314,906
VE = \$682,480
TR = \$1,045,355
DS = \$314,906 + (\$682,480 ÷ \$1,045,355) DS
DS = \$699,791

Since revenue does not reach \$699,791 by the end of Year 1, the practice will not break even by that time. The practice will accumulate \$699,791 of revenue some time between the sixth and seventh month of Year 2. Therefore, the initial goal of break-even by month 13 had to be changed to month 19.

Note that a balance sheet is not completed for this case. A balance sheet could not be completed until the initial investment and support money were approved by the administration. The committee now has all the information necessary to present their plan to administration. The business plan they submitted appears in Chapter 5.

Chapter 5

Gaining the Approval of Administration

Even the best laid business plans will not be meaningful if you cannot gain the approval of administration. Pioneers have echoed a common piece of advice:

> Your plans to establish a practice must be pre-sold to key decision makers long before a formal presentation is made to them. Key decision makers must be predisposed to approve your plans before your proposal is presented.

Discussing the practice with decision makers individually and in advance enables you to listen and learn personal desires, wants, needs, and concerns, as well as desires and needs of the organization. By surfacing needs and responding to concerns, you will be able to determine the approach that will most likely gain approval. You have the opportunity to educate individuals about nutrition services and discuss the potential of the practice personally. People generally have more commitment and ownership for a plan when asked for input. Therefore, seeking the advice of influential people may increase support for your endeavor.

Perhaps the most effective approach is to begin these discussions even before your business and/or strategic plans are formulated. That way, you have the opportunity to develop a business plan that takes the goals, needs, and desires of administration into account. This increases your chances for gaining approval and allows you to seek the approval with confidence. Your level of confidence will be important. Verbal or nonverbal signals that show a lack of confidence could sabotage your efforts.

Once you have gained some support, developed your business and strategic plans, and learned the benefits to and concerns of key decision makers, an informal presentation of your business plan is in order. The most important point to remember is that your proposal must meet your organization's needs. As you develop your strategic plan, keep the lines of communication open by reporting regularly on your findings, either in writing or during a preset meeting. Timing is important. Request approval at a time when your proposal is likely to receive careful consideration.

Although practitioners are usually able to share their enthusiasm regarding the planned practice with key decision makers, pioneers report that careful consideration to the decision makers' viewpoints is often forgotten. This is a critical error. One nutrition practitioner said:

> I couldn't wait for the opportunity to discuss an outpatient nutrition practice with administration. The benefits of such a practice seemed obvious to me. I still have nightmares about how the presentation went. I opened up with a brief discussion about the kind of support we could offer physicians and our ability to improve patient compliance and I noticed the administrators squirming in their chairs. When I asked for questions, I felt like I was bombarded with one question after another. Their primary focus was revenue and referrals to other services. It took us two years to get approval to establish the practice. I think it's because I lost so much credibility during this initial presentation.

HELPFUL SUGGESTIONS

There are some things you can do to increase the chances that your administrators will buy in. Continually stress the benefits of your proposed plan to the organization and the key decision makers. What is the primary value to each? Once you have created a perception of value, prospective clients are more open to listening. Show a willingness to be held accountable for the results proposed in your business plan.

> "If you approve this business plan, I will be responsible for delivering the results contained in this plan. My responsibility will be to ensure that we break even by Month 9, show a profit of $30,000 at the end of Year 1, and a profit of $118,000 at the end of Year 2."

Know your administrator's "hot buttons" and incorporate them into the presentation. One practice knew that their CEO had just stopped smoking. The nutrition counselor was able to incorporate the benefits of a weight maintenance program for those who have recently stopped smoking in her proposal for a weight management program. The CEO became more interested as this topic arose. Networking with board members and other influential people surrounding your administrators, especially his or her secretaries, will lend insight to the administrators' interests. Get the support of influential physicians. If they want the programs you are proposing, your administration will be all ears. Also seek support from other dietitians in your institution.

Sampling is an important tool in any selling process. Invite your decision makers and/or their spouses to sample the services you are proposing so that they can evaluate them. If you know your services are exceptional, this allows the services to "sell themselves" to your decision makers.

Your ability to gain approval and support for establishing the practice relies on the trust, credibility, and rapport you have built up to this point. For example, if administration believes you do not manage money well or that the inpatient nutrition staff you currently manage is weak or unprofessional, the best presentation is not likely to win over these key decision makers. If trust, credibility, or rapport are low, you may want to put your request for approval off until trust, credibility, and rapport can be built. If you expect to control the destiny of the nutrition practice, you must sell your ability to be an effective manager as you sell the practice. Administration commonly considers having the outpatient nutrition function report to a wellness department, rehabilitation center, or even physical therapy department.

Prepare carefully for meetings. Know facts and figures that are important to marketing the program. Anticipate what will be asked, and be prepared with answers. Prior to the presentation with the CEO, present the proposal to the finance officer so that he or she can be prepared with answers to questions on financing, investment, returns, and so on. If you can't answer a question, offer to obtain the information within a short period of time.

If someone else will be presenting, choose your presenters carefully. Consider presenters who will be the most credible, carry the most influence, and be best prepared to handle the presentation. Be sensitive to overpowering your audience with too many representatives from your practice.

Present yourself as a professional and enthusiastic person with a valuable service to sell. Remember, outpatient practices have been viewed as public relations services in many institutions. You must show confidence that the public is willing to buy those services. You may find yourself lecturing rather than selling because you are more comfortable with this form of presentation. This is a trap that may evoke early rejection. Also be careful not to waste time on unnecessary "show and tell." (ADA, 1986) Remember that your audience has no desire to become nutrition experts. Examples of successful programs at similar facilities and samples of materials you will be using will show administrators that you have done your homework.

Probe for understanding and verification. Assume nothing. Then, follow your presentation with a letter of thanks to the administrator. The process of selling ideas to administration is very similar to the process of selling services to worksites. In Chapter 8, under Promoting to Worksites, this selling process is thoroughly reviewed. Refer to that section for additional information. A list of references on negotiating and selling appears in the "Further Readings" section at the conclusion of Chapter 10.

To sustain the support of your administrators once you have gained approval, keep the lines of communication open by:

- Responding quickly to concerns; and
- Determining the decision maker's expectations for reporting results and sending timely reports on the progress of the program.

Overcoming Objections

Throughout the process of exploring this business venture with administration, key decision makers, and those who influence decision makers will identify issues and concerns. There may be a reluctance to discuss sensitive issues or feelings. Your success depends on your ability to bring these underlying issues to the surface. Encourage influential people to raise these objections. You want to know what the concerns are so that you will be prepared to address them when you propose your business plan. Other concerns, yet unspoken, must also be anticipated. In order to gain the commitment and support you seek, you must overcome the objections raised. Develop your business strategies accordingly.

Table 5-1 is a chart of the most common objections. As you read the chart, you will notice three columns from left to right. The first column identifies the objection. The second indicates some of the common ways that decision makers express these objections. The third column suggests some possible approaches for overcoming the objections. Review the chart. As you prepare your plan and your presentation, ask yourself how you would respond if you were confronted with these objections.

THE WRITTEN WORD

The written strategic plan is usually thought of as a document used to persuade investors to support your business venture. In this case, the strategic plan is directed at health care administrators and is a compilation of all of your strategic planning activities. The business plan actually serves two purposes:

1. It communicates your intentions to those who will authorize financial support.
2. It serves as a tool to manage and monitor your business (Mancuso, 1983).

Strategic plans can be written for the start-up of a business or of a single service. The document will change over time with the business.

Like investors, health care administrators will spend little if any time reading the strategic plan prior to your personal presentation. Therefore, all pertinent information must be summarized in five minutes worth of reading time. Yet the

TABLE 5-1 Overcoming Objections

Objections	How the Objections Show Up	Ways to Overcome the Objections
Cost	• You are asking a lot. An outpatient counselor, administrative overhead, office space, phone lines, a quick weight loss program, and other resource materials are a significant investment. • How does the financial return justify the expense? • You're talking in concepts. What is it going to cost and what are the payoffs?" • We can't add full-time equivalents. We have strict guide lines about that."	• We can share some of the current inpatient nutrition resources until the business grows. • All of the initial investment should be returned by the ninth month of operation. That's the break-even point. Profit for the first year will be $20,000. The second year we are estimating a profit of $107,000 and the third year $250,000. • This service will return a profit and it will market the services of other departments.
Limited space	• We don't have clinic space to provide these services. • You wouldn't meet with patients in the cafeteria or food service department, would you?	• Obviously we will need some space, but an office located near any reception area will do. • The radiology department has a classroom that we could share for group programs. • We should be able to start out in the office we are currently using in the cardiac rehabilitation center. No additional space should be needed until the client flow demands an additional counselor.
Not a priority	• For the minimal revenue the department is expected to produce, it is not worth the time or the resources. • Per square foot, we could use the space to provide other healthcare services that could reap a much higher return.	• While the revenue may be low during start up, with proper management, revenues will grow each year. • Additional revenue is not the only reason to provide nutrition services. There are also the added advantages of increased physician services, marketing the institution to the community, and referrals to other departments.

TABLE 5-1 *(Continued)*

Objections	How the Objections Show Up	Ways to Overcome the Objections
Inability to liaison influence key decision makers	• I don't think my boss will like the idea. • I'd have to get the approval of the board. That could be a problem. • You've got my vote, but I will have trouble selling this to the rest of the management team.	• Explore the objections with the subordinate. • Arm the liaison with information that enables him or her to respond to the decision maker's objections. • Network with those who can influence the key decision maker. • Be sensitive to your liaison's position; ask permission to contact the decision maker directly. • If possible, take them both to lunch. • Emphasize the benefits of your services from the decision maker's perspective.
Credibility	• The inpatient nutrition department is a source of discontent with other departments. Your proposal of services relies on their support. How do you intend to gain their support? • You aren't managing the department budget now. You're asking us to risk an investment with little evidence that you can deliver the results you are proposing. • Inpatient dietitians are not well respected by the physicians. How do you intend to gain their support?	• Be prepared with an action plan to address any problem with the inpatient department. • If the credibility of the inpatient nutrition staff is the problem, make a strong distinction between the outpatient and inpatient departments. —Give the outpatient department its own name (e.g., Anyname Nutrition Center). —Hire a new dietitian(s) to staff the department. —Begin a campaign to reeducate physicians and other healthcare professionals to the possibilities and benefits of the services. • Use every tool available to enhance credibility: —Show a track record of results. —Present results of similar practices. —If you are afilliated with a service company, offer to share the risk along with the gain.

TABLE 5-1 *(Continued)*

Objections	How the Objections Show Up	Ways to Overcome the Objections
Skepticism of fluctuations in proposed revenue	• Can the significant fluctuations in revenue from month-to-month really be predicted?	• The experiences of other practitioners in dicates that client traffic reaches a high in September, January, and April and a low June through August. • Certain times of the year, client motivation to address eating habits increases. For example, history shows New Year's resolutions, holidays, bathing suit weather, and seasonal lifestyle changes all result in peak periods.
Institution or physician philosophy	• Protein sparing modified fasting can be harmful, and the eating habits that must be changed to sustain weight loss receive little emphasis. • Only nutrition programs targeted at self-sufficiency will be offered.	• Know the institution's mission, goals, and objectives. • Obviously, the philosophies of your practice must be consistent with the philosophies of the institution and leading physicians. Some administrators will desire a process through which they ensure that the practice will support missions, goals, and objectives.
Pricing	• I'm concerned about the reaction of physicians. The fees you are proposing are equivalent to physician's fees. • Some physicians are going to feel their patients cannot afford the services. They will want them for free.	• Granted, the charge for a general examination by a physician is \$50 to \$100 and we will charge \$65 for an initial session. But during an initial session, we will give each client a full hour of time, as well as printed materials at no charge. The physician may only spend 5 to 10 minutes with each patient. Physicians may raise this objection initially, but with a little explanation we believe their concern can be overcome. • We offer you the results of our market study. Our competitors are charging these fees and getting them.

TABLE 5-1 *(Continued)*

Objections	How the Objections Show Up	Ways to Overcome the Objections
Pricing *(Continued)*		• Research is consistently reaffirming that behavior change takes time. It must occur gradually with ongoing support. Physicians, for the most part, are not nutrition experts and do not have the time to provide the ongoing nurturing and counsel that our clients will need. Ongoing support is extremely costly. Physicians will need to be reminded of this. • At least partial reimbursement will be available to most clients with a physician referral. • Physicians will still have the option to provide minimal nutrition education to their patients who cannot afford ongoing counseling.
Physician support	• Physicians may not refer patients because many of them offer nutrition counseling themselves. • I'm not sure our physicians recognize that behavior change must be nurtured or that it demands a reformation of current methods of providing services. • Inpatient dietitians are not well respected by the physician. How do you intend to gain their support?	• Compliance rates regarding recommended dietary change are staggeringly low. All healthcare professionals must be open to new approaches for the advantage of the patient. • Research is consistently reaffirming that behavior change takes time. It must occur gradually with ongoing support. Physicians, for the most part, are not nutrition experts and do not have the time to provide the ongoing nurturing and counsel that our clients will need. • We have several resources that are calling for new approaches to the compliance program. Among them are recent articles from the *New England Journal of Medicine*. • Our competitors have been successful in getting physicians to buy in. They claim that administration support and a personal visit from the dietitian to develop rapport and explain the advantages was critical to obtaining physician support.

TABLE 5-1 *(Continued)*

Objections	How the Objections Show Up	Ways to Overcome the Objections
Recognizing function as food/ nutrition services responsibility *(Continued)*	• Maybe we should start a wellness department that would offer healthcare services to the well. This service should be offered among other services and managed by the wellness department.	• We advise having each area of responsibility managed by the experts in that field. Even if you choose to market services together to a common market, in this case the community, each should be charged with responsibility for building their own business by addressing the individual needs of their clientele."
	• We are opening a cardiac rehabilitation center and intend to offer outpatient nutrition services as a component of that.	• By having a separate business plan for nutrition services, we are able to specifically address nutrition needs and track specific results. In this way, the contribution of an outpatient nutrition service may be evaluated on an ongoing basis.
		• Nutrition counselors need the support and supervision of managers who understand their needs and problems. We will gladly provide nutrition services to the various programs you suggested. However, resources, reporting, and accountability should be the responsibility of the outpatient nutrition center. There is a greater credibility for the counsel if it is provided by a nutrition professional. Nutrition credentials should be emphasized.

details of the business or service must be documented for further scrutiny over time and for use as a management tool. Hence, the following outline:

I. Cover sheet
   a. Name of proposed business or service
   b. Time period covered by the plan
   c. Date
   d. Authors
II. Table of contents
   a. Major headings
   b. Figures and appendices
III. Executive summary
   a. Statement of purpose

   b. Benefits to the institution
   c. Market
   d. Unique features of the business or service
   e. Financial projections

IV. Business description
   a. Goals
   b. Service descriptions
   c. Product descriptions
   d. Services that will be enhanced

V. Market strategies
   a. Market segments and share
   b. Referral agents
   c. Positioning
   d. Advertising and promotion plans
   e. Competition

VI. Management plan
   a. Staffing
   b. Scheduling
   c. Organization and reporting

VII. Financial plan
   a. Summary of revenues and expenses (profit/loss)
   b. Cash flow requirements
   c. Break-even point
   d. Bail-out signals
   e. Expansion signals

VIII. Appendices
   a. Financial explanations (schedules, bases for calculations, etc.)
   b. Job descriptions/resumes
   c. Other supporting information

The Executive Summary

The executive summary ranks as the single most important component of the strategic plan. Some administrators will base their decisions on the executive summary and your presentation. The executive summary should be designed to entice the administrator to read further. In one to two pages, it will encapsulate the impact, success potential, and necessary resources of the proposed business or service (Rose, 1989).

Emphasize items that are of special interest to the decision makers. Stress the benefits to the organization in the executive summary. Will your services increase patronage of other departments? Will they improve the institution's image with physicians and with the community? Will they generate revenue?

Highlight the unique features of the business or services you will be offering. Explain how you will set yourself apart from the competition and capture the targeted segments. If certain services are considered glamorous at the present time, capitalize on this fact. Health care institutions feel the need to be state-of-the-art. Thus, if cholesterol education programs are available in the country's leading hospitals, sell your administrators on that point.

Unless you summarize your financial expectations in the executive summary, the business is doomed from the start. Administrators want to know what investment is required, the amount of time necessary to recover it, and the profit potential of the business over several years. All of this information can be stated in one to two sentences.

Use present tense, short sentences and short paragraphs (Mancuso, 1983). Bullet points and numbered steps contribute to brevity and ease of reading. A sample executive summary for the Alwell Women's Health Center Case Study follows.

This summary would be accompanied by the business description, marketing strategies, management strategies, and financial projections for those who wish to read further. With this executive summary, only a service/price table, P&L statement and cash flow have been included.

For a list of services, costs, and breakeven analysis, see Table 5-2. For a sample profit and loss projection and cash flow schedule, see Figures 5-1 and 5-2, respectively.

ALWELL NUTRITION CENTER STRATEGIC BUSINESS PLAN EXECUTIVE SUMMARY 1989

Prepared by: J. Doe, Clinical Nutrition Manager
S. Jones, Marketing Counselor

Introduction and Summary

Alwell Women's Health Center realizes that women are taking greater responsibility for their health care. Women want to be informed and involved in selecting methods of treatment when faced with a medical condition. Such trends have created new market opportunities and alternative health care delivery options. Alwell has seized the opportunity to market new services and adapt established services for the needs of women. The Department of Nutrition Services intends to support Alwell's new endeavors through an exciting new outpatient practice.

TABLE 5-2 Alwell Services and Prices

Service/ Start Month	Package Description	Price	New Clients Needed to Meet Goals Year 1	Year 2
Individual counseling (month 1)	Initial (1 hr.)	$60.00	2/wk.	3/wk.
	Follow-up (30 min.)	30.00		
	Initial + 2 follow-ups	100.00		
Prenatal nutrition education (month 1)	2½-hour sessions (part of prenatal classes)	5.00	10/wk.	10/wk.
Weight management (month 1)	2 Individual + 8 1⅓-hr. group sessions (8–14 participants/group)	300.00	130/yr.	150/yr.
Weight management counseling and support (month 3)	6 1-hr./wk. group sessions	75.00 w/ package 15.00 per session	65/yr.	85/yr.
Quick weight loss (month 4)				
Screening	1 hr.	350.00	120/yr.	200/yr.
Program	1 hr./wk. group	450.00 monthly	120/yr.	200/yr.
Adaptive phase	1 hr./wk. group	360.00 monthly	45/yr.	180/yr.
Diabetic counseling (month 6)	4 1-hr. group	100.00	16/mo.	20/mo.
Nutrition counseling for high-risk pregnancy (month 13)	2 1-hr. individual 3 1-hr. group sessions	115.00		16/mo.
Grocery tours (month 13)	1½-hr.	30.00		16/wk.
Box lunch seminars (month 15)	2-hr. group	15.00		40/mo.

The Alwell Nutrition Center would offer its support to the Health Center by developing a focused business, structured to the needs of three target groups of women, providing the greatest opportunity for success and profitability. The benefits to the institution are:

- Increased outpatient profits;
- The competitive edge;
- Attraction of medical specialists;
- Increased visibility and referral to other services; and
- A caring image to the community.

Thorough market research suggests targeting women who are educated (high school graduates and above) in mid- to high income households in the following groups:

ALWELL OUTPATIENT NUTRITION SERVICE CENTER
PROFIT AND LOSS PROJECTIONS

Year 1

	Jan	Feb	Mar	Apr	May	Jun	Jul	Aug	Sep	Oct	Nov	Dec	**Total**
Revenue	4,150	4,150	4,600	15,000	18,250	24,400	28,950	40,075	44,755	44,755	44,755	44,755	**318,595**
Expenses													
Salaries and wages	7,649	7,649	7,649	7,649	7,649	7,649	8,333	8,333	8,333	8,333	8,333	8,333	**95,892**
Office rental	1,000	1,000	1,000	1,000	1,000	1,000	1,000	1,000	1,000	1,000	1,000	1,000	**12,000**
Depreciation	198	198	198	198	198	198	198	198	198	198	198	198	**2,376**
Program expenses	1,193	1,193	1,235	8,229	12,818	18,979	23,178	27,384	27,534	27,534	27,534	27,534	**204,345**
Miscellaneous	1,658	1,458	1,458	1,458	1,458	1,458	1,458	1,458	1,458	1,458	1,458	1,458	**17,696**
Total Expenses	11,698	11,498	11,540	18,534	23,123	29,284	34,167	38,373	38,523	38,523	38,523	38,523	**332,309**
Profit (Loss)	(7,548)	(7,348)	(6,940)	(3,534)	(4,873)	(4,884)	(5,217)	1,702	6,232	6,232	6,232	6,232	**(13,714)**

Year 2

	Jan	Feb	Mar	Apr	May	Jun	Jul	Aug	Sep	Oct	Nov	Dec	**Total**
Revenue	53,350	55,150	57,550	59,350	61,150	62,590	62,920	62,920	62,920	62,920	62,920	63,020	**726,760**
Expenses													
Salaries and wages	10,904	10,904	10,904	10,904	10,904	10,904	10,904	10,904	10,904	10,904	10,904	10,904	**130,848**
Office rental	1,200	1,200	1,200	1,200	1,200	1,200	1,200	1,200	1,200	1,200	1,200	1,200	**14,400**
Depreciation	219	219	219	219	219	219	219	219	219	219	219	219	**2,628**
Program expenses	36,858	38,128	39,928	41,698	43,218	43,218	43,218	43,218	43,218	43,218	43,218	43,225	**502,363**
Miscellaneous	1,424	1,424	1,424	1,174	1,174	1,174	1,174	1,174	1,174	1,174	1,174	1,174	**14,838**
Total Expenses	50,605	51,875	53,675	55,195	56,715	56,715	56,715	56,715	56,715	56,715	56,715	56,722	**665,077**
Profit (Loss)	2,745	3,275	3,875	4,155	4,435	5,875	6,205	6,205	6,205	6,205	6,205	6,298	**61,683**

FIGURE 5-1. Profit and loss projection in Executive Summary.

ALWELL OUTPATIENT NUTRITION SERVICE CENTER
SCHEDULE OF CASH FLOW

Year 1

	Jan	Feb	Mar	Apr	May	Jun	Jul	Aug	Sep	Oct	Nov	Dec	**Total**
Expected revenue	4,100	4,100	4,600	15,000	18,000	24,000	28,000	40,000	44,000	44,000	44,000	44,000	**313,800**
Total cash outflow	60,850	9,634	10,084	16,453	20,242	25,891	29,574	33,773	33,923	33,923	33,923	33,923	**342,193**
Excess of inflow over outflow	(56,750)	(5,534)	(5,484)	(1,453)	(2,242)	(1,891)	(1,574)	6,227	10,077	10,077	10,077	10,077	**(28,393)**

Year 2

	Jan	Feb	Mar	Apr	May	Jun	Jul	Aug	Sep	Oct	Nov	Dec	**Total**
Expected revenue	53,000	55,000	57,000	59,000	61,000	62,000	62,000	62,000	62,000	62,000	62,000	63,000	**720,000**
Total cash outflow	68,042	46,812	51,132	49,852	51,372	51,372	51,372	51,372	51,372	51,372	51,372	51,372	**626,814**
Excess of inflow over outflow	(15,042)	8,188	5,868	9,148	9,628	10,628	10,628	10,628	10,628	10,628	10,628	11,628	**93,186**

FIGURE 5-2. Schedule of cash flow for the Executive Summary.

- Over age 55;
- Working, age 30–45; and
- Pregnant for the first time.

Services that would attract members of these markets, supplement existing outpatient programs, and draw women to the Health Center for various medical needs include:

- Individualized nutrition counseling;
- Comprehensive weight management;
- Educational seminars; and
- Counseling and support groups.

These services would be offered for the medical conditions of high-risk pregnancy, obesity, and diabetes. Many of the service offerings would be suitable for the "well" population interested in improving their nutrition habits.

The revenue projections, represented in the attached financial projections, indicate that this business will break even within the first 19 months with a projected revenue potential of $1,045,355 over 2 years. Profit in the second year is projected to be $61,000. To achieve the desired revenues, an initial investment of $60,000 is required with an additional $5,000/month for the first 6 months. Payback would begin in the ninth month of the first year and be complete prior to the end of the second year.

We believe this proposal provides significant revenue potential and other important benefits to Alwell Women's Health Center. Where more than one hospital exists in a community such as this one, a quality patient education, counseling, and support service can be a significant factor, contributing to the selection of one hospital over another for clients seeking professional services or potential patients for inpatient services.

Business Description

The business description is the next section of the strategic plan. The rest of the document lays out the details of your plan. The business description explains the goals and objectives of the business. Because many of the services you provide may be foreign to decision makers, you must provide descriptions of each service or product. You may also wish to explain how various services will enhance other programs within the institution in this section.

Marketing Strategies

Much of this section can take the form of charts and bullet points. Describe the market segments you intend to serve and what market share you hope to capture.

Estimate the number of physicians/health care providers you expect to receive referrals from. Provide information on how you will position the business to draw this market share. Explain promotional strategies and the rationale behind them.

Management Strategies

How will the business or service run? Describe the staff necessary to provide services. In many businesses, resumes are presented in this section; however, you will only provide resumes if you intend to use existing employees. If you intend to hire new employees for the positions, only job descriptions can be offered.

An intended schedule explains your staffing needs and one of your strategies for gaining clients. This section could be a chart documenting the intended activities of the practice in any given week. Because institutional administrators are not accustomed to the provision of ambulatory care during Saturday and evening hours, you may need to provide rationale for such strategies.

The organization of the outpatient nutrition practice is quite simple in most cases. Administrators will be interested in the supervisory structure of the practice (who reports to whom?). This issue should be resolved with the department heads and administrators long before the strategic plan is written.

Financial Projections

The financial projections section will include finalized copies of the financial analyses you have conducted. If you must explain the assumptions or calculations used to derive the analyses, they can be placed at the end of this section or in the Appendix.

Part 3

Administration

Chapter 6

Administrative Considerations in Establishing the Practice

DEVELOPING GUIDERULES

In dealing with clients, referral agents, and employees, philosophy statements, policies, procedures, and standards of performance must be established to ensure a consistent and efficient practice. Consistency and efficiency are marks of quality that help to build trust and confidence. Adherence or non-adherence to these guiderules will directly or indirectly influence the quality of service your practice renders to its clients. Client satisfaction, profitability, your reputation, and your ability to grow your practice are all affected by quality and consistency.

Policies, procedures, and standards establish a yardstick by which all performance is measured. Without these guiderules, clients, referring agents, and employees do not know what is expected of them; they also do not know what to expect of your practice. Anticipating problems aids in the development of practical policies, procedures, and standards for administering various activities.

Remember, the outpatient nutrition staff is usually small. It is an advantage to be involved enough with your staff on a daily basis to be able to lead them in a sense of common purpose (Albrecht, 1988). However, this advantage is no substitute for structure. Some written guiderules are required to create a smooth organizational process. Many of the issues that are reviewed in this chapter may never be formally printed, but they must be consciously decided and effectively communicated. The act of writing them down forces you to decide how your business will operate day-to-day. Also, it often helps you to clarify your expectations and to manage your practice more effectively.

Some of the guiderules suggested in this chapter are intended solely as an internal guideline. Others will be communicated publicly.

Stating Your Philosophies

For some of us, communicating philosophy is very difficult. Our philosophies are so much a part of our thoughts and feelings, it is often difficult to examine them individually. Obviously, unless we can articulate them, others are not likely to represent them.

Questions to consider in developing a philosophy include:

- Do you support the position that time and ongoing support is necessary for most people attempting to make lasting changes in their eating habits?
- How do you define professional limits?
- Do you encourage self-sufficiency?
- What image do you wish to portray (supportive, professional, etc.)?
- Do you believe group counseling to be a supplement to individual counseling, or will individual counseling provide a feeder pool for group work?

Many of your policies and standards will support the philosophies of your practice.

Policies Regulating the Delivery of Service

To determine how you will go about providing service to your clients, you must first understand what service means. Karl Albrecht, in his book, *At America's Service*, writes:

> *A service is a psychological and largely personal outcome, whereas a physical product is usually "impersonal" in its impact on the customer.* (Albrecht, 1988)

Although most of the current, popular literature written on the service industry applies more easily to large corporations, Albrecht lifts the spirits of the small business person. He suggests that small businesses are more adaptable and have the opportunity to develop their employees on a more personal basis. Therefore, the ability of a small firm to move into a high-quality service mode quickly provides an advantage over the larger competition (Albrecht, 1988).

The first steps in developing a service orientation are your marketing efforts, especially customer-centered market research. However, this customer-centered attitude must carry over into your daily activities in order to maintain a profitable business.

It is often difficult for the nutrition counselor to determine specific customer perceptions of quality nutrition services. Nutrition counselors seldom seek the services of other nutrition counselors. However, we have all experienced some provision of health care service (e.g., appointments with physicians, dental check-ups, x-rays, lab work) that can give us some valuable insight. Your expectations of such service experiences generally include:

- Timely service;
- Courteous communications;
- A feeling of personalization and privacy;
- Sound recommendations and counsel; and
- Professional guidance.

Applying these concepts to the business of outpatient nutrition service follows.

Regulating Time and the Flow of Clients

Creating sound guidelines and policies that support your efforts to use time effectively entails effectively scheduling and managing the flow of clients. These policies and guidelines enable colleagues within the same practice to deal with common situations in a similar manner. Through these efforts, your hope is to ensure that clients arrive on time and prepared for the planned activities. Guiderules encourage clients to share responsibility for maintaining the necessary pace to achieve mutually established goals. They help establish realistic expectations regarding your time commitment and what will be accomplished.

It doesn't take much to throw the schedule into a hectic state. It can be trying to have clients arrive late or unprepared, with unrealistic expectations. "No shows" and cancellations can be just as frustrating.

Timely service is a critical issue of client satisfaction in any service industry. Clients trust you to respect the value of their time and to use this time in the most effective and supportive way possible. Your policies and personal management of time should suggest to the client that you and your staff recognize that his or her time is as valuable to him or her as your time is to you. The following questions are posed to assist you in designing time-regulating policies for your practice.

How will appointments be scheduled?

Many times, clients are scheduled for appointments through the physician's office. This can lead to confusion about times and places. If you choose to allow appointments to be scheduled in this manner, you may want to follow up with a postcard giving some pertinent information. Another option is to ask the physician's staff to give your brochure to referral clients and have the clients call to schedule their own appointments.

Your administrative staff can prepare the client for the appointment by making sure that they have directions to your office and know what to bring with them (physician's prescription, diet records, lab work, etc.) (Helm, 1987). Expectations about payment can also be addressed when appointments are made.

How much time will you need to meet with each client?
It is important that you designate a length of time for the appointment that is realistic because you must become skilled at working within the limits of that time frame. If you base the amount of time on your current skill level or the skill level of the incumbents in the nutrition counseling positions, consider two risks:

1. If the incumbents are not skilled at maximizing time during the session, fewer clients may be seen. This may not be financially feasible.
2. Positions turn over and successful practices expand. This means that the guidelines you establish for the practice must be appropriate for future counselors as well. Your credibility may diminish if you alter services based on the skills of individual counselors, particularly if you do this frequently.

Recognizing these risks, we recommend that you base the length of your appointments on clients' needs and business issues, not current skill levels. Consider norms within the industry (particularly in your marketplace). We recommend that you improve your pacing techniques in order to meet the designated time frame for appointments.

How will you handle walk-ins?
If you do not intend to counsel clients without appointments, it may be helpful to post your policy in the reception area—"By Appointment Only." Also, since physicians often refer clients on a walk-in basis, it is important that they be notified of your appointment policy in advance.

How will you communicate your expectations for the length of the session to the client?
Clients are often surprised and unprepared when they learn, during the session, that you have allocated more time than they anticipated. In some cases, clients may rely on others for transportation and may need this information to make necessary arrangements in advance.

Colleagues and administrative staff who are responsible for scheduling appointments should be trained to review the anticipated length of the appointment at the time it is made. It may be advantageous to include this information in your marketing materials. Also, in communicating your expectations for the length of the sessions, it is wise to emphasize that clients are different and that their needs are often different, so it is not unusual for the length of sessions to vary.

Will you prepare the client in advance about what to expect in the initial visit and in follow-up visits?
Review in advance what will be accomplished during each session. By doing so, clients are better prepared to assist you in meeting the objectives. Preparation may

also reduce the anxiety level of the client, which may contribute to a more productive session.

Again, colleagues and administrative staff who are responsible for scheduling appointments should be trained to review with the client what will be done, any special instructions, the cost of the services, and any applicable reimbursement information. Some clients will not accept nutrition services when they learn about the cost, the extent of reimbursement, or that there is no reimbursement. You cannot afford to have last minute cancellations. Plan in advance, so that this type of cancellation can be avoided.

Some practices have recommended that an orientation package of information be mailed prior to the first visit. Other practices prepare such packages to be given out by the physician's staff upon referral. The package would serve to orient new clients and could be used later for reference. Orientation packages could include:

- A summary of services;
- What to expect;
- Promotional material;
- A request for written physician referral, if applicable;
- Policies and procedures of the practice specific to clients;
- Cost of services;
- Reimbursement;
- Scheduled hours;
- Location of facility (perhaps a map);
- Parking information; and
- Any child care provisions (generally for group activity).

Also suggested is that you discuss with your clients at the close of each session what will be discussed during the following session, how much time you will need, and how soon you should meet (provide an appointment card). Some clients like to participate in this planning process. Others prefer that you guide them. It is critical that you know each client's preferences and expectations.

Could clients complete forms in advance regarding nutrition and family history? Although you will want to review this information with the client, the advance preparation may reduce the amount of time spent gathering information. The information requested requires thought, and the accuracy of the data may be improved due to the additional time expended in advance.

You may want to ask clients to come in 15 minutes early for the initial visit to complete forms if there is no viable way to get the forms to them in advance. You may also want to ask clients to bring in a record of foods eaten during the three days prior to the visit. You could request this at the time the appointment is made.

How can you minimize the amount of unbillable time and the number of interruptions spent on telephone calls?

Since much of your administrative time is consumed with unanticipated phone calls to either respond to client questions or provide follow-up support, it helps to designate a time frame during which you will be available to communicate with clients by phone. Often, health care professionals designate the first or last hour of the workday.

Only calls requiring immediate attention should be taken during other hours. Support personnel should be instructed to screen calls, courteously inform clients of the procedures, take a message, and inform the clients that their call will be returned during the designated hour. This helps you control time and encourages your clients to assist you. If your clients' requests will require considerable time, suggest that they schedule an appointment.

What will you do if a session begins late because the client is late?

You may want to establish a policy or guiderule to deal with this situation. If there is not enough time to accomplish anything meaningful, explain that you will be unable to see the client and ask that he or she reschedule for another time. In a shortened session, you might adjust the clients' expectation for the session and use the remaining time to the best advantage.

If time is available to complete the full session when the client arrives (i.e., time created by a cancellation, break, meal following the session, or the last appointment of the day), you may choose to proceed with the session. Proceeding with the session if the delay will inevitably back up the schedule should be strongly discouraged. This will unfairly penalize those clients who are punctual.

What will you do if a session begins late because you are late?

Although your policies and guiderules should reduce the incidence of backed up schedules, sometimes it is inevitable. Your support staff and colleagues should be able to support you in getting back on track.

Scheduling documentation time between appointments or a break between every few appointments may provide enough time to catch up on hectic days. Clients with similar problems might be counseled together, if both clients agree to do so. Shortening your lunch break may provide the opportunity to catch up.

When you do get behind, inform successive clients immediately that you are behind schedule. Give them the option to reschedule. Clients who have not yet arrived can be contacted by phone and rescheduled, if possible. A colleague may be able to see one or more of the first-time clients. Use caution in exercising this option with clients who have developed rapport with a particular counselor. During group programs with multiple sessions, a counselor may find that he or she will be unable to lead a session. If possible, inform the group in advance and allow them some alternatives. They may opt to postpone the session rather than "break in" another counselor, or you may be able to provide a guest speaker. Giving your clients the power to make such decisions shows that you value their time and feelings.

How will the schedule of appointments be accommodated if you are ill or unable to meet with your clients for any reason?

Clients feel sensitive about meeting with other counselors. A better solution for such clients may be to reschedule. You may have to shift your schedule and add hours to your normal schedule of appointments (e.g., add a Saturday or an additional evening) in order to accommodate your clients.

How will you address "no shows" and confusion about appointments?

The best way to address confusion is to *prevent it.* There are two procedures that nutrition counselors find helpful in this situation:

1. Write appointments down on an appointment card. Either give the card to the client as the appointment is made, or, if the appointment is made by telephone, send the appointment card by mail.
2. Telephone clients the day before the appointment to be sure they are planning to come. You may not choose to do this with all clients. It may produce positive results to do this with new clients and clients who have established a pattern of lateness or cancellations.

A significant number of "no shows" and cancellations may also be an indication that your appointment schedule is not meeting your clients' needs. Providing service during evening and weekend hours may be the answer to your problems. Some medical practices, generally those with client waiting lists, establish policies that are communicated on the initial visit about how frequently delays and cancellations will be tolerated before services to the client will be discontinued.

Some practices require that cancellations be communicated no later than a designated number of hours prior to the appointment. Some practices require that clients pay for the visit if they do not cancel within this time period. In packaged programs (more than one session for one price), clients may receive only a partial refund if they drop out of the program. In medically-monitored weight loss clinics, this procedure is becoming the rule rather than the exception. The hope is that clients will realize the importance of regular monitoring to reduce weight when such drastic measures are taken.

Ensuring Courteous Communication

Communication entails personal conversations, phone calls, and written communiques and encompasses all staff members with whom your clients come in contact. Rudeness and apathy are intolerable to clients and will erode your business potential. Each member of your staff should understand that, regardless of client behavior, they should treat clients with respect. They must communicate in such a way that clients feel understood, valued, and important. Make your clients feel welcome and properly served.

Train your support staff in the proper handling of communications. Your modeling of those techniques with your staff, as well as your clients, will set the standard. Remember, "a picture is worth a thousand words." The more specific you can be with your staff, the better. Describe how you want clients treated in detail.

How will you ensure courteous and professional telephone communications? As telephone contact is often the client's first impression of your business, specify how you want clients greeted. Using the caller's name and providing your own name are excellent ways of personalizing your message and may calm an indignant caller. You must provide your staff and/or answering service with enough information to deal with the majority of calls and enough flexibility to react in a positive way to each call.

In a study cited in Small Business Reports (Business Bulletins, 1987), 5,000 phone calls were placed to various service establishments. Of the calls, 58 percent were answered after the eighth ring; 78 percent of those who answered did not ask the caller's name; 34 percent provided price and hung up; and 11 percent were unable to provide information. Consider setting a standard about the number of rings. For example, "Each call will be answered by the third ring." Some clients may hang up before the fourth ring, and you will lose business if they do.

Although phone calls often arise at inopportune times, try not to act distracted or rushed. If you are truly unable to deal with the call at that particular time, politely offer to return the call at a later time.

Establish a standard for returning phone calls. For example, all telephone calls are returned within 24 hours. Emergency phone calls are returned within the hour. If this is not possible, they should be referred to another nutrition professional so that he or she can return the call immediately.

During periods when you are out of town or on vacation, some means of accepting referrals and directing emergency calls should be established. You may either retain your receptionist or hire an answering service. Calls can often be directed to another department.

If full-time phone coverage is not feasible, an answering machine or answering service may be in order. Answering machines are inexpensive, easy-to-use, and allow you to accept calls during nonworking hours. Some brands allow you to screen calls even when you are available, and messages can be retrieved from any phone with an access code. However, they are impersonal and only provide the caller with limited information.

Although the answering service is more expensive, your callers will be able to gather more information in a personalized manner. In urgent cases, the service can reach you promptly or refer the caller to someone who can help. If you do hire a service, training is a must to ensure that the service represents your practice sensitively and professionally.

How will you ensure courteous and professional written communications?
All written communications should be clear, concise, and positive. Respond promptly to requests for written information, while avoiding any breech of confidentiality. Since the majority of your written correspondence will be with physicians, insurance providers, and marketing prospects, keep your message brief and offer continued service as requested. All written communications should reflect a professional image and should be typed on your letterhead or on professionally printed forms.

How will you ensure that face-to-face communications with clients are courteous and professional?
Books have been written on face-to-face communications. What you say and how you present yourself are the most important determinants of client return. The counselor who is harried by an over-booked schedule and rushes through a client session may very well be pushing profits out the door. The counselor who becomes irritated or angry at the client who always has another "excuse" may lose good word-of-mouth publicity, as well as a client. You cannot allow your personal feelings and judgments, family or work stresses, or personal crises to hinder your relationships with clients.

Instead, treat your clients with respect and empathy. Develop a strong professional image and counseling skills that set you apart from the competition. Remember that effective communication is predicated on effective listening.

How will you ensure that your staff is provided with the most up-to-date information regarding the operation of your practice?
All staff members need to be fully informed regarding the operation of your practice in order to effectively communicate with clients. Updated information must be disseminated on a regular basis.

In small practices, information bulletins, handbooks, and other communiques are rarely used. The information dissemination process is usually more informal. However, regular meetings are strongly suggested. Without some structure in place to ensure that the "right hand knows what the left hand is doing," important information often slips through the cracks, in which case the practice suffers.

Encouraging a Feeling of Personalization
We all like to feel as though we are special and unique. Clients who seek nutrition counseling each have different needs, lifestyles, preferences, influences, and

eating habits. They expect to be treated in an individualized fashion. They expect that their individual lifestyles, needs, preferences, and medical conditions will be understood.

How will you ensure that your clients have a feeling of personalization? Tailoring programs to fit the client, dealing specifically with unique problems, and showing interest in the client's particular lifestyle provides the client with a strong sense of personalization. As you orient and train your staff, you may want to suggest that they learn clients' names quickly and use them often. Follow-up phone calls and/or letters show the counselor's concern for the individual. If you use form letters for follow-up, a brief, handwritten note specific to the client is advisable.

Whenever possible, show a personal interest (e.g., ask about children, ask about vacation, mention something specific to the client's occupation). Verifying your understanding of clients' needs, lifestyles, preferences, cultural influences, and medical conditions shows them that you listen to them. If possible, use computerized nutrition analyses to analyze clients' personal dietary habits.

All of these techniques will help your clients feel that your services are personalized. Advance preparation for each session is critical too. However, you must learn to be flexible and adapt to the situation if it does not turn out as you expect. Let's look at an example.

> John Doe was diagnosed hypertensive by the physician at his HMO. The physician prescribed medication and scheduled him an appointment with the nutrition counselor. The nutrition counselor was sent some basic medical information in advance so that she could prepare for the first session.
>
> When John Doe arrived for his appointment, the counselor looked quite surprised. After verifying the fact that he was indeed John Doe, she explained that the information she received stated John's height as 63 inches (weight: 210 lb.) rather than 6 feet, 3 inches. The counselor corrected the error on her chart, but proceeded with her original plan to educate the client on the dietary regimen for an extremely overweight, hypertensive. She did not ask John about his expectations. Nor did she gather any other personal information on John or his lifestyle. John Doe never returned for follow-up.

Because the nutrition counselor did not evaluate needs, gather information regarding influences or preferences, or adapt the nutrition plan to John Doe's nutrition condition, she lost a client.

Ensuring Sound Counsel and Recommendations

You want nutrition recommendations and counsel to meet four criteria. You want them to be:

1. Nutritionally sound;
2. Consistent with policies and procedures;
3. Consistent with the philosophies of your practice; and
4. Tailored to the needs, influences, financial resources, preferences, expectations, and motivation of individual clients.

How will you ensure that counsel and recommendations are sound?

Sound counsel and recommendations are the product of hiring and training excellent staff members. A thorough screening process before hiring ensures that philosophies are compatible. The interviewer can also look for evidence of the counseling skills necessary to surface and adapt counseling efforts to the personal needs, influences, and preferences of each client. If at all possible, observe each candidate in a mock counseling session.

A thorough orientation and training program helps new staff members understand policies, procedures, and philosophies. Standards for ongoing professional development, including required reading, seminars to attend, peer or supervisory observation and evaluation, and inservice training show the staff that you are serious about sound counsel. An evaluation or monitoring program that incorporates the observation of supervisors and/or peer review can be helpful.

How should questions be handled?

You are expected to offer time for questions. Questions should be encouraged. They enable you to clarify information, correct misunderstandings, become aware of resistance to information or change, and become aware of client skepticism.

Train all members of your support staff to provide accurate information about the operation and locality of your practice. Suggest that they limit their answers to these areas and to refer all nutrition questions to the nutrition counselors. Encourage your nutrition counselors to resist the temptation to give answers to nutrition problems. Instead, guide them to respond to nutrition questions by encouraging clients to resolve their own problems. This will foster self-sufficiency and a greater commitment to the resolution.

If an answer is not known, instruct your staff to offer a resource or to vow that an answer will be found. Following through with such promises is critical.

How will you handle errors or the mishandling of situations?

When you realize you have made a mistake or handled a situation poorly, apologize and correct the error or situation. Stress that blaming other staff members for mistakes sounds defensive. Criticizing prior counselors undermines the practice and, if the client had strong credibility for the prior counselor, the credibility of the new counselor may be undermined.

How will you encourage ongoing counseling, when appropriate?
If you adopt the philosophy that continued counseling provides greater support through the change process, a strategy for encouraging continued counsel is fundamental. Consider honing your counseling skills so that clients will want more. Packaged pricing (e.g., three sessions for one price), incentives, contests, and rebates are effective means of encouraging clients to continue.

A policy to follow up on each client with a brief phone call after a certain number of sessions, as well as when a client does not return can increase the commitment of the client and promote a caring image. A caring relationship may net you great rewards in terms of repeat business. Deciding on strategies to encourage continued counseling in the early stages of your business prevents the need to address the issue of drop-outs later on.

Office Policies and Procedures

If you have clerical/administrative support, policies on office procedures are essential. Phone calls, scheduling, filing, and record keeping should be stated clearly so that they can easily be followed by anyone. Your administrative staff can be an invaluable resource for setting up such policies. You may know how you want correspondence handled, but they have a better idea of the information necessary to guide them in meeting your needs. Below are some basic questions you must address.

How will telephone coverage be handled?
Marketing efforts should not be handled by people who are not properly trained to do so. Determine who will be allowed to quote fees over the phone (all staff, counselors only, manager only). Personal information about yourself or your colleagues is confidential. If you or a staff member are out of town, consider redirecting calls or suggesting a date and time that the call will be returned.

For the most part, you will not want to be disturbed while you are with a client. However, your support staff should be trained to screen calls and determine whether or not the call can wait.

Allow support staff the freedom to provide information in their own words. Prepared dialogues sound like recordings and turn potential clients off.

How will you assure clients of confidentiality?
In the health professions, confidentiality is a given. Stating this fact to your clients allows you to build rapport. Breeches of confidentiality destroy the trust you establish with clients.

Because office staff are responsible for preparing correspondence between the physician, insurance carrier, or other agencies and yourself, their knowledge of confidential information can be great. Many health care providers feel that this issue is so important that they demand that their employees sign a statement of confidentiality. You may wish to express this policy to your clients as a means of building trust.

Your client has the right to see his or her own records or request that they be sent to someone. This fact may affect the words you choose to use when charting. To receive information from or send information to a non-referring physician, you must obtain written permission from your clients. When sending records, photocopies are appropriate. Establish a policy on how confidentiality will be handled and communicated.

Payment Policies and Billing Procedures

If your practice is part of a larger organization, chances are that payment policies and billing procedures will be adopted from the larger operation. In fact, you may find that the financial departments completely relinquish you of such responsibilities, including collection of payment. In such cases, knowing the policies and procedures is necessary so that you and your staff can guide clients properly.

In situations where such a luxury is not available, careful consideration of the handling of money will be necessary. The services of an accountant or controller will reduce your frustrations and insure the fact that you have been thorough in handling financial decisions. The following questions must be addressed before a sound policy can be developed.

Will you establish a set fee for all clients, or will a fee schedule based on income levels be implemented?

A common complaint among practitioners is a lack of consistency in handling nonpaying clients. Some judge a client's ability to pay on appearance, perceived background, or other subjective measures. There may be good reason to offer services at a reduced rate or at no cost. However, it is advisable to consider under what circumstances payment will be excused or lowered. Criteria should reflect financial capability and rely less on subjective impressions.

When will payment for services be expected?

You can request payment for a session immediately following an appointment, prior to the first session of a series, or on a payment plan. A series could be defined as several sessions marketed together.

Many practitioners have found an increased commitment from clients who pay in full before a series begins. Even more effective in maintaining attendance is the policy of refunding a portion of the fee to those with perfect attendance or who meet predetermined goals.

Even when a client is sure that their insurance will cover the cost of your counseling activities, payment should be made according to your policy. Since payment from insurance companies requires six to eight weeks, payment by the client will prevent cash flow problems. Then the client can submit your itemized receipt to the insurance company for reimbursement.

How will you inform clients of your payment policies?

No matter how you expect payment to be made, your clients should know what to expect. A good policy is to make clients aware of your payment plan when they make their appointment. A note about payment may even be printed on the appointment card. Clearly-printed notices are often posted in physicians' and dentists' offices explaining payment policies. Clients appreciate this information so that they are not caught off guard.

What forms of payment will you accept?

Many practitioners find it advantageous to accept a credit card. This is considered a convenience to clients and may actually attract the business of those who have delayed appointments because they lack ready cash. Less resistance to the fee for a series may also result from the acceptance of credit cards (Helm, 1987).

In order to begin accepting credit cards for Visa, Mastercard, and similar credit cards, contact a bank. Most banks will set up your credit card account, rent you an imprinter, and require you to pay a percentage of the deposits monthly, provided your application is approved. The arrangements for American Express are similar; however, you must contact American Express directly to apply for an account.

Payment plans increase your bookkeeping and may decrease your income. Collection of delinquent fees is difficult, and the costs of contracting a collection agency or legal representative can be tremendous. Most practices choose to let clients file for reimbursement themselves. This reduces the paperwork of the practice and prevents lost income if reimbursement is rejected.

If you require clients to file for reimbursement on their own, make it as easy for them as possible. Offer your assistance if they encounter obstacles. It is to your advantage since reimbursement often encourages additional business.

How will you handle payment from worksite programs?

The contract you agree upon should explain the payment policy. Each worksite client organization may have two sources of payment for these nutrition services—company funds and personal employee payment. Regardless of the source, it is best to expect the organization to handle internal collections and to issue a check to your practice.

There are two primary advantages to the organization collecting monies:

1. You don't have to carry large sums of cash.
2. An employer or organization has more leverage than you do to get employees or members to pay or collect on bad checks.

Regarding payment from the worksite organization, some practitioners suggest that you ask for an advance payment of up to 50 percent at the signing of the agreement. Obviously, this must be stated in your agreement as a condition of providing services. Afterward, a monthly payment of two to three installments can be arranged.

Late payment can be a serious problem for your practice. There are three things you can do to discourage late payment from worksites:

1. Request pre-payment. (Some worksite clients will not do this.)
2. State in your agreement that late fees of 1½ to 3 percent per month will be assessed for late payment.
3. Have a credit report done on the prospective client organization before you propose business to them. You probably should not proceed any further in the sales process if their credit rating is low unless full payment, at the time service is rendered, is negotiable.

How will you handle nonpaying clients?

All efforts to avoid billing should be made. If billing is necessary, it should be handled by the institution's billing department. Small medical bills are considered among the most difficult to collect, according to collection agencies. In fact, they suggest that a bill that is unpaid for six months is virtually uncollectible (Helm, 1987).

The quicker you identify delinquent accounts and deal with them, the less money, time, and frustration you will spend collecting them.

Documentation and Record-Keeping Policies

If you work in a medical office or health care institution, you may have medical charts available to you. Otherwise, a method of recording, organizing, and filing client information must be devised. The cost of a chart system may lead you to look for some other ways of maintaining client information. Manila folders, loose leaf notebooks (Helm, 1987), and file cards have all been used effectively for such purposes. Once you decide on a system, your office staff should be able to prepare for a new client effectively.

Documentation and record keeping is much different in the outpatient setting than in the inpatient setting. While the inpatient dietitian uses the chart to communicate with other health care providers, the outpatient nutrition counselor responds to a different set of issues. Documentation is a must in the outpatient setting for three important reasons:

1. It refreshes your memory on client goals and progress when preparing for follow-up sessions.
2. It justifies actions in malpractice suits.
3. It justifies third-party payment.

What client information needs to be documented?

All client visits, phone calls, and correspondence with other health care providers and third-party payers regarding the client should be noted in the chart. The type of information you include in your notes should be adequate for you to recall the counseling or verbal communication that took place. Some items that are important to document for third-party reimbursement can be found in the latter part of this chapter.

You may also want to document clients' reactions to your recommendations and counseling. This information can be helpful in physician feedback and when legal conflicts arise. The way you structure your chart notes is a matter of choice.

How will you structure chart notes?

Clinical dietitians are, for the most part, trained to use the SOAP System of notation. The letters stand for subjective information, objective information, assessment, and plan. This system is used because it is easy for the physician to read and is consistent with his or her charting method. Because you will see most of your clients more than one time, this may not be the best way for you to track your client's progress.

Consider methods of documentation that are comfortable for you. You may find that a narrative is more acceptable under your circumstances. Or you may use one method for the initial session when you are collecting a large amount of information and a different method for follow-up sessions. Some practitioners prefer to make extensive notes, while others are very brief. Consider the amount of time you have available for such tasks. Whatever system you choose, remember to date and sign every documentation note.

What records will you make a permanent part of client charts?

Record keeping is very important. If your clients submit their bills for third-party payment, you must retain copies of the referral form and billing statement. You would also be wise to copy any requests for information or denials from the insurance companies and enter them in the chart. The rationale for keeping such documents is to be able to prove that the services were rendered.

Any written correspondence to or from the physician or other health care professional regarding the client aids you in explaining your actions. These letters and memos can also serve as aids in writing future communications to that professional.

If you have access to medical records and/or lab test results, they can be helpful in assessing needs and charting progress. You must have the client's permission to obtain such information. You must also have the client's permission to use information about them in research. If you offer a waiver for such information, this should also appear in the chart. Although very little regulation has been placed on outpatient nutrition practices in the past, you should assure that your documentation and charting procedures meet any regulatory requirements.

Personnel Management Policies and Procedures

The personnel management guidelines you establish should encourage fair treatment of employees and sound personnel relations and effectively minimize the likelihood of discipline and discharge decisions escalating into successful charges of discrimination, wrongful discharge suits, unemployment claims, grievance, or arbitration. Remember, also, that satisfied employees with a sense of pride in their work will make a personal investment in the success of your practice. Satisfied employees will be the best individual promoters of your business. Conversely, dissatisfied employees may undermine your efforts. Employee concerns must be addressed effectively and immediately.

How will you ensure that the highest levels of performance and productivity be maintained?

The process of ensuring high levels of performance begins with selecting highly qualified personnel. The selection process is reviewed in more detail in a later chapter.

Obviously, in order to perform at maximum productivity, employees must have a clear understanding of expectations. Written statements of philosophy, written job descriptions, and job dimensions help prospective employees to evaluate a position in the interview process, and they help prepare you to select the most qualified employee.

Job descriptions should be tailor-made to describe the specific characteristics and responsibilities of each position and should be revised each time the responsibilities of the position are changed. An example of a job description for a diabetes educator follows.

DIABETES EDUCATOR JOB DESCRIPTION

Principal Function:

Administers, directs, controls, and plans activities related to the operation and future development of the Diabetes Education Program. Is actively involved in marketing nutrition services to the community and the healthcare institution.

Typical Duties and Responsibilities:

Assesses client's nutritional status and designs appropriate diet plan based on the referring physician's information and the assessment made on the patient, as necessary.

Uses effective counseling techniques along with written materials to build rapport, educate, and lead clients to self-sufficiency.

Communicates with physicians and other healthcare personnel by documenting and forwarding assessments of diet counseling, in an effort to establish and maintain effective working relationships.

Develops or acquires educational materials specific to the client class or program, as needed.

Provides community education programs and materials and communicates regularly with community agencies to promote programs and develop rapport.

Participates in staff meetings of the Outpatient Nutrition Department and other departments, as needed.

Maintains accurate records such as billing, patient instructions, and scheduling for outpatient services.

Assists in the development of policies, procedures, and programs related to the outpatient nutrition services.

Assists in the development of quality assurance nutrition monitors related to outpatient nutrition services.

Assists in marketing outpatient nutrition services.

Keeps current with advances in nutrition and diet therapy.

Performs any other job duties as assigned by the immediate supervisor.

Status and Scope:

Reports to Director of Outpatient Nutrition Services.

Works independently following applicable policies, as well as professional standards. Works with a team of professionals. Although the diabetes educator delegates the tasks involved in providing the program, the professionals report to their respective supervisors. Has access to secretarial support, but is not responsible for supervision of any subordinates.

Develops new or revises existing procedures within area of responsibility.

Job requires strong presentation skills, communication skills, marketing expertise, high degree of interactive human relations skill, expertise in counseling strategies/skills, and automobile travel.

Qualifications:

Bachelor's degree in nutrition or related area, registered dietitian, state licensure, and valid driver's license.

Minimum of two years experience as a clinical or community dietitian, including some experience in a variety of counseling and educational activities.

Certified diabetes educator.

Developing job dimensions means taking the time to identify the behaviors that distinguish the most successful performers from mediocre performers in a position.

Then the sets of behaviors are organized into categories that reflect the characteristics needed to excel in a specific position. The concept of dimensions can be clarified by an example of job dimensions developed to accompany the job description for a diabetes educator.

DIABETES EDUCATOR
JOB DIMENSIONS

Decision Making

Analysis: Relates and compares data from different sources, identifies issues, secures relevant information, and identifies relationships. Understands and interprets nutrition data.

Assesses nutritional needs of clients by analyzing nutrition history, medical records, food consumption, lifestyles, motivation, and environmental, social, and personal influences.

Interprets oral feedback and staff and client satisfaction survey questionnaires to determine which aspects of our services should be continued or enhanced and which require corrective action.

Assists in various studies in response to JCAHO or other government regulatory agencies, administrator, or direct supervisor's recommendations to provide information and answers for particular problems.

Reviews different product lines based on set criteria to recommend the most suitable product for the purchase of new equipment, computer software, nutritional products, and so on.

Observes role models and determines how successes were achieved.

Analyzes efficiency and effectiveness of nutrition counseling operations, including the flow of information from client and referring agent.

Anticipates and interprets physician's questions and concerns.

Analyzes diet order prescriptions to determine validity.

Analyzes performance of clerical support staff.

Decisiveness/Responsiveness: Readily makes decisions, renders judgments, takes action, or commits oneself and/or the practice or institution in response to changing conditions, requests, or needs. Gathers necessary information and decides on and takes action quickly. Does not procrastinate.

Pays personal attention to the needs of clients.

Immediately responds to administrator, physician, or client requests, complaints, or problems with action or statement of intended action. Actions are generally of high priority and aimed at visible results, resolution of the problem, and satisfaction of individuals.

Makes 'quick' decisions with little deliberation, and takes immediate action in response to day-to-day problems and emergency situations.

Confronts important issues and problems.
Recommends healthcare facility's needs relative to outpatient diabetes care.
Keeps supervisors informed about actions taken and results.

Judgment: Makes rational and realistic decisions that are based on logical assumptions and that reflect factual information and consideration of organizational resources. Takes reasonable risks. (Judgment refers to the *quality* of decisions.)

Provides correct nutrition information and suggests appropriate approaches for changing behavior.
Offers approaches to clients that consider environment, culture, social, and psychological influences, needs, personal preferences, and motivation for incorporating new eating behaviors into their lifestyle.
Decides how to handle client complaints, taking into account the needs of the practice and the client.
Recommends revenue-generating programs to supervisor or administrator.
Understands the missions of the institution and practice, distribution of authority, chain of command, and politics. Takes appropriate steps to get things done or make requests.
When making important decisions, consults superiors, peers, subordinates, or others who might provide valuable information or insights about situations.
Maintains confidentiality and exercises discretion in sharing appropriate information with others. Does not speak negatively about the institution, the practice, its employees, or other healthcare professionals.
Thoroughly researches alternative solutions to problems before making recommendations to supervisor and staff.
Determines individualized approaches as for making recommendations to physicians.
Establishes priorities for meeting client needs based on diagnoses, observed behavior, level of care, relative importance, and time constraints.
Keeps commitments realistic and achievable.
Determines appropriate educational material for clients.
Refers clients to appropriate persons or agencies if the advice they seek extends beyond professional boundaries.
Makes commitments to accomplish tasks and projects only for which he or she has appropriate resources and authority.

Leadership Skills

Delegation: Makes effective use of competencies and time of subordinates. Allocates decision making and other responsibilities to the appropriate subordinates.

Sees that staff have proper training and resources to accomplish tasks for which they are responsible.
When delegating work, explains:

- Purpose;
- Expected results;

- Deadline for completion and priorities;
- How the task fits into other work in the clinic and contributes to overall objectives; and
- How performance will be measured and followed up.

When delegating, communicates confidence in staff to do the work effectively.

When delegating work, solicits staff's ideas on ways to accomplish tasks.

Appropriately allocates work among staff, considering relative workload and competency. Equitably distributes desirable and undesirable tasks.

Assigns project work based on business plan goals.

Education, Training, and Development: Improves the knowledge, skills, and competencies of clients, physicians, and community through information dissemination, counseling, training, and development activities.

Prepares clients to differentiate between supermarket items and foods presented on restaurant and fast food menus.

Encourages program staff to offer suggestions for new programs or methods of accomplishing goals.

Develops and conducts inservice education sessions (including materials) and presents journal articles and nutritional research for other dietitians, medical staff, and other staff.

Uses visual and graphic aids to educate clients.

Conducts community nutrition education programs.

Provides nutritional counseling and education to clients.

Leadership: Utilizes appropriate interpersonal styles and methods in guiding individuals and groups toward task accomplishment.

Is accessible to staff and provides feedback and direction to staff on a regular basis.

When implementing a new program, meets with staff to describe overall objectives, explain each individual's role, and obtain their commitment in accomplishing the objectives.

Remains abreast of nutrition changes and trends and the strengths and weaknesses of competitive diabetic education programs.

Establishes challenging, measurable, and attainable goals.

Facilitates resolution of conflict in a quick and constructive manner.

Maintains high visibility and exposure within the practice and the institution.

Leads or actively participates in institution's or professional committees.

Acts as "image-maker," responsible for creating a positive image for the institution and the profession.

Schedules hours of operation to meet client needs.

Communication Skills

Oral and Written Communication: Conveys information and ideas to individuals and groups, in person, on the telephone or in writing through effective oral, nonverbal, and tonal expression and effective writing.

Speaks and writes clearly, specifically, concisely, confidently, and assertively.

Uses correct grammar, punctuation, spelling, and sentence structure.

Changes complexity and style of speech and writing according to level, education, and background of individuals with whom the diabetic educator is communicating. Uses correct and appropriate vocabulary.

Effectively uses illustrations (pictures, charts, graphs, role plays, etc.) to amplify understanding.

Makes eye contact when speaking with others and uses facial expressions, hand gestures, and body language effectively.

Plans, organizes, and rehearses important oral communications (presentations, meetings, etc.).

Presents accurate written information in a neat, attractive, concise, and well-organized format.

Obtains feedback from others prior to sending out important written communications to ensure that the target audience will understand the message as it is intended.

Writes:

- Activity reports;
- Reports to superiors, sharing results of projects;
- Brochures and newsletters;
- Training materials and lesson plans for inservice and nutrition instruction;
- Menus;
- New forms for interdepartmental use;
- Memos to physicians, nurses, and so on;
- Correspondence;
- Progress notes in client records;
- Speeches;
- Nutrition care plans and goals; and
- Responses to inquiries concerning nutrition care.

Oral Fact Finding/Listening: Attends to and accurately understands the oral communication of others. Records, remembers, and uses data so obtained.

Admits when he or she does not understand information or directions and asks for clarification.

Writes down important comments or requests, especially when action or follow-up is necessary.

Listens to obtain specific and accurate details of comments, suggestions, problems, and complaints to:

- Get ideas to improve service;
- Identify and resolve any problems; and
- Monitor status of activities within department.

Listens to obtain specific and accurate details of client comments, suggestions, problems, and complaints to:

- Appropriately respond to requests;
- Identify and resolve problems or complaints; and
- Learn ways to improve service and visibility to department.

Asks appropriate questions and listens carefully to obtain information (likes and dislikes, lifestyle, medical history, disabilities, etc.) from clients to:

- Surface underlying issues that could impact client's behavior changes;
- Recommend nutrition plans;
- Meet medical and nutritional needs;
- Meet needs and personal tastes; and
- Develop nutritional goals.

Records specific information and specific action to be taken.

Obtains feedback and probes for verification that he or she accurately understands what others say.

Obtains important information through discussions with medical and professional staff.

Seeks information to learn what the client and staff expects from the nutrition counselor and how the counselor is performing against those expectations.

Listens to and is receptive to feedback from staff.

Organizational Skills

Monitoring/control: Monitors and/or regulates the counseling process, tasks, or activities of subordinate's job activities and responsibilities. Takes action to monitor the results of delegated assignments or projects.

Reviews client satisfaction surveys to be aware of client feelings toward the nutrition education and counseling services and to resolve any indicated complaints or problems.

Monitors revenue generation of programs and results.

Develops forms and systems to monitor programs.

Assists in establishing and monitoring the quality and appropriateness of client care through a quality assurance program.

Assists in establishing and monitoring policies and procedures to meet regulatory and JCAHO standards of nutrition care.

Regularly meets with staff, individually or collectively, to review and upgrade day-to-day operations and special assignments.

Participates on various interdepartmental committees to establish policies and procedures and follow up on interdisciplinary problems and issues.

Establishes policies designed to:

- Regulate the delivery of service;
- Regulate time usage and the flow of clients;
- Ensure sound counsel and recommendations; and
- Ensure customer satisfaction.

Planning and Organizing: Establishes a course of action for self and/or others to accomplish a specific goal; planning proper assignments of personnel and appropriate allocation of resources.

Organizes reports, paperwork, manuals, and other information to facilitate quick retrieval and avoid loss.

Organizes oral presentations, using appropriate charts, audiovisual media, written materials, and so on.

Develops lesson plans for inservices and nutrition education presentations for clients, staff, community groups, and so on.

Allows necessary lead time to meet deadlines or due dates.

Focuses time on important issues. Efficiently schedules own time and activities through the use of such tools as daily "to do" lists, calendars, and so on.

Develops strategic and business plan for diabetes programs.

Uses pacing techniques to increase the pace of client discussion to collect less information and avoid being sidetracked, or to reduce the pace of the discussion to collect more information.

Plans time effectively to provide adequate opportunity for self-improvement.

Plans other commitments around patient workload.

Interpersonal Skills

Rapport Building/Sensitivity: Makes positive initial and continuing impact. Able to meet people easily, to be liked, to get along well with people, to put them at ease, and to quickly build rapport through proactive development of close relationships. Understands and shows consideration for the feelings and needs of others. Acts in ways that show awareness and concern for image projected to others and impact of behavior.

Effectively builds and maintains clients' self-esteem.

Maintains professional appearance. Dresses appropriately.

Makes effort to include staff in decision-making process when formulating new ideas and procedures.

Through words and actions, conveys respect and a sense of genuine caring toward clients.

Avoids conveying judgement of client behavior.

Interacts regularly with physicians and other healthcare professionals through informal conversations and formal meetings. Understands political environment of institution and uses appropriate channels of communication to accomplish goals.

Develops trust, credibility, and rapport with clients and their families during individual and group nutrition consultations.

Deals effectively with difficult clients, accommodating them when possible.

Acts in ways that show understanding of individual needs of clients.

Willing to admit mistakes; takes responsibility for actions.

Acknowledges people by name.

Pays personal attention to special requests from clients.

Keeps supervisor informed about day-to-day operations, department needs, problem situations, and upcoming events through regular formal and informal meetings.

Chooses settings for counseling and education that are professional, private, quiet, and comfortable.

Prepares clients in advance for educational and counseling activities.

Assists physicians on special projects to establish and maintain professional rapport.
Acknowledges others' points of view when presenting his or her own.

Nutrition Counseling Skills: The process of offering individualized guidance so that the client acquires the expertise to self-manage his or her own nutrition care.

Recommends techniques and approaches for addressing nutrition concerns that encourage self-sufficiency.
Guides clients to suggest solutions to their own problems.
Focuses counseling activities on helping the client "own" and "commit to change" his or her nutrition problems before suggesting techniques and approaches.
Involves clients in goal setting.
Breaks long-term client goals into smaller incremental steps.
Emphasizes the benefits of change from the client's viewpoint.
Identifies barriers to behavior change and assists clients to find ways to overcome them.
Utilizes appropriate behavior change techniques.
Suggests that the client utilize appropriate behavior change techniques.
In the termination phase of counseling, takes measures to prevent and prepare clients to deal with setbacks.

Group Facilitation Skills: Leads groups toward the accomplishment of a specific purpose by guiding discussion and lecturing, utilizing techniques that enable group members to apply the information offered, whenever possible.

Balances individual priorities with group priorities, and the amount of new information offered with opportunities to practice new behaviors.
Draws out ideas, feelings, and experiences, and encourages participants to share, air concerns, and raise questions.
Ensures that the thoughts, ideas, and experiences of participants are recognized and supported.
Ensures that the viewpoints of all group members are respected.
Guides debate, discussion, role-plays, case studies, exercises, and the establishment of group groundrules.
Builds and maintains the self-esteem of group members.
Ensures that conflict provides an opportunity to reexamine issues, rather than cause defensiveness or protectiveness.
Assists group members to be open to accepting an array of potential solutions.
Helps group members integrate new information with old beliefs.
Surfaces and works to correct misconceptions.
Attempts to reconcile disagreements.
Acts as "mouthpiece" for group feelings, feeding back the feelings or tenor expressed by the group.
Maintains group cohesion and attempts to keep lines of communication open.
Applies adult learning theory to structuring active learning experiences.
Helps group members set standards for how the group will function.

Monitors group activities and assesses the reactions of the group.
Keeps the group activities on track.
Manages inappropriate participant behavior.

Persuasiveness: Utilizes appropriate interpersonal styles and methods of communication to gain agreement or acceptance from others.

Emphasizes the benefits of changing behavior to clients.

Reinforces client behavior change through positive feedback, consequences, and rewards.

Persuades medical staff, organizational client, or superiors to accept or adopt new ideas or methods by:

- Presenting relative advantages;
- Having all facts and accurate information;
- Communicating confidently, assertively, and with sensitivity;
- Using creative communication to instill interest; and
- Speaking enthusiastically and persuasively.

When promoting services to clients and healthcare professionals, emphasizes the benefits of utilizing the services from each individual's viewpoint, stressing a track record of success.

Appears on TV and radio talk programs to promote the registered dietitian and the diabetes educator as nutrition experts.

Plans responses to possible opposition when presenting an idea or product.

Personal/Motivational

Adaptability: Maintains effectiveness in varying environments, tasks, responsibilities, or groups.

Readily adapts to changing priorities, and readily changes daily plan and routine to meet unexpected demands.

Remains flexible and realistic in terms of meeting set goals within specified time frame.

Performs duties of other staff members when necessary.

Initiative/Innovativeness: Actively attempts to influence events to achieve goals; self-starting rather than passive acceptance. Takes action to achieve goals beyond what is necessarily called for; originates action.

Generates imaginative approaches to resolving nutrition related problems with clients.

Determines ways to create rather than respond to customer flow.

When notifying superiors about a problem, also suggests solutions.

Continually tries new ways of doing things to improve profitability, productivity, efficiency, quality, and client relations, or to reduce expenses.

Customizes and enhances programs to fit institution's needs.

Continually seeks opportunities to increase revenues by marketing services in creative ways.

Develops and suggests ways to standardize and simplify work processes.

Initiates community outreach programs.

Develops, suggests, and implements new diabetes programs and services to generate income and enhance the image of the institution.

Job Motivation: The extent to which activities and responsibilities available in the job overlap with activities and responsibilities that result in personal satisfaction.

Derives satisfaction from having responsibility of all aspects of nutrition counseling programs and having a high degree of autonomy and authority.

Enjoys developing and implementing programs and procedures.

Enjoys serving as nutrition expert and providing nutrition services to clients and the community.

Enjoys opportunity to be creative in developing and marketing fee-for-service programs.

Enjoys being recognized as a valued member of the healthcare team.

Enjoys working in a continually changing environment and on a wide variety of tasks.

Demonstrates a genuine sense of caring for clients and enjoys providing services to meet their nutritional needs.

Derives satisfaction when clients change behavior, with positive effects on their health status.

Enjoys interaction with people on both a business and social level.

Enjoys public speaking activities, such as television appearances, guest speaking, lectures, and so on.

Wants to achieve goals and changes quickly.

Continually desires to learn and know more.

Enjoys involvement with food and nutrition.

Self-Development Orientation: Initiates actions to further improve skills and performance proficiency. Active efforts toward self- development.

Stays informed of technological changes.

Attends professional continuing education activities to remain current and informed.

Reads journal articles.

Solicits and is receptive to constructive feedback.

Actively participates in local, state, and national professional organizations.

Work Standards/Attention to Detail: Sets high goals or standards for self. Dissatisfied with average performance. Has concern for all areas of performance, no matter how small. Makes extra efforts to ensure that all work is completed and meets high standards.

Models high work standards through personal example.

Continuously evaluates client care services and looks for ways to improve service and generate income.

Never satisfied with status quo, even when client or superiors are.

Works extra hours when necessary to handle workload and day-to-day operations, meets project deadlines, assists in special events.

When doing any kind of work, tries to achieve results that are better than those previously achieved by self or others.

Writes thorough, specific, accurate, and concise progress notes in clients' records.

Remains technically current and proficient.

Insists on ensuring compliance to quality assurance and regulatory requirements.

Meets commitments.

Displays honesty and integrity in dealing with others.

Professional Knowledge and Proficiency: Acquires, understands, and applies technical and professional information and skills.

Knows purchasing procedures and available products.

Knows how to market healthcare nutrition services.

Demonstrates understanding and application of sound nutrition knowledge to various disease states, physical conditions, and prevention of chronic illness.

Demonstrates ability to read and analyze client medical records.

Is able to recommend balanced, creative menus for clients.

Demonstrates knowledge of administrative procedures relevant to a nutrition office.

Thoroughly understands department's policies and procedures.

Familiar with human resources policies and procedures.

There are several other things you can do to maximize productivity. Upon hire, it is advisable to continue discussion about performance expectations by reviewing written policies, procedures, standards of conduct, and standards of performance. Assign and thoroughly train employees for job responsibilities.

Once expectations and performance measures are clearly understood, encourage open communication. Welcome recommendations and be responsive to them. Observe and monitor performance regularly. Offer direction, support, appreciation, and ongoing performance feedback. Conduct exit interviews that are designed to gather recommendations for improvement.

Research shows that formal performance evaluations are valuable, but they are no substitute for everyday, ongoing performance feedback. Performance feedback is the single most important factor affecting employee productivity. Develop a performance evaluation program that provides frequent opportunities for performance feedback. Keep in mind that all these productivity-maximizing suggestions apply equally to professional and administrative staff. Each position and each employee deserves careful consideration.

How can you ensure that nutrition practitioners will not leave your practice and take their clients with them into another practice?

Consider an employment contract. Employment contracts may limit an employee's ability to leave your practice and take current clients with them. Be sure to consult legal counsel regarding the appropriateness of an employment contract.

Other action on your part may also discourage this. Emphasize the strengths of the practice in all promotions and appropriate communications. Specifically, emphasize:

- Affiliations and endorsements of physicians and the institution;
- Resources that might otherwise not be available;
- Proven track record of success;
- Years the practice has been operating if the number of years encourages a successful impression; and
- Location/convenience.

Encourage opportunities for your clients to get to know and build rapport with other members of your staff. Invite them to preview sessions, holiday celebrations, or an event like a "come meet our staff cooking class."

Most importantly, give your staff members little reason to want to leave. Maintain good employee relations and keep communications open. Be flexible in meeting their needs. Let's face it—their rapport with you may be the single most important interest. If employees like and respect you and appreciate how you treat them, they usually respond in kind. Not wanting to affect your practice or jeopardize their relationships with you is a powerful deterrent.

Some benefits don't cost you anything, but the value to the employee is great. Flexible scheduling and job sharing, if appropriate, are two good examples.

Some practices have offered clients two or three free sessions to transition them to a new counselor, recognizing that the counselor will need time to get to know the client's needs and lifestyle before the counselor can reach the same level of effectiveness.

How will new clients be assigned in practices with more than one nutrition counselor?

As additional counselors are added to the staff to handle an increasing number of clients, some intervention may be necessary on your part to ensure that the workloads of your counselors are appropriate. You must be sensitive to several issues. Some clients and physicians may request a specific nutrition practitioner. This is not always possible. You don't want any counselor to be so bogged down with clients that there is no time to promote the practice. Some may discourage additional business if they feel they are too busy to handle it.

If counselors are compensated for building revenues, interference from another counselor may threaten their earnings potential and sound employee relations. As you set your policy, you may want to consider asking your counselors for input on the best way to assign clients, or consider assigning clients on a take-turn basis. You might also consider assigning clients based on medical condition, nutrition expertise of the counselor, or availability of the counselor (e.g., if clients want appointments on Thursday evening, they would see the counselor who works at that time).

It is perfectly reasonable to tell clients who are referred to an overloaded counselor that the counselor is not taking new clients at this time; however, you would be happy to schedule an appointment with one of his or her colleagues.

How will you ensure that your compensation program is effective?
Salary and benefits are important to attract and retain highly qualified employees for your practice. Generally speaking, the greater the demand for specific professions in your community, the higher the compensation package must be. To determine an appropriate compensation program for your practice, learn about competitive compensation programs. You can conduct a survey, interview employees, watch the classified advertisements, and network to gather this information. Consult with the institution's human resources director before doing so, and keep him or her abreast of your findings.

Because most new practices are working with tight budgets, how you allocate available compensation money is critical. Consider a base wage, benefits, and, if appropriate, incentives. Some nutrition professionals may be willing to grow their income along with the practice. Consider offering a salary base with commission earnings or bonus potential. Tying the success of the practice to the success of the practitioners is wise.

How will you ensure that a professional dress code be observed by all employees?
Ensuring that dress reflects professionalism and enhances credibility is important. There are two suggestions offered:

1. Establish a policy that is communicated prior to the selection of employees.
2. Model a professional dress code.

Dress codes are often avoided because discussing them can be uncomfortable. Dress codes are not in themselves sensitive issues. Confronting an employee about inappropriate dress *is*. Communicating clear expectations upon hire is much easier than hurting an employee's feelings by confronting inappropriate dress later. Be as specific as possible in defining your dress code. Be sure your dress code establishes dress expectations for men and women.

How will you ensure that disciplinary action and discharge is handled appropriately?
Just as it is a manager's responsibility to communicate, guide, and train employees to enable them to be successful, it is also a manager's responsibility to offer corrective guidance when they do not succeed. All disciplinary action, counseling sessions, performance problems, changes in the status of an employee, and terminations should be administered in accordance with written policy and written

standards of conduct. They should be well-documented and factually supported. Your disciplinary practices must be applied consistently to all employees whose records or actions involve similar infractions or misconduct. Disciplinary procedures must be consistent with the institution.

A formal disciplinary procedure should be established and spelled out in advance to all employees. For example, you might establish a two warning system—one verbal, one written. Keep in mind that discharging an employee without a written warning encourages poor employee relations and is generally not viewed favorably by the courts or administrative agencies.

LEGAL AND ETHICAL CONSIDERATIONS

All outpatient nutrition counselors should review the legal and ethical responsibilities of their work. This information can be gathered from the legal authorities affiliated with your employer. Here are some of the common legal questions confronting practitioners and the resource people who may be able to provide answers.

Questions	Resource
What legal issues are involved with naming the practice?	Lawyer
What licenses and certifications are needed to provide outpatient services in this state?	Lawyer/State ADA
Do current insurance policies fully cover the outpatient nutrition practice, or are adjustments needed?	Lawyer
What measures should be taken to protect against malpractice suits?	Lawyer
Which legal contracts are appropriate for the practice? How should they be designed?	Lawyer
How do legal guidelines regulate the selection and management of employees?	Lawyer
How should materials be copyrighted/trademarked?	Lawyer
What form of record keeping do you recommend for client documents? Professional communications?	Lawyer
What form of record keeping do you recommend for personnel records?	HR Director
Do I need to charge sales tax for services, products, and materials? How do I administer this?	Accountant
How is credit established for the business?	Accountant

What form of record retention do you recommend for finances? | Accountant

Some of these issues deserve further review.

Malpractice Liability

As the number of outpatient and private practice nutrition counselors rise, so do the chances of nutrition counselors being sued for malpractice. Malpractice is the part of the law of torts that compensates individuals for injury or loss caused by the actions of another. Malpractice is based on a negligence theory. In other words, the professional negligently performed (or failed to perform) the professional services for which he or she was contracted. The assumption is that individuals—in this case, nutrition counselors—while performing their professional duties, must conduct themselves in a non-negligent manner that will not cause harm or injury to others. Even if you are affiliated with an institution, you can be sued for malpractice as an individual professional. Understanding the elements of a medical malpractice suit and your responsibilities as a nutrition professional can protect you against a malpractice suit (Cross, 1988).

A medical malpractice suit contains four elements that must be satisfied for the plaintiff to be awarded compensation:

1. Proof that actual injury occurred. The plaintiff must have had symptoms that are documented.
2. Proof that a relationship of duty existed between the two parties. Appointment slips, signed diet instruction slips, and canceled checks can all be used as evidence that diet instructions or recommendations were given by a particular nutrition counselor.
3. Proof that the health professional performed a breach of duty. The question that must be answered is, "Did the nutrition counselor provide the care and skill that is expected of any competent practitioner in the same field under similar circumstances?"
4. Proof that the actions of the health professional caused the injury. This includes failure to act on the part of the practitioner. The plaintiff must prove that the actions of the practitioner alone caused the injury (Cross, 1988).

Protecting yourself and your practice against malpractice liability involves some very important steps:

- Possess the requisite education, training, and expertise in the area for which you provide services.
- Acquire any licensure, certification, or registration recognized or required by the state in which you practice.

- Remain current in the field of nutrition.
- Know the limits of your expertise, and refer clients to other health care professionals when their needs go beyond your professional limits.
- Obtain a physician referral for any instruction related to a medical condition or screening results.
- If you believe a prescription or diet order is erroneous, call the physician for a correction, and follow up in writing to document the change (Cross, 1988).
- Document all services rendered.
- Obtain written permission to use client information in research and to send information to physicians.
- Obtain malpractice insurance. Information on purchasing such insurance follows.

Liability Insurance

Several forms of liability insurance are available, depending on the type of practice and services you provide. Seek legal advice on your need for coverage beyond that offered by the institution. All practitioners should carefully examine the insurance policies they are considering before making a purchase. The terms you may encounter and their definitions follow:

- Professional liability—The type of insurance that protects you against real or alleged acts of malpractice or omissions in professional duties. If you have employees, you are also responsible for their actions and can purchase insurance that covers them.
- Comprehensive general liability—The type of insurance that protects you against liability for contracts in the conduct of your business, injuries to employees while working, fire damage to rented or leased structures, copyright infringement, advertising, bodily injury, and property damages that are not associated with your professional services.
- Non-owned automobile liability—Protection against claims made on automobile accidents involving your employees when using their personal vehicles for business purposes.
- Amount of coverage—How much the insurance company will pay on a single claim or total claims per year.
- "Claims made" policy—Under such a policy, the insurance company will cover costs only if the policy is in effect when the suit is filed. Notification to the insurance company of the claim must be made within a certain time frame (Cross, 1988).
- "Occurrence" policy—The insurance company will cover costs, as long as the policy was in effect at the time the incident occurred, no matter when the claim is made.

Legal Agreements

Several forms of legal agreements can be made. The method of presenting and finalizing an agreement depends on the risks involved and your relationship with the party with whom you are making the agreement.

An agreement is generally considered to be legally binding if it contains the following three components:

1. There is an offer made by one party that is accepted by the second party.
2. The parties making the agreement must be of sound mind, authorized to enter into the agreement, and cannot be minors.
3. The agreement must be for the purpose of a legal pursuit.

Note that verbal agreements are not mentioned. Caution should be taken to avoid verbal agreements that are not placed in writing later. Although they are not easy to prove, verbal agreements can be legally binding. The following forms of agreements are those that you will most likely use.

Letters of Agreement

Written agreements take the form of bids, letters, proposals, and contracts. Probably the most common form of agreement made for nutrition services is a letter of agreement. A letter of agreement is a contract; it is just a less formal way of expressing a deal. A letter of agreement may be developed as an extension of a proposal (ADA, 1986).

A letter of agreement should address the following points:

- Services/products included in the agreement;
- The responsibilities of each party;
- How, when, and where services will be provided;
- Price;
- Fee schedule and billing procedure;
- Additional provisions;
- Time period of the agreement; and
- Procedures for termination of the agreement (Helm, 1987).

Both parties should sign a letter of agreement. You should consult a lawyer to discuss provisions that should be covered in the agreement. If you are working within an institution, legal advisors are most likely available to you.

Contracts

When there are greater risks, larger amounts of money, or more responsibilities involved, a formal contract is advisable. In nutrition counseling, a formal contract is most often used when a practice is making an agreement with an independent counselor. Formal contracts are also recommended for agreements with large corporations and when services will be provided over a long period of time (ADA, 1986).

"Contracts should be practical, easily understood, and complete enough to protect your reasonable interests." (Helm, 1987). Contracts are time consuming and can be expensive. Although you will require the services of a lawyer to prepare the contract, you should know which needs and concerns you wish to include in the contract before consulting your legal expert. Explain that you need an agreement that will fully and fairly protect each party's interests.

Content Considerations for Legal Agreements

No matter which type of agreement you choose to use, there are many provisions or legal considerations you must ponder. The following considerations apply to a variety of situations:

- Cross hire clauses (physicians/worksites hiring counselor away from institution).
- Noncompetition clauses.
- Are there restrictions or specifications about location?
- How may changes to the original contract be made?
- Liability.
- Unforeseen events (death, plant closings, acts of God).
- Work for hire agreement.
- Confidentiality.
- Ownership of materials.
- Future expansion of services.
- Employee/client grievances.
- Billing procedures.
- Permission to act on worksite premises.
- Payment/collection of fees.
- Cancellation terms.
- Access to medical records.
- Appropriate communications/documentation.

Proprietary Rights

Any material or product that is copyrighted, trademarked, or patented belongs to the person or organization who owns the copyright, trademark, or patent. Under copyright laws you must have permission to use quotes, graphics, and charts from copyrighted or written works. Also, be aware that materials you produce as an employee of an organization are the property of that organization. Therefore, you must have permission to use those materials for any purpose unrelated to the organization.

Code of Ethics for the Profession of Dietetics

The American Dietetics Association House of Delegates has adopted a Code of Ethics for the Profession of Dietetics that neatly summarizes a policy of conduct for all nutrition professionals. That document is published here with the permission of the American Dietetic Association.

Preamble

The American Dietetic Association and its credentialing agency, the Commission on Dietetic Registration, believe it is in the best interests of the profession and the public it serves that a Code of Ethics provide guidance to dietetic practitioners in their professional practice and conduct. Dietetic practitioners have voluntarily developed a Code of Ethics to reflect the ethical principles guiding the dietetic profession and to outline commitments and obligations of the dietetic practitioner to self, client, society, and the profession.

The purpose of the Commission on Dietetic Registration is to assist in protecting the nutritional health, safety, and welfare of the public by establishing and enforcing qualifications for dietetic registration and for issuing voluntary credentials to individuals who have attained those qualifications. The Commission has adopted this Code to apply to individuals who hold these credentials.

The Ethics Code applies in this entirety to members of The American Dietetic Association who are Registered Dietitians (RDs) or Dietetic Technicians Registered (DTRs). Except for sections solely dealing with the credential, the Code applies to all American Dietetic Association members who are not RDs or DTRs. Except for aspects solely dealing with membership, the Code applies to all RDs and DTRs who are not ADA members. All of the aforementioned are referred to in the Code as "dietetic practitioners."

Principles

1. *The dietetic practitioner provides professional services with objectivity and with respect for the unique needs and values of individuals.*
2. *The dietetic practitioner avoids discrimination against other individuals on the basis of race, creed, religion, sex, age, and national origin.*
3. *The dietetic practitioner fulfills professional commitments in good faith.*
4. *The dietetic practitioner conducts himself/herself with honesty, integrity, and fairness.*
5. *The dietetic practitioner remains free of conflict of interest while fulfilling the objectives and maintaining the integrity of the dietetic profession.*
6. *The dietetic practitioner maintains confidentiality of information.*
7. *The dietetic practitioner practices dietetics based on scientific principles and current information.*
8. *The dietetic practitioner assumes responsibility and accountability for personal competence in practice.*
9. The dietetic practitioner recognizes and exercises professional judgment within the limits of his or her qualifications and seeks counsel or makes referrals as appropriate.

10. *The dietetic practitioner provides sufficient information to enable clients to make their own informed decisions.*
11. *The dietetic practitioner who wishes to inform the public and colleagues of his or her services does so by using factual information. The dietetic practitioner does not advertise in a false or misleading manner.*
12. *The dietetic practitioner promotes or endorses products in a manner that is neither false nor misleading.*
13. *The dietetic practitioner permits use of his or her name for the purpose of certifying that dietetic services have been rendered only if he or she has provided or supervised the provision of those services.*
14. *The dietetic practitioner accurately presents professional qualifications and credentials.*
    a. *The dietetic practitioner uses "RD" or "registered dietitian" and "DTR" or "dietetic technician registered" only when registration is current and authorized by the Commission on Dietetic Registration.*
    b. *The dietetic practitioner provides accurate information and complies with all requirements of the Commission on Dietetic Registration program in which he or she is seeking initial or continued credentials from the Commission on Dietetic Registration.*
    c. *The dietetic practitioner is subject to disciplinary action for aiding another person in violating any Commission on Dietetic Registration requirements or aiding another person in representing himself/herself as an RD or DTR when he or she is not.*
15. *The dietetic practitioner presents substantiated information and interprets controversial information without personal bias, recognizing that legitimate differences of opinion exist.*
16. *The dietetic practitioner makes all reasonable effort to avoid bias in any kind of professional evaluation. The dietetic practitioner provides objective evaluation of candidates for professional association memberships, awards, scholarships, or job advancements.*
17. *The dietetic practitioner voluntarily withdraws from professional practice under the following circumstances:*
    a. *The dietetic practitioner has engaged in any substance abuse that could affect his or her practice;*
    b. *The dietetic practitioner has been adjudged by a court to be mentally incompetent;*
    c. *The dietetic practitioner has an emotional or mental disability that affects his or her practice in a manner that could harm the client.*
18. *The dietetic practitioner complies with all applicable laws and regulations concerning the profession. The dietetic practitioner is subject to disciplinary action under the following circumstances:*
    a. *The dietetic practitioner has been convicted of a crime under the laws of the United States which is a felony or a misdemeanor, an*

essential element of which is dishonesty and which is related to the practice of the profession.

b. The dietetic practitioner has been disciplined by a state and at least one of the grounds for the discipline is the same or substantially equivalent to these principles.

c. The dietetic practitioner has committed an act of misfeasance or malfeasance which is directly related to the practice of the profession as determined by a court of competent jurisdiction, a licensing board, or an agency of a governmental body.

19. The dietetic practitioner accepts the obligation to protect society and the profession by upholding the Code of Ethics for the Profession of Dietetics and by reporting alleged violations of the Code through the defined review process of The American Dietetic Association and its credentialing agency, the Commission on Dietetic Registration. (ADA, 1988)

REIMBURSEMENT FOR NUTRITION SERVICES

If your nutrition services practice engages in one-on-one or group counseling, you will need to be aware of the reimbursement policies of insurance carriers and establish a payment system. The extent to which you become involved with assisting clients in obtaining maximum reimbursement is a matter of preference. However, since individual clients rely on reimbursement for full or partial payment of nutritional and other medical services, greater involvement will enhance revenues and the success of the practice.

Reimbursement of nutritional services was once scarce. Today, more and more insurance companies are recognizing the value of nutritional care and are considering reimbursement for qualified services. The movement toward more widespread reimbursement is attributable to changing attitudes and opinions by insurance carriers and the persistence of pioneer nutrition practitioners. Also, consumers, recognizing the value of proper nutritional care in reducing insurance costs, request coverage as a part of their medical plan. To a great extent, individual practitioners have furthered the cause by working to educate insurance carriers about the value of their services. Reimbursement trends are a direct result of continued hard work and effort by nutrition professionals to achieve greater recognition.

Establishing a Reimbursement Policy

Several good resources are available on implementing a payment system. The following stepwise approach is a compilation of ideas from those resources (Consulting Nutritionists in Private Practice, 1988; Earl, 1988; Murray, 1985; Wellman and Fox, 1990):

Dear Insurance Carrier:

Clinical observations have long suggested a connection between obesity and a variety of illnesses, both physical and psychological. In February 1985, the National Institute of Health (NIH) convened a conference to review the most recent findings by experts in the fields of nutrition, nutritional biochemistry and metabolism, endocrinology, internal medicine, gastroenterology, and so forth, to determine the health implications of obesity. (A copy of this report is available upon request.)

The findings of the NIH Conference strongly suggest a connection between obesity and cardiovascular disease, coronary artery disease, and a variety of other medical problems, including increased mortality rates for medical problems not directly related to obesity.

The health care professionals at Anytown Hospital are greatly concerned about the findings of the health debilitating consequences of obesity. In response, Anytown Hospital, in collaboration with Anytown Laboratories, a leader in human nutrition, have developed a Level II weight loss program for the obese. (Generally speaking, obesity is defined as 20 percent or more above desirable body weight.)

The program, which we have called "Take Off," is a medically supervised approach to the treatment of obesity. It combines a balanced, low-calorie diet with behavior modification, nutrition education, and an exercise regimen. It operates under close supervision of an Anytown Hospital team, consisting of a medical physician, registered dietitian, behavioral psychologist, nurse, and exercise physiologist.

During the weight loss phase, the patient will be on a 600 to 800 calorie per day meal replacement powder produced by Anytown Laboratories with vitamin and mineral supplementation to meet 100 percent of the RDA's requirement. Once goal weight is achieved, the patient enters a refeeding phase that includes a balanced diet for weight maintenance. Patients continue to be monitored during the behavior modification and nutrition education phase that follows the weight loss phase. Patients will be admitted to the program by physician referral.

As each program is individually tailored to the patient, the cost will vary, based on total weight loss required and other clinical considerations; however, the basic cost is as follows:

- Phase I
  Clinical services: $450.00 per four visits for medical evaluation services, as well as behavior modification and nutrition education.
  Dietary supplement: $10.00 per day

FIGURE 6-1. Sample introductory letter to insurance carrier.

Duration: Normal program will be 3 to 5 months for Phase I at one, 2-hour visit per week.

- Phase II
  $20.00 per session for weight maintenance behavior modification and nutrition education.
  Duration: Lifetime at one 1-hour visit per week.

So that we may give patients the proper information, please fill in and return the attached questionnaire concerning insurance coverage and procedures to be followed in applying for reimbursement. Please use the enclosed self-addressed, postage paid envelope.

Sincerely,

Enclosure

FIGURE 6.1 *(Continued)*

1. Gather information on client insurance coverage. Determine "payer mix." If none of your clients are medicare recipients, you need not spend large amounts of time learning the medicare system and regulations.
2. Learn as much as you can about nutrition services coverage of the third-party payers you are most likely to deal with. This step is managed through mail surveys, personal phone calls, and networking with other health care professionals. A sample introductory letter to insurance providers and a sample questionnaire follow (Figs. 6-1 and 6-2). Sometimes, the knowledge that third-party payment for your services is being made speaks for itself.
3. Establish a rationale and plan to guide implementation of a payment system, including goals, objectives, rationale, and strategy. Your strategic plan, as explained in Chapters 3 and 5, fulfills this step.
4. Identify, define, and describe services provided. This is a critical step to achieving reimbursement. All invoices must be submitted with a list of services rendered and narrative descriptions. Use lay terminology in your descriptions, not technical health care jargon.
   Detail every task you complete, then determine which procedures may be reimbursable. Preventive medicine is not generally covered by insurance companies. Evaluation and treatments are considered active care and may be covered. The business services department of your institution should be able

QUESTIONNAIRE

1. What is your company's policy regarding physician-referred Level II weight loss programs?

   ____

   ____

   ____

2. In Phase I, charges for clinical services will be separate from those for the dietary supplement. Will your company cover the cost of the dietary supplement?
   Yes ☐ No ☐
3. Please describe forms, reports, and so on, necessary to effectively handle communication between your company and Anytown Hospital and to expedite reimbursement to the patient.

   ____

   ____

   ____

Company Name:____

Insurance Representative:________________________________
(Name)

Phone Number:______________________ Date:__________________

FIGURE 6-2. Sample questionnaire for insurance carriers.

to assist you in determining codes to match your services (if the codes exist for nutrition care).

5. Establish fees for each identified service. You must create consumer demand for third-party payment; this can only be achieved if you charge a fair price for your services. Although your fees have been established through your strategic planning, veterans of fee-for-service planning advise you to validate your fees. This can be accomplished with the help of your business advisor or by contacting the local fiscal Medicare intermediary. Ask for a copy of the current prevailing and customary fee schedule for internal medicine and physical therapy.
6. Establish a payment system. Whether you bill the client and encourage them to submit the insurance claim or bill the third party directly is your decision. However, Medicare, Medicaid, and Worker's Compensation cases in particu-

lar require billing the third-party payer directly. Be familiar with the policies of the payers you expect to deal with.

7. Develop a billing statement and counseling referral form. Your billing statement should be personalized with the necessary information about your practice. A local printer should be able to print your statement with enough carbon copies to meet your business needs. The client will need a copy of the physician referral to submit with the claim. To aid in the reimbursement process, this form should include the patient's diagnoses.

   The sample billing statement (Figure 6-3) illustrates the information that most third-party payers require. On the statement, you will note the term, "ICD-9-CM codes." These codes are the identification numbers used by health care providers to classify diagnostic and surgical procedures. Some common ICD-9-CM codes that relate to nutrition are:

Fatigue 780.7	Weight Loss 783.2
Weight Gain 783.1	Malnutrition 263.9
Pregnancy 648.9	Allergies 477.9
Atherosclerosis 414.0	Hypertension 401
Anemia 285.9	Hypoglycemia 251.2
Diabetes Mellitus 251.2	
Gestational Diabetes 648	
Hyperlipidemia 272.4	Diverticulitis 562.11
Diverticulosis 562.10	

   Medicare/Medicaid reimbursement forms must be filed by the medical facility or physician. The billing department will provide you with the latest information on reimbursement from Medicare and Medicaid.

8. Process charges and bill appropriate parties. Remember to place a copy of the bill in the client's record.
9. Document services rendered, including information on type of service, frequency of use, time required, cost, and outcome. Try to anticipate the documentation that third-party payers will request before they will act on a claim. The following documentation is imperative:

   a. Physician's order for nutrition services;
   b. Diagnosis assigned by physician;
   c. Treatment plan;
   d. Expected duration of treatment;
   e. Information on progress;
   f. Objective "benefits of service";
   g. Signature of professional; and
   h. Professional's licensure or registration number.

PLEASE RETURN THIS FORM TO THE RECEPTIONIST

PREVIOUS BALANCE	PATIENT NAME

For insurance, complete below and submit to your carrier.

Ins. Co. ______

Grp/SS # ______

Subscriber: Name ______

Employer ______

Patient: Birthdate ______ Male Female Relationship to subscriber: Self Spouse Dependent

Other Ins. & Policy # ______

Referring Dr. ______

Facility Name and Address

Consultants Name

Federal Tax I.D. # ______

Credential # ______

Insurance:

DATE OF SERVICE ______

PATIENT ______

Address City, State Zip ______

Phone ______

SAMPLE

*UNITS OF SERVICE	VISITS	FEE
	Comprehensive	
	Limited	
	Brief	
	Re-assessment	
	Nutrition Analysis Comprehensive	

*1 UNIT = 15 MINUTES

TODAY'S CHARGES ______

Fatigue	780.7	Hypoglycemia	251.2	Gastroenteritis	558.9
Weight Loss	783.2	Diabetes Mellitus	250	Hepatitis	573.3
Wt. Gain	783.1	Gest. Db.	648	Peptic Ulcer	533.9
Malnutrition /	263.9	Hyperlipidemia	272.4	Spastic Colon	586
Pregnancy	648.9	Hyperthyroidism	242.9	Arthritis	716.9
Allergies	477.9	Hypothyroidism	244.9	Bursitis	731.9
Atheroscelosis	414.0	Menopausal Syn.	627	Degen. Disc Disease	772.6
Edema	782.3	Headache	784	Degen. Joint Disease	715.9
Hypertension	401	Amenorrhea	626.0	Gout	274.9
Myocardial Infarction, Acute	410.9	Abdominal Pain	789.0	Musculo-Skeletal Pain	781
		Diarrhea	558.9		
Asthma	493.9	Diverticulitis	562.11		
Anemia	285.9	Diverticulosis	562.10		

Please make check payable to:

______
Nutritionist's Signature

FIGURE 6-3. Sample billing statement (reprinted with permission from Consulting Nutritionists in Private Practice Dietetics Practice Group.)

10. Monitor payment and reimbursement to evaluate the success in receiving reimbursement and to provide assistance to clients in obtaining maximum coverage. If you bill the third party directly, they will send notification of payment or denial. Therefore, a system can be established with your business office to audit payment. If the client submits the claim, you must develop a system for reporting such information. Some practices provide clients with a prepaid postcard to return when the claim is paid or denied. The process usually takes 90 days; therefore, you may want to consider telephone follow-up.
11. Aid clients in resubmitting denied claims. Follow up with any requested information. You may want to submit a letter that explains the cost/benefit of nutrition service and the specific outcome criteria of the case. Changes in clinical measures, such as reduced weight, cholesterol, or blood glucose and increased hemoglobin, are outcome criteria that appeal to insurance providers.
    You may not achieve immediate results in convincing the insurance carriers to reexamine a denied claim. However, the contact and discussion will help to turn opinions. The goal is to obtain reimbursement for nutritional services on a broader basis now and in the future.
12. Educate users by marketing nutrition services, working toward a better understanding as to the value of nutrition services. Plan actions to gain support from physicians, administrators, and third-party payers, as well as clients.

Factors Affecting Reimbursement

A major obstacle to obtaining direct reimbursement is that most state insurance codes do not, at the present time, include dietitians as certified providers. Therefore, a provider number cannot be obtained. Amendment of insurance codes is achieved through the state legislative process. Furthermore, dietitians, in most instances, cannot get provider numbers (licenses) and, therefore, cannot get direct reimbursement from the third-party payer. Listings of certified providers is usually established by a state's insurance code and regulated by a board of insurance or rate-setting committee. However, organized efforts are currently underway in states and at the national level to change this situation. Every dietitian can play a part in these efforts.

During the 1987 legislative session, an amendment to the Texas State Insurance Code was passed to include the licensed dietitian among other health care professionals already included in the Code as certified providers. This was the first legislative victory of this type in the nation, providing a legal basis for reimbursement. This law does *not* make reimbursement for nutrition services mandatory in Texas, but establishes a legal avenue for reimbursement if such coverage is included in group health policies.

The American Dietetic Association, through its Division of Government Affairs and its Nutrition Services Payment System (NSPS) department, collects data on the status of state insurance laws. If you cannot find the answers to your reimbursement questions in the listed references, contact your state NSPS representative, the Dietetic Practice Group, or the Division of Government Affairs, American Dietetic Association (Consulting Nutritionist in Private Practice, 1988).

Direct negotiation with insurance companies is preferable to legislative action, due to the time and expense involved in achieving success through legislation. Each practitioner will face a different set of variables in obtaining reimbursement. Coverage of nutrition services by third-party payers varies from state to state, insurance company to insurance company, plan to plan, and policy to policy. Commercial carriers do not appear to approach nutrition care services by a single standard. Most policies fail to specifically mention approval or denial of coverage for nutritional services. The specifics of the policy must be examined or perhaps tested to determine if those services are covered.

One important reason why there is such a variation in coverage of nutritional services is lack of consumer demand to have nutrition services included in coverage. Therefore, encouraging your clients to seek reimbursement for your services is imperative. When clients submit such claims, insurance providers realize that a demand exists.

Several factors seem to contribute to success in obtaining reimbursement.

Nomenclature Nomenclature, the way services are described, is key. Description of services should be brief and general. The term "consultation" is preferred over counseling services and programs. Most services will fall into this general category. However, many carriers prefer to use the term "nutrition care services," instead of listing specific services (Earl, 1988). Do not use the words "diet," "weight loss," "nutrition education," or "counseling" (ADA, 1985). Insurance companies seldom pay for "monitoring." They may pay for "follow-up care" to evaluate the effectiveness of treatment protocols.

Physician's Order A physician's order is required for all known instances of reimbursement for nutritional services. Include this order along with the standard bill and insurance forms. Medicare and Medicaid will pay for nutrition services only if the dietitian is employed by the physician, the service is an integral part of the physician service, and the physician provides direct personal supervision. Hospital outpatient departments can receive reimbursement for services through Medicare/Medicaid if the services are an integral part of the physician's diagnosis and treatment (Earl, 1988). The diet prescription, including the patient's diagnoses, documents that diagnosis and treatment plans were determined by the physician.

Cost/Benefit Documentation Cost/benefit documentation is necessary to demonstrate that a service provides the patient/client with a specific benefit that will offset the cost of the service and also provide a cost savings to the client, institution, and third-party payer. Documenting the value of services (i.e., the cost/benefits and effectiveness) requires a vigorous and sustained effort. Through documentation and follow-through, the value of nutrition services can be demonstrated (Dougherty and Gilmore, 1989). Clinical outcomes that have been known to justify reimbursement include decreased serum triglycerides and cholesterol, decreased blood glucose or urea nitrogen, decreased weight, percent body fat, or blood pressure, and improved hemoglobin, serum albumin, or immune response. Figure 6-4 shows a sample Statement of Cost/Benefit.

To: ______________________________

Subject: Insurance Coverage for ______________________________

was referred to ______________________________
for Nutritional Counseling. Following is an information statement to clarify the rationale for the referral of this patient.

Nutrition intervention is a vital component to primary treatment in medical and health care. Individuals are frequently referred to the Registered Dietitian for nutritional assessment and counseling. The referring physician realizes the cost-benefit of nutrition management by the practitioner trained in this specialty, the Registered Dietitian. As a skilled professional, the Registered Dietitian has been trained in accredited universities and medical centers for implementation of nutrition prescription. The Registered Dietitian practitioner has also had extensive training in educational techniques for effective patient adherence and behavior change.

From the cost-benefit perspective, a visit to a Registered Dietitian for nutrition counseling, tailored to the individual's eating habits, life-style and nutrient needs, is much less expensive for long-term control, compliance and disease management. These poor results are evidenced when inflexible preprinted diet sheets and vague advice are the primary mode of corrective, maintenance and preventative nutrition counseling.

Reimbursement for treatment and health maintenance can prevent and control unnecessary and inflated medical costs to your company.

______________________________ ______________________________

Registered Dietitian Physician

FIGURE 6-4. Sample letter to be sent to insurance company if payment is refused. Resubmit bill with this letter typed on letterhead. (Reprinted with permission from Consulting Nutritionists in Private Practice Dietetics Practice Group.)

Provision of Forms Providing forms that are ready for signature and mailing are helpful in aiding your client to obtain reimbursement.

Addressing Private and Commercial Carrier Concerns Although cost/benefit is important to all third-party payers, private and commercial carriers are also concerned with issues such as their policy and services, cost to purchasers, profitability of the package of services, and what services the competition (especially HMOs) provide. Any information you can give them on these issues will increase your reimbursement claims.

Educating Administrators of Capitated Insurance Plans Nutrition services are consistent with the goals of most HMOs and PPOs. Here again, cost effectiveness and clinical benefits are key selling points. Contracting with capitated plans provides a steady source of income. These plans are more likely to buy into preventive nutrition programs, as their preventive care benefits set them apart from other third-party payers (Earl, 1988). Self-insured plan providers are also more likely to buy into preventive care. The information in Chapter 8, "Selling to Worksites," applies to capitated and self-insured plans as well.

Chapter 7

Executing Business and Marketing Plans

EXECUTING PLANS

Starting up a new practice or program is the transition point where your plans are placed into action. The key is to manage various tasks or short-term activities simultaneously, in a smooth transition. You also want to establish a foundation of sound management practices that will culminate in a quality practice.

Because the "how to's" of start-up are mapped out in the planning stage, a review of start-up activities risks redundancy. With that concern in mind, only those start-up activities that have not been previously mentioned or need further development are discussed in this chapter.

This stage of establishing your practice is crucial. Success in the implementing phase relies on your ability to keep your antennas up and adjust your start-up plans as indicators or experience dictate the need. Even if you have done an excellent job of planning and organizing, you will encounter surprises. You may find that your assumptions were inaccurate, or unanticipated obstacles may arise. Once you have organized your start-up activities according to your business and marketing plan, the primary rule of execution is: When unforseen hazards or opportunities arise, be prepared to adjust your course of action quickly.

Organizing Start-up Activities

Since start-up presents a challenge in managing and coordinating several activities, many practices have used a start-up checklist as a guide. When organizing a start-up checklist, you might consider developing categories of activities, such as administrative concerns, staffing, facilities, and so on. Then list all the activities to address under each category. Assign an expected completion date and a person to be responsible for the activity. You may find it helpful to record the actual completion date as well. Recording the actual completion date for each activity points out those activities that still demand attention. Keep in mind each service or product you plan to offer and what will be required for its initiation.

The start-up checklist shown in Figure 7-1 will help identify and track these activities. This start-up checklist is categorized by groups of activities.

Some practices use a similar checklist to organize and coordinate all activities, including business and financial planning. Because it is difficult to know which activities need to be included in the checklist before you determine your strategies, a checklist for start-up activities is recommended. A start-up checklist is not to be substituted for thorough and effective communication with all members of the start-up team regarding individual roles, expectations, standards, or goals. Instead, it can assist you in keeping the start-up team informed.

Setting Up Facilities

In planning your strategies, you selected a location that would position your practice to meet your goals. Now you must take care of the details. If you are renting space, you will be concerned with the location of the office within the building, leasing, utilities, and deposits. You must learn who is responsible for obtaining housekeepers and security and what parking arrangements are available. A practice within an institution also will most likely need to inform the housekeeping and security departments of their needs. They may also need to determine what overhead allocation will be charged to the practice.

In either location, telephone installation should be a high priority. Careful consideration should be given to the options for telephone service. Learn what services are available to a small business and the cost; then, weigh the benefits against the cost. Consider the number of lines necessary to accommodate your practice over the next two years, to avoid added installation charges as your practice grows.

Again, look to the future when making decisions to remodel. A practice that outgrows their space biennially stands to lose time and profits. Remodeling is better done when clients are not being counseled. It is distracting and detracts from your image.

Employee Selection and Staffing

Hiring is one of your most critical performance areas. Your practice cannot flourish without the selection of the "right" people properly placed. In a nutrition practice, personnel are business assets. Each employee represents the practice to the public, current clients, prospective clients, companies, organizations, and other employees.

START-UP CHECKLIST

Expected Completion Date	Activity	Person Responsible	Actual Completion Date
	Facilities		
________	Locate office	________	________
________	Allocate overhead	________	________
________	Determine meeting requirements	________	________
________	Locate meeting place	________	________
________	Install telephones	________	________
________	Order supplies	________	________
________	Order equipment	________	________
________	Check parking facilities	________	________
________	Advise security of needs	________	________
________	Advise housekeeping of needs	________	________
________	Arrange for remodeling	________	________
________	Arrange for furniture	________	________
________	Set-up office	________	________
	Staffing and Personnel Management		
________	Determine staffing needs/ scheduling	________	________
________	Prepare organizational chart	________	________
________	Prepare job descriptions	________	________
________	Review wage structure	________	________
________	Review benefit program	________	________
________	Develop training program	________	________
________	Develop orientation program	________	________
________	Establish performance evaluation system	________	________
________	Recruit staff	________	________
________	Review responsibilities	________	________
________	Assign start-up activities	________	________
	Communication		
________	Schedule and conduct staff meetings	________	________
________	Review business plan and marketing plan with staff	________	________

FIGURE 7-1. Start-up checklist for an outpatient nutrition practice that has already received approval from administration.

Expected Completion Date	Activity	Person Responsible	Actual Completion Date
___	Review job descriptions	___	___
___	Review policies and procedures	___	___
___	Establish weekly goals with staff	___	___
___	Establish reporting system with administration	___	___
___	Develop client communications	___	___
___	Develop performance evaluation system	___	___
___	Develop referral and feedback system	___	___
	Marketing Program		
___	Place yellow pages listing	___	___
___	Order business cards	___	___
___	Order letterhead and envelopes	___	___
___	Develop and arrange start-up marketing program (external)	___	___
___	Mailings	___	___
___	Posters	___	___
___	Brochure	___	___
___	Publicity	___	___
___	Press releases	___	___
___	Promotional items	___	___
___	Public appearances	___	___
___	Attend medical staff meeting	___	___
___	Meet with key physicians individually	___	___
___	Develop and arrange start-up marketing program (internal)	___	___
___	Notices	___	___
___	Newsletter articles	___	___
___	Staff meetings	___	___
___	Committee meetings	___	___
___	Develop fee structure	___	___
___	Discounts	___	___

FIGURE 7-1. *(Continued)*

Expected Completion Date	Activity	Person Responsible	Actual Completion Date
______	Allowances	______	______
______	Payment terms	______	______
______	Billing procedures	______	______
______	Policy for nonpaying clients	______	______
	Program Development		
______	Purchase packaged programs and materials	______	______
______	Develop written program	______	______
______	Develop and print handouts	______	______
______	Develop and print support materials	______	______
______	Develop enrollment form	______	______
______	Develop nutritional assessment form	______	______
______	Schedule programs	______	______
______	Select program names	______	______
______	Prepare program description or brochure	______	______
	Administration		
______	Design reports and forms:	______	______
______	History and Assessment Form	______	______
______	Diet Plan	______	______
______	Progress notes for counselor files	______	______
______	Consent for Treatment Form	______	______
______	Waiver for research or mailing info to physician	______	______
______	Billing and Payment Forms	______	______
______	Develop internal records and filing system	______	______
______	Personal records	______	______
______	Client records	______	______
______	Set up computer (programs and files)	______	______

FIGURE 7-1. *(Continued)*

Expected Completion Date	Activity	Person Responsible	Actual Completion Date
________	Obtain procedures for internal reporting or computer software	________	________
________	Financial reports	________	________
________	Payroll records	________	________
________	Expense report	________	________
________	Petty cash	________	________
________	Identify suppliers	________	________
________	Establish written policies and procedures	________	________
________	Billing procedures	________	________
________	Payment policies	________	________
________	Bad-debt procedure	________	________
________	Hours	________	________
________	Scheduling procedure	________	________
________	Investigate third-party reimbursement	________	________
________	Obtain list of local insurance companies	________	________
________	Develop questionnaire	________	________
________	Contact insurance carriers to determine coverage	________	________
________	Set up procedure to monitor reimbursement	________	________
________	Develop procedure for follow-up contact	________	________
________	Determine inventory levels	________	________
________	Develop reorder procedure for supplies and materials	________	________
________	Establish filing system	________	________
	Ongoing Planning		
________	Develop method to monitor effectiveness	________	________
________	Ongoing client feedback	________	________
________	Ongoing competitive analysis	________	________
________	Incident log	________	________
________	Fiscal management	________	________
________	Develop reporting form for administration	________	________

FIGURE 7-1. *(Continued)*

Much can be learned in the area of staffing and employee selection from pioneers in the field. During ARA's interviews with institutional outpatient practitioners, many staffing and selection war stories were shared. The common pitfalls are worth reviewing.

Rotating members of an inpatient staff to cover the outpatient demands.
Rotating nutrition counselors through the outpatient practice has proven detrimental to nutrition practices. Once a client establishes rapport with a counselor, his or her success in changing behavior often hinges on the continuation of that relationship. Clients are reluctant to trust and open up to more than one counselor, and counselors must often start from the beginning to fully understand the client's progress. Therefore, the counseling process is stinted and often terminated when more than one counselor is involved.

This factor also suggests that turnover is destructive to a practice. A change in counselor can mean lost clients. For this reason, compromising in the selection of a nutrition counselor is *not* an option.

Splitting a dietitian's time between inpatient and outpatient services.
To reduce the investment in outpatient nutrition services, outpatient practices were often begun with one dietitian splitting time between inpatient and outpatient duties. These dietitians found that the demands of each service and the needs of the clients varied significantly. Therefore, incumbents were not able to devote the attention necessary to one or both functions. Often, appointments conflicted with the urgent requests of the medical staff, and outpatient appointments were canceled or shortened to meet such demands.

Inundated workloads provided little incentive to increase customer traffic. In fact, an inundated workload might have provided a disincentive. The incumbent reported to two different supervisors in many cases, influencing how priorities were addressed. All of these factors contributed to the frustration of the dietitian, limiting his or her desire to "own" the responsibility to grow the business.

Therefore, this alternative is best avoided. If this approach is used, the success of both functions hinges on proper training and preparation of the incumbent. The responsibilities and accountabilities of each function must be assigned when the function begins. Measures of performance must also be established.

Hiring nutrition professionals who are unprepared for the demands of an outpatient practice.
It is important to recognize that the skills and techniques necessary to be an effective outpatient counselor are very different from those used by inpatient counselors. The six primary selection errors that pioneers have echoed are hiring nutrition counselors who:

1. Are predisposed to educating;
2. Lack the sophisticated counseling skills that outpatient clients demand;
3. Lack the sophisticated interpersonal skills necessary to manage and promote the practice and "sell" oneself;
4. Lack business and marketing knowledge and savvy;
5. Are not willing to invest the number of hours that start-up demands; and
6. Are not willing to work a schedule that will meet client needs.

It is particularly easy to make these poor hiring decisions in the start-up phase because the interviewers are often unaware of the demands of the practice until they are encountered. Even when they are aware, the pool of experienced outpatient nutrition counselors who have received training in counseling or business skills is limited.

Transferring a dietitian from inpatient to outpatient.
Dietitians are often transferred from inpatient to outpatient services because the assumption is made that a competent inpatient dietitian will automatically be a competent outpatient dietitian. Incumbents in the inpatient positions are attracted to this move, and, in some cases, the outpatient position may provide a career track and an opportunity for promotion. They often fail to recognize the differences between inpatient and outpatient nutrition counseling. To complicate the problem for administrators, the pool of experienced, competent outpatient dietitians may be limited.

The fallacy that a competent inpatient dietitian will automatically be a competent outpatient dietitian is worth exploring. Herein lie the primary considerations:

1. Inpatient counselors too often have the mindset that clients should be given as much information as possible in one session. On an inpatient basis, one session may be all there is. Thus, the return of a patient is sometimes interpreted as a failure to meet the client's needs. Consequently, the inpatient nutrition counselor sometimes discourages return business. This mindset can be destructive to the practice.
2. Research shows that behavior change occurs over time and that lasting change comes from gradual change (Zemke and Zemke, 1981). The inpatient nutrition professional provides diet information. His or her role from the patient's perspective is to educate. The outpatient nutrition professional influences behavior change in a stepwise approach. He or she views the role as that of change agent. This requires additional training and experience.
3. Some nutrition professionals who entered the field because of their desire to be "helping" professionals often view business and financial objectives as a conflict with their value systems.
4. The demands of the day-to-day worklife between the two functions are different. In addition to the new skills required, measures of performance and

> accountability are greater. The scheduled hours of work must be flexible, and some evening and weekend hours must be included. Each outpatient dietitian must be comfortable shifting gears throughout the day, intermingling group and individual activities. Many dietitians have found the design of this type of workday too stressful.

If an inpatient dietitian is hired for the outpatient position, the food service director or other managers may expect the counselor to perform both inpatient and outpatient duties, especially before the practice has a chance to grow. Such demands may limit the opportunities to grow the practice.

A specific job description can clarify the differences between the inpatient and outpatient positions. It may also justify the need to hire a counselor outside the inpatient practice, both to administrators and to the inpatient staff. In one particular case, the inpatient counselors in a hospital had an unrealistic picture of outpatient counseling. They felt that the job would be easier and would require less flexibility in hours than their current positions. Once the clinical manager developed the job description for the outpatient position, many of the counselors realized that, not only was the schedule more varied than their current position, the responsibilities included areas beyond their training or interests.

Sometimes a different title can help make the distinction between positions. If you consider this, do so cautiously. Several states now regulate titles along with the practice of dietetics and nutrition counseling. Contact your state dietetic association in order to determine the licensure and advertising regulations of the state in which you intend to practice.

If you are considering hiring nutrition professionals from within, take an honest look at physicians' and nurses' perceptions of the current inpatient staff. You will not be able to count on the referrals of the medical staff to keep your business going if a strong rapport does not exist with current inpatient dietitians. If physicians do not recognize the impact or contributions made by current inpatient dietitians or the credibility of inpatient dietitians is low, the outpatient practices will have an added barrier to success. Sometimes a new face and upgraded credentials will help overcome negative perceptions and the objections lodged by medical staff resisting the associated costs for what they have come to expect as free services.

Unrealistic expectations of the position.
If the job assignment exceeds what is possible for the incumbent to accomplish, the incumbent may become discouraged, frustrated, or disillusioned. The incumbent may experience "burn-out" and, in turn, become ineffective, in an attempt to fulfill all job responsibilities as assigned. Employee turnover and lowered morale may result. Even if the counselor stays, the responsibility to serve more clients when the current number of clients is too much to handle may cause the nutrition

practitioner to discourage business consciously or unconsciously. Good performance may be punishing. If the workload is overwhelming and help is not on the way, what incentive is there to continue to build a clientele? These factors are the precursors to lost or dissatisfied clients.

Another problem with unrealistic expectations is that priorities may not be addressed. Most often, employees gravitate to the parts of the job responsibility with which they feel most comfortable. Most outpatient dietitians feel comfortable educating clients and handling the administrative aspects of their work. Conversely, they feel least comfortable with the financial, marketing, and sophisticated counseling skills demanded of today's outpatient nutrition counselors. Neglecting the latter responsibilities usually results in little or no growth.

The earlier you determine a need for support, the better your chance is of reducing burn-out and frustration from an overloaded schedule, waiting lists, and possibly the loss of business. Identify early in the planning process the point at which new staff must be added. If possible, get advanced approval from administration for additional staff dictated by client flow. This plan offers incentive to the incumbent practitioners to grow the business and reduces the chance that the practitioner will become buried and ineffective before he or she can objectively determine the need for more help.

If you are not in a position to hire an employee or if you need time to sell a new position to administrators, you may be able to contract with a nutrition consultant to work part-time during the interim. Remember though, you want to avoid changing counselors after the first session. Therefore, consider an overlap in time between terminating your contract with a nutrition consultant and beginning a new staff counselor.

Particularly when practices and positions are new, job responsibilities may not be distributed in an optimum way. Keep in mind that each counselor will require time for counseling, as well as time to prepare for counseling activities. In addition, time must be allotted for documentation, feedback and follow-up, administrative responsibilities, marketing, and development of new programs. Pioneers report that underestimating these administrative responsibilities is a common and serious mistake.

Influencing First Impressions

Judgments about your services will be made on first impressions of you, your staff, the environment, and the session. This is especially true with service offerings because prospective clients must make a determination about the service without being able to touch or examine a tangible item. They will search for signs or indications of the quality and value of the service. As the practice and its reputation grow, attracting new clients will require less effort (Helm, 1987).

You and Your Staff

To promote a good impression prior to the client's first visit, support staff must handle telephone calls appropriately. Phone receptionists should be congenial, provide specific information on the practice, and offer accurate directions to the facility. Visits by the outpatient nutrition counselor to inpatients also creates a favorable impression.

Once clients arrive for the first session, how they are dealt with will determine whether they will return. The way you approach and communicate with clients will reflect upon your practice. Your staff should exhibit knowledge, sensitivity, and enthusiasm. The initials, R.D., behind your practitioners' names are not enough to sell your practice. Credibility is developed by actions as much as by credentials. Encourage nutrition counselors to show confidence and support recommendations with factual information. Meeting deadlines, keeping appointments, and starting sessions on time are all visible signs of professionalism that build credibility.

Nutrition counselors are role models. Consequently, it is important that they demonstrate good eating habits and a healthy appearance. The appearance of you and all members of your staff must be professional and comfortable. Appearance, however, is more than attire. Posture, eye contact, handshake, and body language should all convey a positive, concerned, self-assured attitude (Helm, 1987).

Your clients measure the effectiveness of counseling in two ways—the result of the counseling efforts and the way their nutrition counselor relates to them. They are concerned with the answers to questions like:

- "How will this counselor affect my ability to make changes?"
- "Do I trust this person?"
- "Am I comfortable talking with this person?"
- "Can I understand what I'm learning?"
- "Are my problems understood?"
- "Am I being treated as an individual with individual needs?"

Your practice is in a good position to attract and retain clients if clients can answer "yes" to these questions.

Media appearances, interviews, and public presentations require skill and self-confidence. Obviously, the skills required to be an effective public speaker cannot be reviewed comprehensively in this book; however, there are a few basic points for the person making the appearance to remember. Be well prepared to make a presentation and answer questions on the topic requested. Television news interviewers may contact you the day of the interview. Ask for some time, even if only an hour, to prepare. Ask for questions in advance, or provide interviewers with appropriate questions.

If time allows, practice. You may even ask colleagues to critique a "dry run" of your presentation. You can also learn from watching or listening to yourself on tape so that you can polish your next presentation.

Impressions of the Session

Assuming that the counselors are qualified nutrition professionals, the quality of their sessions from the client's perspective depends on their counseling skills. This book cannot substitute for a comprehensive training program on effective nutrition counseling skills. However, certain aspects of counseling make a critical first impression. These impressions may determine whether clients will continue to use your services. Encourage counselors to:

- Prepare clients in advance. Help to create realistic expectations. Review time commitments, the counseling process, clarification of roles, policies and procedures of your practice, confidentiality, cost of services, and reimbursement considerations, either before or during the first session.
- Probe for each client's expectations of both the nutrition counseling process and the counselor early in the process.
- Build sufficient rapport so that clients feel comfortable opening up and divulging sensitive information.
- Let clients know that counselors have a genuine interest in getting to know them.
- Explore clients' needs and influences to help them integrate information into their lifestyle.
- Build self-esteem and encourage clients to become self-sufficient. Resist the temptation to give answers; guide clients to resolve their own problems.
- Actively listen. Offer undivided attention to all clients.
- Seek clarification of vague or confused client messages. Confused messages may be a sign that important information is being withheld.
- Withhold judgments of clients' behavior. Criticizing or showing disapproval of client behavior may diminish rapport, set counselors up as authoritative figures, and shut down communication, particularly within the subject areas that are sensitive. Instead, show empathy and understanding.
- Watch the use of words like "should and shouldn't." They communicate a dictatorial and authoritarian attitude that works against closeness, rapport, and self-sufficiency.
- Answer questions directly.
- Be sure each client's individual needs are satisfied, and vary approaches according to their needs.
- Adjust the delivery of information to the learning and understanding of clients.

Giving the Appearance of Prosperity

As you develop a business, the reputation of your practice will speak for itself and much of your advertisement will become word of mouth. Until that time, appearances will be important.

Create physical signs of success through locale, office decor, and dress. Offices in medical complexes suggest success better than clinics or offices in kitchens.

Office space need not be lavish, but should be private, clean, comfortable, and tastefully decorated with easy access. The impression someone gets walking into the office will be as lasting as the office itself. Privacy is mandatory in developing rapport with a client and establishing a professional image. Meeting rooms should be comfortable, of a good general appearance, provide ample room, and include furniture that will serve the needs of clients.

In Chapter 3, "Determine Key Strategies," the possibility of "well" clients being reluctant to visit the hospital or clinic setting is mentioned. If this is where you will locate the practice, compensate by using a private, warm, homey, yet professional setting for your model in decorating your facilities. Contrast your decor with the sterile, cold, functional images most people associate with health care institutions. Carpeting or rugs and attractive wall hangings will go a long way to soften up the institutional look. If possible, wood furniture or fabric chairs rather than metal will also provide a warmer, more comfortable ambience.

When you are just getting started, create an atmosphere that appears successful. Beyond dressing in a professional manner, appear busy. Give clients a choice of several appointment slots rather than telling them the calendar is free. Avoid long breaks in public view. Pricing your services to suggest that they are of high quality implies success. You must be reasonable in pricing; however, people want to feel they are getting the best, and the best is often judged by price (Helm, 1987).

Provide professionally printed materials, whether marketing tools or educational information; they can enhance your business. Graphics, print style, and white space all add to the professional image your materials convey. Create the image you wish to portray with a consistent logo and style on your business cards, letterhead, printed materials, physician reporting procedures, and proposals.

Developing Programs and Support Materials

Expect a large portion of time to be devoted to developing programs and the materials that support them. Before you begin this endeavor, thoroughly investigate the materials available to you.

Developing your own nutrition programs and materials allows you to personalize your services and products. These programs and materials will be consistent with your philosophies and style. Therefore, they will be easy and enjoyable to use. The time invested by yourself and your staff may increase your investment in the practice and provide greater job satisfaction. You may find that certain materials are unavailable for purchase, leaving you no choice but to develop something. However, development of presentations, handout materials, monitoring tools, and promotional vehicles is very labor intensive. If counselors need training to develop and provide particular programs, costs will rise even higher.

Purchased programs provide resources and expertise, while reducing the time that self-developed programs require in interaction with typesetters, printers, computer specialists, and so forth. Costs are easier to track with purchased programs, since the time of development, resources, and materials are bundled into one price. The slick promotional campaigns of the larger corporations that make such programs and materials their business may make selling the program to administrators, worksites, and clients easier. In fact, if you plan to offer a service that can be supported with preexisting materials and training, why reinvent the wheel?

Printed nutrition education materials on a variety of subjects abound in the health care market. Sophisticated, very low calorie diet (VLCD) programs for obese clients offer everything from training and promotional tools to monitoring, accounting, and tracking systems. Although purchased programs and materials can be expensive, they may save you valuable time.

Consider purchasing all or part of the components necessary for a particular service. For instance, one outpatient nutrition practice that focused their efforts on eating disorders found good materials on general nutrition at an affordable price. But, less was available on some of the more specific topics to be dealt with, such as "Eating and Stress." Therefore, the practice purchased handout and audiovisual materials on nutrition basics and developed their own materials for the more specific topics. So that the printed materials provided to clients would look as though they all belonged together, the practice purchased binders imprinted with their logo. Both purchased and self-developed materials carried the practice logo, and the print shop used a style similar to the purchased materials when laying out the handouts, brochure, and educational posters.

Before purchasing a program, look critically at the available programs, to select one that fits your needs. The features to investigate include:

- The basic principles and methods of presenting the program. Do you agree with their philosophy?
- Available training. Is there enough for you to use the program effectively? If training requires time with the company's personnel, will they come to you or must you travel? Is training part of the cost of the program?
- Ongoing support. Will it be offered? If yes, at what charge?
- Support to prepare and present marketing plans. Is it needed? Is it available?
- Success of the program. Has the company tracked the success of the program? Will the commercial organization continue to track success in sites where the program is in use?
- Appearance of the materials. Do they have a professional look? Are they easy to read/understand? Do they cover pertinent information?
- Accounting and tracking systems. Are such systems established for the program, or will you have to establish them yourself?
- Promotional materials available (camera-ready ads, news releases, etc.). Have they been developed? Do they meet the needs of your practice?

When developing programs and support materials, it is important to focus on the needs of the audience by addressing material to the reading and understanding level of your audience. Most good healthcare literature for the public is written on a 6th grade level. This means that vocabulary, choice of words, and the print size must be carefully considered. Keep your message simple and as brief as possible. Cultural and social influences, financial resources, and personal preferences must be taken into consideration.

Effective nutrition programs and services incorporate strategies that take into account how adults learn. Adults seek out learning experiences to solve a specific need or problem. They will not learn something just because someone says they "should." They must have a personal use for the knowledge or skill. Adults become impatient with too much theory or background and prefer straightforward "how tos" that offer immediate application of the information. Therefore, adults learn best by doing.

Because adults tend to personalize failure and allow it to affect self-esteem, they take few risks in the learning process. Adults tend to trust their own experiences and the experiences of others to which they can relate. So weaving experiences into programs strengthens the learning (Ross, 1987) and provides an avenue to integrate new information with what they already believe.

Adults learn best if key points are presented in many different ways through many sensory channels. Asking clients to assist in designing the curriculum of a program strengthens the learning process. Autonomy and self-resolution of problems is important, since it encourages adults to become self-sufficient (Ross, 1987).

PROMOTING YOUR PRACTICE

Anytime a new business is formed or new services and products are initiated, some strategy must be developed to communicate your intentions to your market audience. These communications are called promotions, and a variety of promotional vehicles are available to you. The key to success in selling your services is determined by your selection of appropriate vehicles that speak directly to the target market at a time when they are most likely to buy. As your practice grows and becomes well established, you will be able to rely more heavily on word-of-mouth. But, some promotional efforts will always be necessary in order to maintain an active practice and promote new services. First, you must gain an understanding of the various means of promoting your practice. Then you will be prepared to maximize your returns on promotional efforts.

Promotional Vehicles

The seven categories of promotional vehicles that will be reviewed are:

1. Naming your practice;

2. Publicity;
3. Networking;
4. Advertising;
5. Nutrition fairs;
6. Sales call; and
7. Direct mail.

Although numerous promotional vehicles are available, these seven categories seem to be the most useful in outpatient nutrition practices. Marketing experts, advertising agencies, and public relations departments can be invaluable in developing the promotional vehicles you choose.

Several promotional vehicles will be examined closely. To determine which one(s) will most effectively build the practice, you must understand your target market, appropriate messages, and your resources. These will be discussed immediately following promotional vehicles.

Naming Your Practice

The first consideration in promoting the practice is naming it. Names help form a link to the services they represent. The name will be the first point of contact with prospective clients, as well as the first chance to establish an impression in their minds. Select names that are consistent with a professional image—descriptive, generic, and easily understood. Avoid names that conjure up negative thoughts. For instance, what image might be conveyed by the following name?

"Outpatient Nutrition Clinic"

Many people associate sickness and hospitals with the word "patient." Clinic is often paired with welfare. Hence, your name can sabotage your practice. Consider the following name:

"Greater Philadelphia Nutrition Center"

Prospective clients are more likely to think of nutrition services for well people, with no income perceptions.

Naming your practice to link yourself with an institution may provide even more credibility. For instance, "University Hospital Center for Nutrition." Healthcare institutions wield a large amount of credibility in the community. When consumers are asked where they would go to be referred to a nutrition expert, their second choice (physicians being first) is the hospital. Therefore, your practice will be considered more credible if you are recognized as part of the institution.

Publicity

Publicity is used to gain exposure to the marketplace, familiarizing people with your name, practice, and services. Because the public eye does not know how to discriminate between sound nutrition services and quackery, publicity gives you the opportunity to increase their awareness. Unfortunately, weight loss centers and other nutrition-related businesses have engaged in advertising and publicity, thus holding significant name identification. You, therefore, must look for all chances to establish your practice in the community through public and media appearances, presentations, organizational involvement, and writing activities.

Your greatest challenge to obtaining publicity is getting your foot in the door. The media is attracted to unusual or creative ideas. They also have nutrition concerns of their own. Offering free counseling to a media representative may not only get your story covered, but also get a testimonial from a community celebrity. If you have the opportunity to speak in public, be sure your name and affiliation are given and, if printed, spelled correctly. Make your points clear to avoid misquotation. Also, don't hesitate to offer your expertise and support for their future needs. Follow your interview with a thank-you note, a business card, and a list of topics about which you are able to speak.

Press kits are one way of attracting attention. They will stimulate media interest in your work. This type of communication is useful to help promote new products and services, speaking engagements, innovative concepts, or activities that you are engaging in. The kit includes such items as:

- A press release;
- Sample products;
- Brochures;
- Copies of publicity (articles, ads, and critical reviews);
- A short biographical sketch; and
- A photograph of staff members, an activity, or a product.

The information should be concise, descriptive, and distinctive. You may want to explain why the public or the media audience will be interested.

A public relations department within an institution will often help you prepare and distribute press kits. They already know the appropriate contacts. The use of information depends greatly on the beliefs and attitudes of the media representative who receives it. Food, consumer, or lifestyle editors are good contacts. Their names can usually be obtained from the media office's telephone information operator. A sample press release can be found in Figure 7-2.

Writing and publishing articles can be personally rewarding and provide exposure to the marketplace. It helps to establish your professional staff as experts in their fields. There are a variety of places where material can be submitted:

- Newspapers (both regional and local);

Tower Memorial Hospital
2001 KEYSTONE AVENUE • CHESTNUT HILL, PA • 19106

NEWS RELEASE

EATING TIPS FOR OLDER AMERICANS

Contact: Katie Wilson
(215) 238-5910

As the elderly segment of our population grows in size, the need for good nutrition education for this group grows in importance. To help aid in this nutrition education effort during May, "Older Americans Month", dietitians at Oceanview Nutrition Center will present the following educational facts and suggestions.

Changing bodies - Changing needs
One of the greatest physical changes undergone by the elderly concerns the proportional change in the body's composition - from less muscle and bone to more body fat. The effect of this shift in the body's make-up means that the elderly require fewer calories, since body fat does not expend energy at the same rate as muscular tissue.

Additionally, the elderly's lower activity level decreases their daily caloric requirements even further. And, though fewer calories are required on a daily basis, the elderly's need for nutrients remains largely unchanged. This lowered need for calories combined with unchanged nutrient requirements can lead to many nutritionally related problems.

As a measuring stick for charting caloric needs, nutritionists estimate that for each decade after the age of 20, our daily caloric needs decrease by 2 to 8 percent - depending on an individual's lifestyle and physique. Unfortunately, many elderly persons ignore this fact and continue to eat like a much younger person. Result? Obesity and all the resultant health complications.

Still other elderly persons cut back on their calorie intake so drastically that they deny themselves needed nutrients. Result? Dangerous weight loss and possible vitamin and mineral deficiencies.

Nutritional balancing act
An elderly person must learn to determine their individual caloric needs, while maintaining a diet rich in all necessary nutrients. This can be achieved by avoiding junk foods, which are high in calories and low in nutrients, while consuming adequate amounts of food from the four basic food groups which are nutrient-rich.

In particular, the elderly must make an extra effort to eat fresh fruits and vegetables and other fiber-rich foods. Unfortunately, many elderly individuals avoid these fiber-rich foods because they are experiencing difficulties in chewing. This results in sluggish digestion and a possible dependency on laxatives.

Daily exercise also plays a vital role in the nutritional balancing act by stimulating the appetite and burning calories. Exercise is also known to help fight depression and boredom, conditions which can cause serious eating problems.

Calcium needs
Calcium is a particularly important component of the elderly person's diet because of the dangers of osteoporosis, a bone-thinning disease which affects one in four women over the age of 60. The problem of osteoporosis can be prevented, or lessened in severity, by consuming adequate amounts of calcium, vitamin D and phosphorus. However, many elderly individuals commonly consume far too much phosphorous and too little calcium, thereby aggravating the bone loss which is the main symptom of osteoporosis.

To avoid the dangers of calcium deficiencies, the elderly are urged to consume calcium-rich foods such as milk, yogurt, cheese, sardines and canned salmon (with bones), collard greens, cooked spinach and broccoli on a daily basis. Calcium supplements should be taken only after consulting a physician. If you need help to apply this information to your everyday lifestyle contact:

Oceanview Nutrition Center
555 Byer Road
East Hampton, NY 10010

FIGURE 7.2 Sample press release to be sent to the media.

- Newsletters (employee, health, community, school, etc.);
- Handout materials for health fairs and presentations;
- Trade publications; and
- Magazines.

Choose printed media that will reach your target markets and write to that audience. Leave technical and scientific information for professional journals. Choose topics that are timely and somewhat controversial, to spark interest. Limit your information so that it can be read in a short time.

Community exposure is good publicity. Get involved in community organizations or civic groups. Offer yourself as a speaker to various organizations, such as parent-teacher associations, schools, American Society for Personnel Administrators, senior citizen groups, local libraries, and professional organizations.

Nutrition month activities can be extremely helpful in gaining some name recognition. Offer your posters, handout materials, demonstrations, and presentations at local grocery stores, physicians' offices, schools, community organizations, and fitness centers. Attract the attention of media to cover and write about events that you are hosting. You might even ask for a proclamation from the mayor. That will surely get you in the news!

Networking

One of the ways that you can stay ahead of trends, learn how businesses operate, and become influential and well known in the marketplace is through networking. Networking means to establish informal communication and support from people who are associated with your target markets and who can "open doors."

You already have some networks established, such as the local dietetic association, civic or philanthropic groups to which you belong, and the people you currently interact with in your work. You can build a stronger network by volunteering some time with groups that increase visibility.

For instance, a particular outpatient nutrition counselor volunteered to help with activities for the American Heart Association's Food Festival. She did some demonstrations in grocery stores where she was visible to many people in the community. As a result, the local Association invited her to a fund raiser where prominent members of the community would be present. She was able to meet many influential people at this gathering and followed up on many of her conversations with a letter and business card. Through these efforts, the nutrition counselor received several physician referrals, four speaking engagements, and is now on the board for the local Heart Association, where she can continue to nurture helping relationships.

Networking doesn't just happen. It requires a conscious process of planning, acting, and reacting. Some of the most successful people in the field of nutrition actually set networking goals to strengthen and maintain their position and future endeavors (Ross Professional Development Series, 1989). Remember that networking is a two-way street. You and your staff should be selective about the activities you involve yourselves in so that they will be profitable to you. Also, be willing to help others in your network when you are able. A good example of this is your opportunity to refer your clients to other professionals who direct referrals to you. Specifically, you might reciprocate with referrals to physical therapists, cardiologists, social workers, and so on.

One of the most valuable sources of publicity and indirect referral is the inpatient dietetic staff. This effort may begin by networking with the inpatient staff and develop into a routine procedure. The following conversation between an inpatient dietitian and her patient offers insight on just how an inpatient nutrition counselor can help the outpatient nutrition practice.

> **Inpatient Counselor:** Mr. J., I understand that you are leaving us tomorrow. I know you still have many questions and concerns about the high-fiber diet Dr. K. recommended. Things will be different when you get home. You'll be feeling more relaxed and more able to concentrate on your eating habits. Then you will probably have a lot of questions about the foods you eat. As I mentioned earlier, making change takes time and you'll need support. I'd like to suggest that you see our outpatient nutrition counselor. We would need to get a referral from Dr. K., but you could see the dietitian at a time when you are better prepared to focus on your diet. You've got a lot on your mind, and you won't have all the interruptions we had yesterday.
>
> **Mr. J.:** Sounds like it might be helpful. Is it expensive?
>
> **Inpatient Counselor:** Not really. Why don't I ask the nutrition counselor to pay you a visit before you leave. She can fill you in on the details, and, if you're interested, we'll contact Dr. K. for a referral and make you an appointment.

Suggesting that the outpatient nutrition counselor visit inpatients regularly may seem time consuming. However, if the counselor is allotted three hours per week for marketing and uses all of that time visiting inpatients, he or she could attract as many as 12 new clients per week. In cases where this technique is not useable, the inpatient dietitian could provide names, addresses, and phone numbers to the outpatient nutrition counselor so that a follow-up could be made.

Together, the inpatient and outpatient nutrition staff can develop a "survival kit" that the patient will use until the outpatient nutrition counseling begins. The kit may be anything from a week of preplanned menus to some basic tips on the prescribed diet. This process reduces the frustration of the inpatient dietitian who feels that the patient leaves the hospital inadequately prepared to comply with the diet. Also, the outpatient nutrition counselor reaps the benefit of a steady flow of new clients.

Advertising

Whereas publicity and networking are generally recognized as cost-free or low cost promotional techniques, advertising of any kind will demand a price. When developing an advertising strategy, you must be extremely sensitive to the methods that will provide you the greatest amount of exposure to your target market for the lowest cost.

Advertising techniques provide incentives that encourage people to purchase products or services. The underlying premise is that once people use a good product or service, they will become loyal customers if it satisfies a need. Thus, promotional techniques are directed toward cultivating new business and keeping old business. Certain methods of promotion work best with particular targets or distribution channels.

Choose advertising techniques that focus directly on target markets or distribution channels. For instance, if the target market consists of people undergoing cardiac rehabilitation, you can most effectively promote your program through physicians (particularly cardiologists), the American Heart Association, and inpatients. Launching a full scale media campaign will reach a large audience that includes cardiologists and cardiac rehabilitation clients. However, much less expensive promotional techniques that reach only cardiologists and hospital inpatients would probably draw in more clients.

On the following pages, you will find descriptions of various advertising vehicles.

Preview Sessions Preview sessions give potential clients an opportunity to sample your services, your products, and the style of the nutrition counselor. This vehicle is used primarily for group education and group counseling programs. A preview session is simply an overview of the program you are offering in the form of a personal presentation. It can be open to the public or offered by invitation and can be advertised through community publicity, referral agents, or direct mail. The greatest advantages of preview sessions are personal contact, limited cost, the ability to register clients for the program(s) on the spot, and the opportunity to use all the senses (sight, smell, taste, touch) in promoting the program. Preview sessions also pinpoint an interested portion of the target market.

If you choose to provide preview sessions, be flashy. This is the time to "show off." Above all, limit the presentation time and the scope of information, to prevent giving the audience all they need to know without purchasing your services. Presenters should impress the audience with the benefits of nutrition services and show them how individual needs will be addressed. Make preview sessions interactive to maximize the opportunity to involve participants and build rapport.

Printed Advertising Printed advertising requires thought and planning. Unless printed advertisements attract the attention of potential clients, they will not be read. There is a big difference between typed or photocopied materials and those that are typeset and printed professionally. Your marketing or public relations department may have professionals on staff, or you may contract with professionals who can help you develop attractive printed advertisements that will be read.

Another resource is the print shop within your facility. The print shop supervisor can explain their capabilities in terms of print styles, graphics, paper, and number of colors they can print. Even if you prepare the written content of the advertisement, utilizing these resources will professionalize your materials and eliminate that "homemade" look.

To work effectively with printers, typesetters, and/or graphic artists, prepare yourself for the first meeting. Collect advertisements, brochures, and so forth, so that you have an idea of what can be done. Also, be prepared to explain the target market and the objectives of the advertisements and how they will be used. This information will allow the printing experts to select the most effective mediums to use.

When you meet with the print expert, ask to see similar work that he or she has done to determine quality and style. Demand an estimate of cost and time. A schedule can be developed to delineate responsibilities and set deadlines for each stage of the project. The schedule should include time for you to proof materials at each step of the process. Schedules increase the commitment to work within a time frame and legitimize your "nagging" calls if materials are not reviewed.

A wellness center trying to downplay their past reputation as a sports medicine clinic had new brochures printed. They altered and reviewed proofs of the written copy for the brochure, but failed to look at the illustrations. On the cover of the final brochure was a marathon runner just completing a race. The center learned an important lesson: *Always proof copy, format, and illustrations.*

When selecting graphics and clip art, consider the style of print and colors you have chosen for paper and print. Pictures of food seldom look appetizing in black and white or blue and pink. Pictures of plants have become the standard of health food vendors and vitamin companies, and are, therefore, a poor choice. If the content of the message is fairly serious, choose more realistic graphics, photographs, or sketches of people for instance. Save the cartoons for programs you hope will seem fun.

Yellow Pages Listings Yellow pages listings were rated one of the most effective advertising tools by nutrition counselors in outpatient practices. In fact, consumer surveys show that the public views the yellow pages as the most appropriate medium for healthcare advertising (Haschke, 1984). When people don't know where to find services, the yellow pages are their major resource. Be sure to list your practice where it will be found easily. Listings under "Nutritionists" and "Weight Control" have been fairly successful. In addition, you may ask the institution, clinic, or physicians you are affiliated with to list your practice under their names. A white pages listing for your practice is free of charge. Charges for yellow page listings vary from place to place, but are considered affordable by most practices. Two samples are offered in Figures 7-3 and 7-4.

Brochures Brochures are a very effective means of communicating general information about the practice and program offerings. They are easily distributed

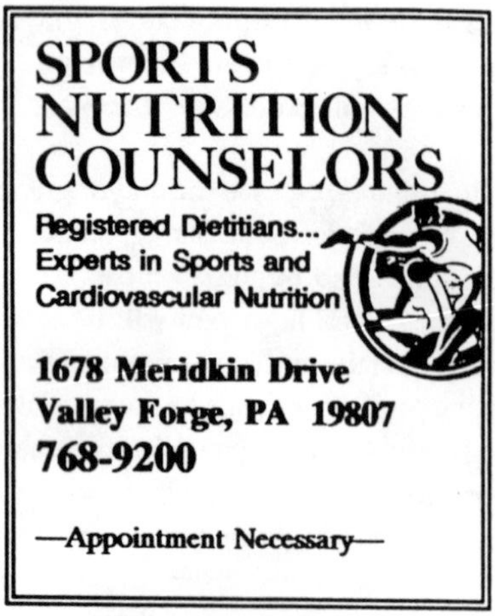

FIGURE 7-3. Sample yellow pages advertisement with graphics.

Riverdale Nutrition Experts

For Total Family Care

- Weight Control
- Special Diets
- Infant & Child Nutrition
- Diabetes Counseling
- Prenatal Counseling
- Speakers on Nutrition

By Appointment Only:
Registered Dietitians
421 South Drive
New York, NY 21401

685-4000

FREE PARKING

FIGURE 7-4. Sample yellow pages advertisement without graphics

and useful for any target audience. Your brochures should include a description of the practice or program, credentials of the staff, and functional information (hours, address, phone number, and contact name). A statement of purpose, list of program benefits, and brief client testimonial will give potential clients the impetus to learn more.

Avoid publishing charges in brochures, as they may quickly become outdated and the enticement for prospective clients to call for more information may be price. Printing counselors names may also date the brochure, as counselors can change. Some brochures are developed with a slot for a business card.

The flier (Figure 7-5) was prepared as part of the patient discharge packet. Although it will be placed in every packet, it is targeted at persons who leave the hospital on modified diets and those with a special interest in nutrition. It attracts the client's attention by voicing the frustration of not knowing how to follow the prescribed diet once discharged from the hospital. It also identifies the benefits of making dietary changes to reduce symptoms and hospitalization. The phone number provides the opportunity for action, and the practice name ties it to the institution for greater credibility. This flier could be printed on a fine grade, colored paper, using black ink, and it could be an inexpensive, eye-catching advertisement.

Newspaper Advertising Newspaper advertising is probably the most commonly used media. Placement and ad content are of prime importance. The newspaper representative can provide demographic information for the various sections of the paper. For example, advertising in the sports section is appropriate if you are attempting to attract athletes, while ads in the food or lifestyle section are more likely to be read by women. Information may also be available on the demographics of daily versus weekend readers. You must determine where you will gain the greatest exposure, based on the target market.

Newspaper ads must be distinctive, uncluttered, and concise. It is important to choose a page that is filled with articles, rather than other ads. White space, print style, and art work attract attention to the ad. If the ad will cover a fourth of a page or more, professionals should be hired to design it.

Investigate weekly and small daily newspapers, as well as larger papers. Although the small newspapers have fewer readers, their readers tend to be more loyal and read a greater portion of the pages. At various times, newspapers will publish medical or fitness supplements that can be ideal for advertising some services. Some sample advertisements follow.

The first ad (Figure 7-6) grabs the audience through the initial statement relating to their needs. It speaks directly to the senior population trying to prevent or control chronic illness. To increase the effectiveness of this ad, it should be placed in a section of the paper they would most likely read. If the tour is offered on "Seniors Day" at the supermarket, that is an added feature.

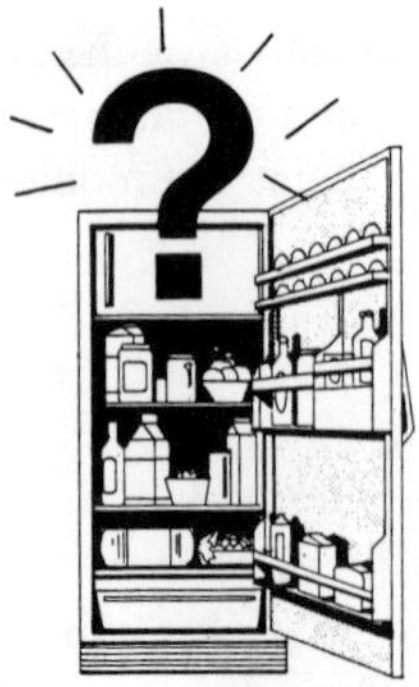

GOING HOME? NOW WHAT?

Changing your eating habits can lessen the symptoms of many illnesses and greatly reduce your chances of returning to the hospital. But, how will your diet fit into your daily lifestyle?

Special nutrition experts can help you take control of your eating habits without drastic changes in the way you want to live.

Special diet experts offer personalized and group counseling on:

- Prescribed Diets
- Medication/Food Interactions
- Blood Sugar Monitoring
- Nutrition and Exercise.

Sessions led by:
Certified Diabetes Educators • Registered Dietitians • Nurses • Pharmacists • Exercise Specialists

For more information or to schedule an appointment call 782-4000

Tower Memorial Hospital
NUTRITION CENTER
2001 KEYSTONE AVENUE • CHESTNUT HILL, PA • 19106

FIGURE 7-5. Sample flier advertising the outpatient nutrition services of the institution to be place in discharge packages.

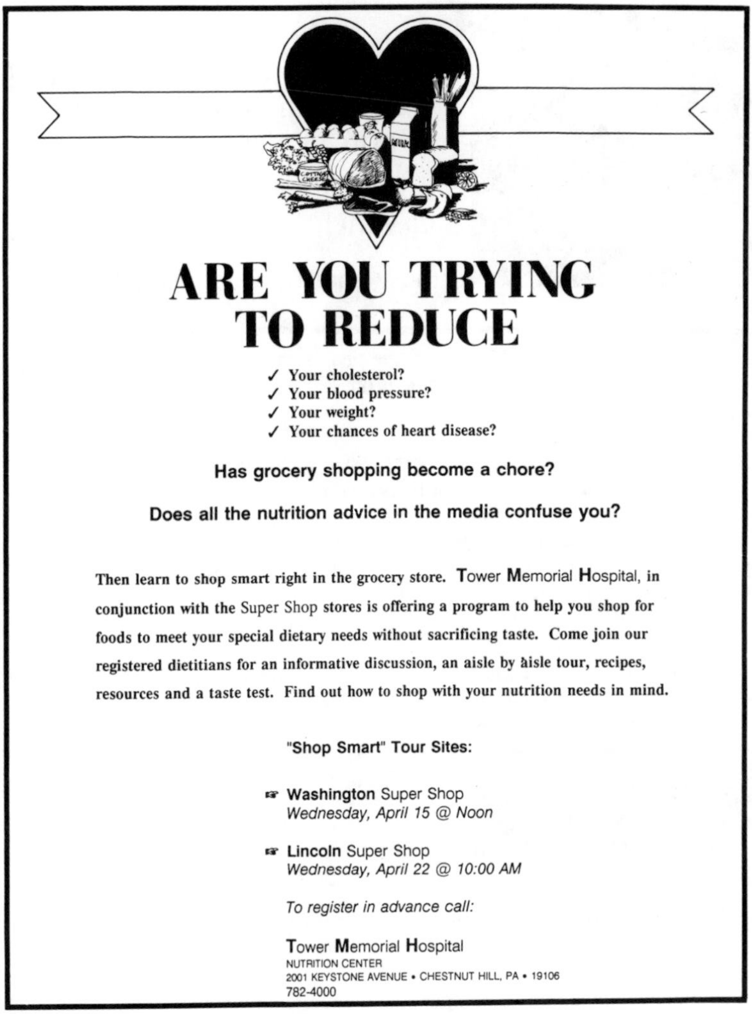

FIGURE 7-6. Sample newspaper advertisement for a grocery store nutrition tour targeted at senior citizens.

The second ad (Figure 7-7) speaks to the audience through humor. But it gets right at the heart of the overweight working woman's dilemma—"How do I lose weight without giving up my busy work and social schedule?" The benefits of looking good and social acceptance are stressed. Again, placement and timing of the ad will impact its success.

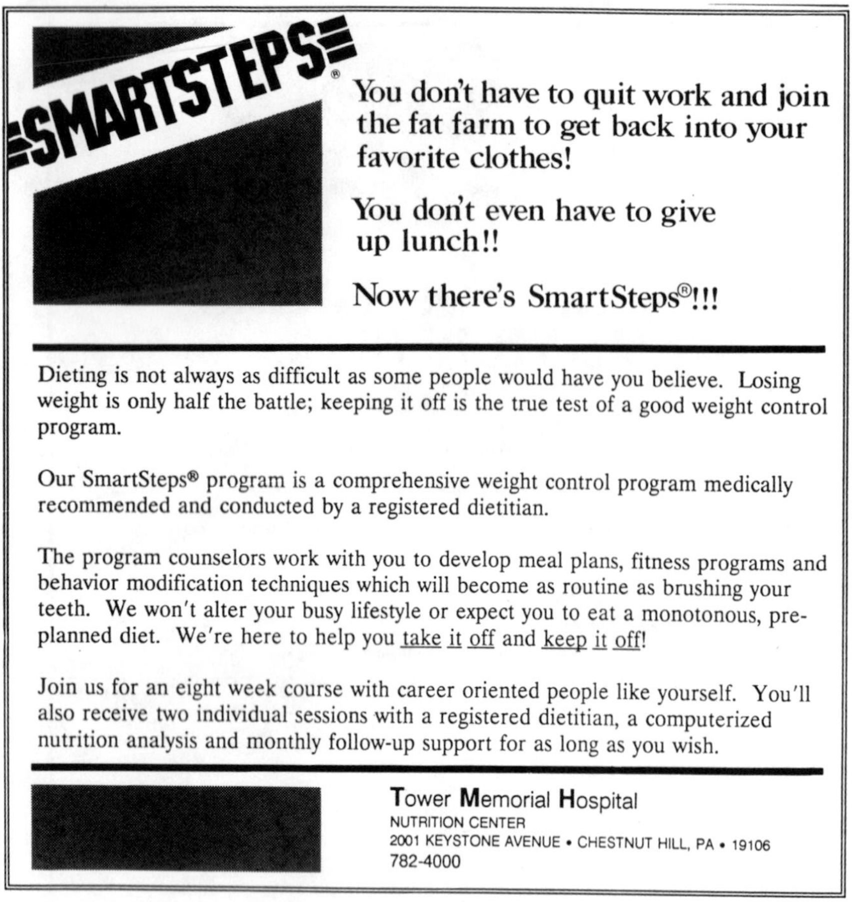
SMARTSTEPS®
You don't have to quit work and join the fat farm to get back into your favorite clothes!
You don't even have to give up lunch!!
Now there's SmartSteps®!!!
Dieting is not always as difficult as some people would have you believe. Losing weight is only half the battle; keeping it off is the true test of a good weight control program.
Our SmartSteps® program is a comprehensive weight control program medically recommended and conducted by a registered dietitian.
The program counselors work with you to develop meal plans, fitness programs and behavior modification techniques which will become as routine as brushing your teeth. We won't alter your busy lifestyle or expect you to eat a monotonous, pre-planned diet. We're here to help you take it off and keep it off!
Join us for an eight week course with career oriented people like yourself. You'll also receive two individual sessions with a registered dietitian, a computerized nutrition analysis and monthly follow-up support for as long as you wish.
Tower Memorial Hospital
NUTRITION CENTER
2001 KEYSTONE AVENUE • CHESTNUT HILL, PA • 19106
782-4000

FIGURE 7-7. Sample newspaper advertisement for a weight reduction program targeted at working women

Promotion Incentives Promotion incentives provoke curiosity and draw people in for a sample of your products/services. Such things as coupons, discounts, contests, "giveaways," and gift certificates fall under the realm of promotional incentives. Before using these techniques, you must carefully examine the outcome. These techniques are widely used and may be associated with bargains and lower quality goods. Use incentives that will maintain a professional image and produce the intended results.

Figure 7-8 illustrates a coupon that was printed on the back of a grocery receipt to promote grocery tours. Although stating benefits is virtually impossible in such a small space, the coupon does offer the benefit of reduced cost. Benefits of the tour can be highlighted better if the counselors who provide the tours also promote this program through posters or through other services. To use the cash register tape for advertising requires that you speak to the customer service representative for the particular store.

"Giveaways" and "leave behinds" are frequently used to remind prospective clients about your services. They are also advertisements to others who might see them. Useful items are often left with physicians or key decision makers at the worksite. They are also provided at health fairs, grocery store promotions, and nutrition booths in various locations. Although "giveaways" have traditionally been products, free services can also be used. "Giveaways" are most effective if they are items related to the nutritional concepts you wish to convey or be associated with. To increase the association between the gift and the practice's name, either have the items printed with the name of your practice and phone number or include a business card.

SHOP 'N SAC COUPONS SAVE YOU $$$

—$5.00 OFF—

HEALTHWISE
SUPERMARKET SAFARI

Tour the aisles and learn how
to make healthy food choices!!

See customer rep for details

Offer good thru MM/DD/YY

FIGURE 7-8. Sample coupon for a reduced price on grocery tours.

Promotional gifts can be costly, so you must weigh the potential results against the expenditure. Often, suppliers will provide these items for promotional purposes free of charge to nonprofit organizations or regular customers. Ideas of appropriate giveaways can be found in Table 7-1.

Contests Contests can be used as an advertising medium or as an incentive to remain in a program. Worksite contests have been used very effectively. They are relatively inexpensive; in fact, nutrition practices often charge for weight loss competitions and use part of the payment as prize money. If you offer a weight loss competition, set very specific criteria. Otherwise, you may not be promoting sound nutrition concepts. A particular nutrition practice used the following guidelines.

Nutrition Competition Guidelines

1. A team consists of four members.
2. Each member pays $30.
3. All members are weighed at the start, and body fat is measured. Then a weight goal is set by the participant and the nutrition counselor. Weekly weight-ins are monitored by the nutrition counselor.
4. Nutrition counseling is provided weekly to all teams in a group setting.
5. Points are given for:
   a. Attending group sessions
   b. Exercising at the worksite
   c. Losing weight of ½ to 3 lbs. per week.

TABLE 7-1 Nutrition and Health Giveaways

Nutrition Related	Fitness Related	Others
Nutritious foods	Exercise classes	Pencils
Counseling sessions	Exercise consultations	Item in gift shop
Preview sessions	Exercise equipment	Car sun visors
Restaurant meal	Gym bags	Mugs/cups
Cafeteria meal	Shoe laces	Key chains
Cookbook	Wrist wallets	Balloons
Nutrition book	Headbands	T-shirts
Fruit basket	Wristbands	Calendars
Refrigerator magnets		Bumper stickers
Sample seasonings		Health classes:
Free screening:		Lamaz
Body fat		CPR
Nutrition analysis		
Cholesterol		
Blood sugar		
Free follow-up		
Recipe cards		

Points are lost for:
a. Gaining weight
b. Hindering other team members from achieving goals.
6. The team with the most points gets their $30 back and $30 more per member.
7. All employees who lose weight will be recognized publicly.

Contests, games, and competitions also serve to stimulate interest in nutrition and ultimately in nutrition services. Such promotions suggest that nutrition isn't boring and regimented and that your programs are active and entertaining. Ideas that have been effective include:

- Cook-offs of nutritional foods;
- Planning the perfect meal;
- Recipe contests;
- Scavenger hunts for nutrition information with clues in newsletters, grocery stores, worksite, or institutional facilities;
- Poster contests;
- Guessing calories, fat, or fiber in a specific food (one practice placed a giant muffin in a cafeteria and had a "guess the fiber content contest"); and
- Team competitions to select the most healthy lunches at work.

When using competitions, further interest can be sparked by offering free sessions as prizes and providing brochures to all participants.

Nutrition Fairs

Nutrition practitioners find that health and nutrition fairs yield varying results. They can be a very effective way to disseminate information and draw interest to nutrition. They also have some lasting value because people will take home information about the practice. On the other hand, booths at health fairs and nutrition fairs can be an expensive promotional activity with limited return. The space, equipment, and material are not the only costs incurred. You and your staff also lose the time you could be using in profitable activities.

If you do decide to participate in a health fair or provide your own nutrition fair as a promotional activity, get specific information about the health fair before you decide to participate.

- What groups are participating? Are they offering sound advice and selling reputable products?
- Will the location of the fair draw the clientele you hope to attract?
- Will the location of the booth and the physical surroundings reflect well on the image of the practice?
- Will your participation (or lack of it) send a message to the community?
- Does the booth/display reflect the image you wish?

Use the opportunity to create a need for nutrition counseling by providing screening. Body fat, cholesterol, and fitness screening are very popular, as is computerized nutrition analysis. Effective visuals (fat models, thinning mirrors, games and quizzes, etc.) stimulate interest in your services. Using videos, celebrity support, live testimonials, pictures, and printed materials will enlighten people on the various services the practice provides and the benefits they offer.

To draw people to your services, provide sign-up sheets, drawings for prizes that include a free service, and discount coupons for services. Sending them home with a reminder of the practice, such as fun giveaways with a significant message, might encourage them to call you in the future.

Choose sites for nutrition fairs that will reach the largest number of prospective clients possible. Note, however, that large numbers are not as important as reaching people who will use your services. A nutrition fair at a shopping mall may put you in contact with the masses, but you may receive more business by locating the fair in a business office complex.

Rather than using nutrition fairs as a promotional activity, you may want to consider selling them as a service. In the worksite setting, you may sell the nutrition fair to organizational decision makers so that it can be used to promote nutrition programs to employees. The more interest you can spark through the nutrition fair, the larger the number of employees you can attract to the practices. This, in turn, reflects well on you and your staff's ability to motivate people, a quality that worksite administrators will appreciate.

Sales Call

The *sales call* is a vehicle you are all familiar with, as many businesses sell products and services in this manner. In essence, the sales call entails contacting potential clients by phone and informing them of your services, start-up dates and times, special packages, and prices. You may even register clients by phone to strengthen commitment. Although the sales call may seem totally inappropriate for use in the healthcare field, it has a place. Consider phone call sales for follow-up on hospital inpatients, nutrition fair participants, or participants in screening programs.

Direct Mail

When personal contact is not feasible, direct mail is an option. Direct mail advertising, not to be confused with mail order selling, includes any form of advertising that is sent through the postal service.

The advantages of direct advertising are:

- It is very selective, limiting waste circulation.
- The advertiser selects the target audience.

- The advertiser controls all decisions related to timing, placement, and acceptance of the advertising.
- The ad campaign can begin or end at a moment's notice.
- Few distractions compete with the advertisement at the moment it is received.
- It allows the buyer to take action, by including business reply cards, registration cards, and so on.
- It provides an easy method to measure performance through reply cards, coupons, and so on.
- It limits the exposure of your competition to your promotional efforts (Cohen, 1972).

The disadvantages are:

- Low readership—A consumer attitudes study (Direct Mail Advertising Assoc. 1965) showed that only 30 percent of the sample thoroughly read direct mail and 25 percent discarded their direct mail ads unopened. Although 60 percent have at some time purchased products or services through direct mail, only 7 percent did so frequently.
- The cost per unit of circulation is high, and the cost per inquiry or sale is even higher (Cohen, 1972).
- Lack of professional quality printed materials usually creates a perception of "junk mail," which reduces credibility.

How is direct mail best used? Direct mail advertising proves to be most effective for:

- Welcoming new clients;
- Winning back inactive clients;
- Capitalizing on special events;
- Announcing new services;
- Distributing samples and coupons;
- Building good will; and
- Building employee morale.

Research shows that direct mail is only effective if the potential client perceives the need at the moment they read it. Timing is critical.

How are mailing lists generated?

Mailing lists can be developed through your own clients and the clients of your institution or affiliates. Lists can be developed through public sources of information, such as telephone directories, birth lists, voting lists, and Who's Who (Cohen, 1972). Worksite organizations can help you build your list by offering contacts with their business associates. Very specific lists can be purchased, rented, or exchanged; however, this service can be costly.

What costs are involved in direct mail advertising?
Direct mail encompasses many cost factors. The price of producing the mailer from copy and layout to paper and printing varies, depending on how elaborate a mailer you envision. Mailing cards are usually the least expensive direct mail advertisement, while booklets and folders tend to be the most expensive (Cohen, 1972). In many cases a cost is incurred for the mailing list that can be as high as 50 cents per name. If the mailer must be stuffed in an envelope and posted, the price of labor must be added. Third class postage can be used for direct mail and is cheaper. However, first class mail is delivered more quickly and stands a greater chance of being read (Cohen, 1972).

All of these costs must be considered when choosing direct mail. To determine the cost per inquiry of your advertisement, divide the total cost by the total number of inquiries you receive. Some important pointers to bear in mind when preparing direct mail advertising include:

- Contact the services of professional printers to prevent an appearance of "junk mail."
- Check with your local post office for regulations on size, style, and form of direct mailers.
- Personalize the advertisement to increase readership. Computer letter programs can be used to place specific names in the salutation and text, as well as personalizing the heading and generating mailing labels.
- Establish immediate interest through strong consumer benefits or a pertinent question.
- Offer one basic idea, simply and logically.
- Give the reader impulse for action by including reply cards, samples, or coupons, or by offering free preview sessions or invitations to special events.
- Maintain your mailing list by regularly adding names, eliminating duplicates, and correcting errors (Cohen, 1972).

MAXIMIZING RETURNS ON YOUR PROMOTIONAL EFFORTS

Four primary decisions underlie the effectiveness of all of your promotional efforts. You must decide:

1. Which promotional vehicle(s) and methods of distribution will best reach your target audience(s)?
2. What will inspire your target audience to take action?
3. How do you best use each vehicle to communicate your message and persuade your audience?

4. How will you allocate limited resources for promotion to maximize your return on the investment (for example, money, time, and advertising space)?

Which promotional vehicles will best reach your target audience?
Look closely at the demographic information on your chosen target(s). Determine which promotional efforts will be most visible. Brochures and pamphlets in a physician's office will not increase your clientele if you are targeting amateur and professional athletes, whereas posters and brochures in local health clubs might. If your target market envelops people who work the 9 A.M. to 5 P.M. shift, consider advertising on a radio station that targets the same market, during the hours the majority of this group is listening.

Determine the greatest interests or concerns of the target market. If your potential clients are business people, your advertisements will most likely be read if they are in the financial section of the newspaper. Or better yet, send them a fitness/nutrition article from a business publication along with your brochure.

The more personal contact you can make in promoting your services, the more likely you are to attract clients. Speaking at community meetings and making yourself available for questions will spark greater interest than a form letter or a newspaper advertisement in most cases. Choose vehicles that allow you to make personal contact or that single out individuals. For instance, when promoting a new service to past clients, send them cards on their birthdays, with a brief personal note.

Brochures can only be effective if they are distributed in places where they will be used. Your best approach is to deliver brochures personally and to sell to the people who will be distributing them on your services. For the most part, a stack of brochures laying on a table in a waiting room will be ignored, whereas one presented by a nurse or fitness specialist will be studied.

What will inspire your target audience to take action?
Determine what will inspire your target audience to take action. Celebrity endorsements or testimonials make a great impression on a variety of people. However, the backing of a physician or academic institution may have greater impact with professional people. Discounts are often used with employees and senior citizens. They can also be effective to draw in family members or large groups, and as an incentive to bring a friend. Special offers (two for one, door prizes, and drawings) and coupons are best limited to specific groups rather than large, generic populations.

Printed advertisements must grab the reader's attention if they are to be noticed. Provocative phrases and flashy graphics entice the reader to open the brochure and learn more about the program or practice. The brochure front (Figure 7-9) is a good example.

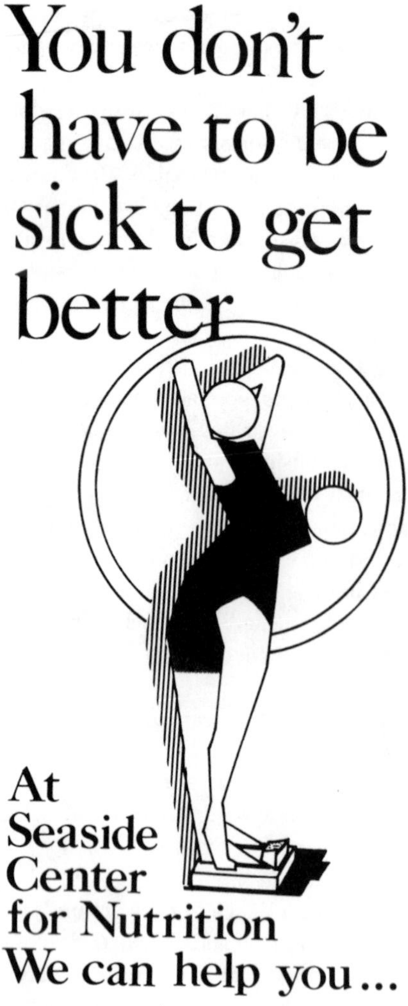
You don't have to be sick to get better
At Seaside Center for Nutrition
We can help you...

FIGURE 7-9. Sample brochure front intended to catch the eye of potential clients.

What catches the eye of a potential client is very different from what catches the eye of a worksite decision maker. The front of a brochure that appeals to this audience might look like Figure 7-10.

ARE YOU AWARE THAT:

- Corporations pay $97 billion for health-care per year.
- More than 65% of worksites with 50 or more employees offer wellness activites. 17% of these programs offer nutrition education.
- 90% of top executives say they try to watch their diets to improve overall health.
- Over 40% of Americans are overweight to a degree which negatively affects their health.
- Cancer risks can be reduced by as much as seven times through diet alone, saving your health dollars.
- The American Heart Association estimates the costs of treating cardiovascular diseases at $78.6 billion.

FIGURE 7-10. Sample front of a brochure targeted at worksite decision makers.

How do you best use each vehicle to communicate your message and persuade your audience?

Emphasizing value is key. Whether your promotional efforts are aimed at the prospective client or at the physician or organization, success depends on promoting the benefits of your services to the user. As stated earlier, you must know your audience well before launching a promotional campaign. Your role is to help clients and referring agents see just how your programs and services help to satisfy their needs.

Often features are confused with benefits. It is important that the distinction be clearly understood:

- A *feature* is a description or a characteristic of a product or service.
- A *benefit* is its value to the client or the need that has been satisfied.

Some examples follow:

Example #1
FEATURE:
Our nutrition counselors are all registered dietitians.
CLIENT BENEFIT:
Clients receive accurate, nutritionally sound guidance.

Many prospective clients do not understand the value of having a registered dietitian provide nutrition counseling. But most clients know that they are seeking accurate, nutritionally sound guidance. Remember, your clients aren't experts in the nutrition field, and your promotional efforts must show the value of your services to them.

Example #2
FEATURE:
Monthly follow-up sessions are offered for group nutrition programs.
CLIENT BENEFIT:
Clients receive ongoing guidance and support for dietary compliance.

This example was taken directly out of a newspaper advertisement. Only the feature was stated. It is easy to see how a potential client could overlook the value of follow-up sessions if the advertiser assumed the benefit was known.

Both features and benefits are important to your promotional efforts. However, sometimes, due to limited money, time, and space, you must make choices about which words will send the most valuable message. As is the case in the last two examples, benefits can often stand alone, but features are rarely effective without benefits. Promoting features without emphasizing benefits weakens your appeal. This is a common mistake.

Knowing the target audience is extremely important in promoting benefits. A brochure developed specifically to interest organization decision makers in offering nutrition services to their employees might include the copy in Figure 7-11.

Benefits to the employees would also be important; therefore, the brochure might also include the copy in Figure 7-12.

High-quality, professionally prepared brochures are the rule for this market. Accompanying this brochure might be a business card and an invitation to a luncheon or a letter stating the intention of the nutrition practitioner to telephone soon.

Take major steps towards improving employee health and reap the benefits of:

- Reduced disability
- Reduced costs of retraining
- Reduced absenteeism
- Improved employee morale
- Improved company image
- Reduced injury
- Increased porductivity

FIGURE 7-11. Benefits of worksite nutrition programs as they might be perceived by decision makers.

We find that people are genuinely interested in improving their nutrition habits in an effort to:

- Improve health and well-being
- Reduce risk of chronic disease

— Heart disease
— High blood pressure
— Cancer

- Improve their physical image as well as their self-image
- Increase stamina
- Control chronic conditions

FIGURE 7-12. Benefits of worksite nutrition programs as they might be perceived by employees.

If you think that a feature of your service is of benefit but the prospective client does not, usually one of two things has happened:

1. Failure to communicate *how* the feature is of benefit.
2. Failure to understand what the client perceives to be of benefit.

Each market segment and client will have different needs. So, as you promote the practice, the benefits you emphasize must shift, depending on the audience. During your market research, you must identify the perceived needs of each target market. You must also be sensitive to changing needs over time. Business pressures, new technology, changes in the marketplace, and identification of new problems or new therapies change the needs of the client. Examples of potential benefits for different market segments are listed in Table 7-2.

Here is an example of how one practice promoted the same service to two target markets differently.

A nutrition practice offered computerized nutrition analysis in a worksite program. One program dealt with business executives and the other with factory workers. The following promotional messages were used for each group.

Business Executives

"You wouldn't sell a product without analyzing the market...Don't sell yourself short. Computerized nutrition analysis can:

- Lower your blood pressure
- Reduce stress
- Increase energy
- Improve your blood cholesterol profile"

Factory Workers

"What you eat can be the difference between:

- Catching the bus and catching up with the time clock.
- Bench pressing your weight and struggling to lift your lunch box.
- The life of the party and the party pooper.

Get in on the secret of healthy eating. Contact your nutrition counselor."

Promotional design and layout are key too. You want to design the promotions so that they reach out and capture the attention of the audience. You want to encourage the audience to go to the phone and call without hesitation. This may be accomplished through visual images, a catchy tune, a memorable hook line, a coupon, your choice of words, artwork, and borders or white space properly placed. Obviously, promotional design requires specific expertise and talent.

TABLE 7-2 Potential Benefits of Outpatient Nutrition Counseling Services By Market Segments

Market group	Benefits of outpatient nutrition services
Organizational clients (those providing worksite programs)	• Improves employee morale • Increases productivity • Reduces turnover • Reduces worker compensation claims • Reduces insurance claims • Reduces absenteeism • Reduce injury
Physicians, dentists, and clinics	• Markets the practice • Increases accuracy in nutrition instruction to patients • Increases revenue potential • Provision of more comprehensive medical care • Reduces physician's time to personally provide nutrition instruction • Promotes a caring image to clients • Increases credibility
Individuals	• Increases likelihood of correcting nutrition problems • Improves health • Improves self-image • Prevents need for lifetime medication • Improves control over chronic conditions • Prevents chronic disease • Establishes an ongoing support system
Healthcare organization	• Markets the healthcare organization • Increases revenue potential • Improves productivity with better utilization of staff • Reduces costs by using resources more effectively • Enhances clinical programs • Attracts physician referrals

You may want to seek the assistance of marketing experts to ensure that promotions bring a flow of clients through the practice that enables you to achieve the results you anticipate. Advertising agencies often offer promotional assistance free of charge if you purchase advertisements through them. Solicit support from other departments for promotional efforts. The marketing and public relations staff can be extremely helpful when developing promotional strategies and materials for use outside the institution. Within the institution, call on the expertise of human resources, patient education, wellness, and social services departments.

How will you allocate limited resources (money, time, and advertising space) to maximize your return on the investment?

The answer to this question depends on your situation. Consider:

- Which services are most beneficial to promote? Which are most profitable?
- Which groups within the target market are the largest?
- Which service(s) will provide the most repeat business?
- Which approach will broaden the referral base most quickly?
- Will certain services attract a feeder pool for other services?
- Will the majority of your clients find the practice through referral agents, or will they have to find the practice on their own?
- Is the target market well educated about nutrition? Do your promotions need to sell the value of nutrition along with your services?
- Do you have name identification, or must it be developed?
- Is the target market well informed regarding the availability of services?
- How much promotion can be done jointly with the institution or affiliates?
- How much advertising will the institution or affiliates do for you?
- How much free promotion can you obtain through publicity and networking?
- What kinds of promotional techniques are your competitors using? How successful are they?

The answers to these questions should help you determine how to allocate time, promotional dollars, and advertising space. Compromising your professional image is not an option for cutting costs. If your resources do not provide for well written, professionally printed, and visually appealing ads and materials, then promote your services through personal presentations. Your own enthusiasm will be more effective than poorly prepared ads.

It is important to recognize that the answers to these questions are based on considerable speculation on your part. That is why you must monitor closely the return on these promotional investments. Be sure to gather information from each new client on how they became aware of your services, and train each staff member who answers the telephone to ask for the same information of each prospective client calling. Have the information recorded in a log. This data should indicate which promotional efforts are reaping the best results.

Promoting to Clients

Although most outpatient nutrition counselors strive for a physician referral on every client, many times it is more effective to promote services to individuals and seek a referral later. When selling to individuals, you compete directly with commercial programs and products. Therefore, you must promote a professional image that sets the practice apart from overnight diet pills and hair analysis. In addition, your promotional efforts must educate the public on the value of your services and the difference between sound nutrition and quackery.

Public speaking is one of the best options for promoting to individuals. Other ways of reaching people personally are through demonstrations in grocery stores, health fair booths, county fair booths, nutrition month promotions, community cholesterol screenings, and visitation of hospital inpatients. When you or your staff cannot personally promote your services and products, other forms of publicity are the next best thing, as many people are more comfortable with healthcare providers giving information than selling their services and products. Effective publicity vehicles include radio and television talk shows, community calendars, news interviews, press releases, newspaper articles, and participation in Dial-a-Dietitian.

Advertising mediums must be considered carefully in the aspects of cost, placement, audience, and exposure time. Printed mediums have the advantage of longer exposure, the ability to disseminate more information, and, in many cases, low cost. Television and radio ads are more expensive and shorter in length, but have the advantages of repetition, large audiences, and more select placement. Using a celebrity who has successfully completed your program can be advantageous in advertising, as well as using testimonials from successful clients.

Consider the target market(s) when choosing places to speak, display, offer brochures, advertise, or do demonstrations. Printed materials, displays, and posters are well received by grocery stores, welcome wagons, libraries, physicians and dentists, YMCAs, county extension offices, health clubs and spas, and sports bars.

One practice found a local grocery store chain to be very effective in promoting services to senior citizens. Once a month, on "senior discount day," they did demonstrations in the stores. They also advertised via posters, displays, and flyers in grocery bags on a regular basis. For the cost of printing and materials, the store manager gave them permission to print coupons on the back of cash register tapes. Since the promotions benefited the stores as well as the nutrition practice, the store often published the dates and times of demonstrations in their weekly grocery ads.

Organizations that are receptive to speaking engagements include senior citizen, homemaker, and school association. You might also obtain speaking engagements from community health programs, adult education programs, schools, and church groups. If your institution has a speakers bureau, make them aware of the topics that you and your staff can address. One practice developed their own nutrition speakers bureau for nutrition month. They sent letters to schools and community organizations. The response was so great that presentations continued well beyond the month of March and the publicity brought in many new clients.

Although your first concern in worksite organizations is selling to executive management, you must also prepare a promotional campaign for the employees. Support of industrial nurses and physicians can set you up with a direct referral system. Displays or advertisements in the cafeteria or breakroom, on bulletin boards, and in the in-house fitness center tie your services to familiar settings in the workplace. Getting the word out about service offerings can be accomplished through payroll stuffers, employee newsletters/mailings, and free overview sessions. Gimmicks, such as family discounts, contests, nutrition fairs, cooking demonstrations, and free screenings, stimulate interest and show the audience that nutrition can be fun.

An open opportunity for promotion to individuals lies within the healthcare institution. Not only can inpatients be easily informed of your services and products, but visitors to the institutions can be introduced to the services and products as well. Promote your services in the institution through:

- In-house TV ads or programs;
- Brochures in admission or discharge packets;
- Information from inpatient dietitian;
- Displays and promotions in:
  - Cafeteria
  - Gift shop
  - Lobby
  - Elevators
  - Waiting rooms;
- Open houses;
- Ads on prepackaged foods sold in the cafeteria;
- Messages on patient satisfaction surveys;
- Patient tray pamphlets, tents, or placemats;
- Cooking demonstrations;
- Handouts on nutrition and/or recipes with services and products listed; and
- Inpatient classes—cardiac rehabilitation, diabetes, breastfeeding, and so on.

Another captive audience is your existing clientele. Make brochures of your services available to them. Place informative posters in your waiting room and office. Offer incentives to bring a friend to class or refer a friend for services. Through such efforts, word-of-mouth advertising and return business will grow. In fact, your clients may even attract referrals from their healthcare providers better than you can.

Promoting to Referral Agents

While referrals can come from anywhere, there seem to be four primary sources:

- Physicians;
- Dentists;
- Other healthcare professionals; and
- Former and current clients.

Each of these sources can provide a steady flow of clients into your practice. Consequently, you want to persuade as many members of these groups as possible to recommend your services.

Throughout the text, both client satisfaction and promoting to individual clients have been reviewed. This section will focus on the unique aspects of promoting to physicians, dentists, and other healthcare professionals.

Soliciting Physician Support

Because 90 percent or more of outpatient nutrition clients are referred by physicians, it is important to describe some of the specific issues involved in selling your practice to the physician. During focus groups conducted with physicians throughout the country, specific concerns regarding outpatient nutrition practices were raised. These concerns included:

- The need for better follow-up and feedback to the MD;
- The desire for control over patient services;
- Easily accessible locations of services and flexible scheduling;
- Cost to the client;
- Tailoring and adapting nutrition plans to individuals; and
- Clinical studies or data proving the efficacy of programs.

As a rule, these physicians were not aware of the scope of services that outpatient nutrition counselors could provide. Many of them, however, were interested in offering nutrition services in their offices with the major concerns being space, cost-effectiveness, the need for more staff, and profit potential. Let's look at some specific ways to interest physicians in outpatient nutrition services, whether you are promoting your own practice or attempting to contract directly with the physician.

Establishing a Need

You can attract physician attention very early in your marketing efforts by probing their interest in nutrition programs and their beliefs about the nutritional needs of their patients. In so doing, you can more effectively match services and needs, as well as demonstrate your respect for the physicians' opinion. There are several ways to involve physicians in developing programs:

- Survey for patient needs or to learn the physicians' attitudes toward a program you are planning.
- Use focus groups to gather physician opinion and support.
- Get involved in staff meetings (Kernaghan and Giloth, 1984).
- Investigate the unique interests of specialists (e.g., cardiologists, nephrologist).
- Some institutions have liaisons between the hospital and the physicians who will promote your services to the physicians.

Caution must be exercised in choosing physicians for this effort. Some counselors have found that, if the programs were not established according to the physicians' wishes, those physicians would not refer clients. In fact, their influence is so great that they can discourage others from using your services. Therefore, if you choose to use physicians as a sounding board, select those with whom you have strong relationships and those you can count on to be open minded.

Getting Physicians' Attention

The biggest hurdle in selling the physician is making contact. Physicians are busy people. Mail and sales representatives are often handled by their receptionists and nurses. You may be able to interest the physician's staff in your services and use them to influence the physician. Let's look at some successful approaches to reaching the physician.

- Offering to bring lunch to the office has allowed some practices time with the physicians and their staff. Food tends to be a great enticement, especially when it is provided in a convenient place.
- Buffets in the doctors' dining room, refreshments in the physicians' lounge, and special teas provided at appropriate times in common meeting places have all been used to capture physician interest. If you can't get the physician to come, try inviting his or her administrative staff.
- Letters of introduction are important. Too often they are not read by physicians. Two things aid their effectiveness:
  - You must develop clever ways to deliver your message if you want it to be heard. For example, one particular outpatient practice tied helium balloons to the letters and brochures written to introduce a new service. The letters were placed in the physicians' mail boxes at the hospital one morning with all the attached balloons floating near the ceiling. Needless to say, this outpatient practice got the physicians' attention.
  - You must emphasize the benefits to the physician and individual clients. See Figure 7-13 for a sample letter.

- Refer clients to physicians and send the physician a letter of referral.
- If you cannot reach the physician personally, market to the office staff. A practice

ANYTOWN NUTRITION CENTER
111 N. FIRST STREET
MONMOUTH, IL 61462

Date

Paul Johnson, M.D.
Medical Plaza–Suite 10
500 M Street
Monmouth, IL 61462

Dear Dr. Johnson:

Anytown Nutrition Center is proud to announce a new alternative in nutrition counseling and education for your clients. Association with our quality nutritional counseling practice gives you the ability to provide more comprehensive medical care to your patients. Referrals reduce the time it takes for you to personally provide nutritional instruction, and you will still be able to monitor your client's progress through the feedback you will receive, at timely intervals, throughout the counseling process.

Our recent survey indicated that physicians in this area desired an outpatient nutrition practice that offered:

- Nutrition counseling tailored to the needs and lifestyles of individual patients;
- Nutrition services that "get results";
- Continuous feedback to physicians; and
- Affordable services.

Our services are designed to alleviate these concerns. And our nutrition programs are offered at convenient locations. With your referral, most of our nutrition services are reimbursed.

Our team of registered dietitians have specialized in nutritional management of outpatient and well clients. Mary Smith, M.S., R.D. completed a Fellowship in obesity and eating disorders last year at Anytown Medical Center, and Jane James, R.D. has served on the Board for the American Heart Association for two years, helping them provide sound nutrition promotions to the community. We offer experience and professional skills to serve your patients and clients within the community.

The enclosed brochure explains the variety of nutrition counseling programs that Anytown Nutrition Center can offer your clients. I will call next week to arrange an appointment, at your convenience, to further discuss how we can serve your unique needs. I look forward to meeting you and working with your patients.

FIGURE 7-13. Sample letter introducing new service to physicians.

```
Sincerely,


Nora Phillips, R.D.
Outpatient Nutrition Manager

Enclosure
```

FIGURE 7-13. *(Continued)*

provided a buffet luncheon and invited both physicians and their staff. The nutrition counselor commented that her contacts for referral were with staff people, anyway, and that they increased after the buffet.

Soliciting a Physician Advocate

Your credibility among the medical community will increase considerably if you can find a well-respected physician to support your programs. Although research shows that a formal relationship with a physician advocate is more beneficial, an informal relationship can be useful as well. If you do not already know of physicians who might assume this role, you might locate them through the following sources:

- Chief of the medical staff;
- Medical directors of clinical departments (family practice, orthopedics, cardiology, etc.);
- Hospital department heads;
- Nursing supervisors who have contact with medical staff; and
- Local medical society (Kernaghan and Giloth, 1984).

In many health promotion organizations, a medical director is employed. However, less formal arrangements can be made. You might use a physician advocate to:

- Be a liaison between the practice and the medical community (Kernaghan and Giloth, 1984). In this capacity, the physician would:
  - Speak on your behalf at meetings;
  - Introduce you or a member of your staff as a speaker at meetings;
  - Endorse letters of introduction; and
  - Talk informally with physicians about your efforts.
- Act as a chairperson or member of committees that affect the use of the practice and programs.
- Promote the program by first participating in it and then allowing the use of his or her name for advertising and testimonials.

- Be directly involved in developing promotional efforts.
- Preview or review programs and materials.
- Orient new physicians to the program offerings.

To reciprocate, you can act on behalf of the physician by serving on committees or boards, referring patients, and advocating organizations with which he or she has strong ties.

Communicating with Physicians

As stated earlier, physicians are busy people. Therefore, they are not interested in large amounts of printed material, nor do they enjoy lengthy presentations. When presenting information on your program to physicians, be brief and concise. Target your promotional efforts on specialists and practitioners whom you feel will truly be interested in your services. There are several issues that traditionally interest physicians. Be sure to cover the following points:

- Price.
- Reimbursement for services by major insurance providers.
- Patient satisfaction survey information. (If you have data that suggests that patients are interested in your services or have been satisfied with your services, physicians will more likely buy in.) (Kernaghan and Giloth, 1984)
- Statistics on trials or past successes.
- Results that show higher compliance rates than those currently published.
- How follow-up and feedback will be handled.
- The necessity for physician and office staff involvement.
- How you will achieve compliance.

Messages in physician newsletters are helpful if they are clever or interesting. Use the services of graphic artists and marketing experts or input from supportive physicians to develop your message or article. Physicians are particularly appreciative if you somehow title your message so that it speaks to the target audience (Kernaghan and Giloth, 1984).

A practice might use a classified ad style to announce a new nutrition program for cardiac rehabilitation patients. The bold heading for the ad might read, "Cardiac Rehabilitation Support Services," thus attracting the attention of cardiac surgeons and general practice physicians. Speaking at physician meetings and educational programs can be important ways to create program recognition. See the section on "Communicating Your Message" for more information. Medical rounds sometimes offer the opportunity for pharmaceutical representatives to display literature. You might be able to display your materials at the same time, especially if they apply to that particular day's rounds (Kernaghan and Giloth, 1984).

Hand-delivered brochures and sample materials will allow office staff and physicians to associate a face with the practice. You may consider something to leave behind that is associated with the concepts of the practice. The following example shows a very effective way of capturing physician attention.

The following items were sent to physicians' offices:

- Week #1—A small packet of nuts with this card attached:
  "Nut (nut) n. 1. a dry, one-seeded fruit consisting of a kernel, often edible, in a woody shell. A very concentrated source of many nutrients including the B vitamins, phosphorus, calcium and magnesium."
- Week #2—A small packet of metal nuts (as in nuts and bolts) with the following card attached:
  "Nut (nut) n. 2. a small, usually metal block with a center threaded hole for screwing onto a bolt. Totally lacking in nutritional value, but suggesting that the services of health providers have a supportive relationship."
- Week #3—A gag nut can with spring loaded snakes attached to the following card:
  "Nut (nut) n. 3. a foolish, crazy, or eccentric person, seldom (and especially not in this case) due to poor nutritional habits."
- Week #4—A package containing a tin of nuts, a brochure, sample materials and a letter of introduction with the following business card attached:
  "Nut (nut) n. 4. the abbreviation for nutrition counselor, one who facilitates the change of eating behaviors in clientele who wish to reduce the risk of chronic illness while enjoying the nutritional, cultural and social pleasures which food provides." (The name, address, and phone number of the practice was printed on the reverse side.)

All physicians received a follow-up letter thanking them for their participation in this "nutty" promotion and reminding them of the services the practice offered.

Overcoming Physician Objections

There are several crucial barriers that you must overcome with physicians:

- The resistance to referring patients to a practice that they perceive overcharges. Many physicians have reacted unfavorably to fees that are perceived to be similar to or the same as their own.
- The feeling that their patients cannot afford the services. They want the services offered free.
- Past impressions of clinical dietitians.
- Lack of recognition that behavior change must be nurtured and demands a reformation of current methods of providing services.
- Lack of recognition of the counselor with a nutrition degree as the nutrition expert.

The first barrier can only be overcome if you can speak directly with the physician. You must get the physician to compare apples with apples. Granted, the charge for a general examination by a physician is $50 to $100 and you want to charge $60 for an initial session. But you are offering the client an hour of counseling time plus printed materials at no extra charge, and the physician may spend only 5 to 10 minutes with each patient. State your case clearly, and offer information on reimbursement if you have access to it.

Hopef... nformation on reimbursement and the value perception you ... ıp overcome the second barrier. Show a genuine concern for ... patients are paying for healthcare, and sell your program as a ... for further healthcare costs. After all, if the client with heart ... motivated to comply with the dietary recommendations, the chances ... attack will decrease.

... third barrier is one that you will overcome by presenting the practice and programs as something totally removed from inpatient services. If the physician has a good relationship with the inpatient dietitian, capitalize on that image. If not, present yourself and your staff as positive, professional, and flexible. Your greatest promoters in dissolving such barriers are your mutual clients.

Selling new methods you are employing in nutrition counseling is the solution to the fourth barrier. Back your words with sound research. Show the compliance rates for traditional programs, along with expert opinion on nutrition counseling as an ongoing process. This is a barrier that is much easier to overcome once you are established and can show results. In the beginning, one good physician advocate can dissolve this barrier more successfully than you can.

The biggest campaign you will undertake is that of educating the physician about who your professional staff really is and why your services are substantially more beneficial to his or her patients than printed materials, self-teaching programs, or other support staff providing nutrition education. Physicians seldom know what a dietitian's training or background is. More importantly, they don't know what services you provide or how you provide them. Keep in mind that printed materials, self-teaching programs, and other support staff providing information all target nutrition education. If your services include counseling, there is no competition. Point this out. Use your four years plus of education, your registration, your licensure, your experience, and current statistics on compliance to convince them. And most importantly, allow your professional image to speak for you.

Soliciting the Support of Dentists

Dentists may seem to fall into the same category as physicians in terms of selling nutrition services. However, experience shows that most dentists have a keen interest in nutrition and are often more willing and able to learn about your services. Therefore, emphasis should be placed on the benefits of your services to the dental practice as well as to dental patients. Prevention is of utmost importance to dentists and can be used as a major selling point. They will also be interested in how your practice can help clients cope with chewing problems. Again, price, reimbursability, compliance, and patient satisfaction will be key issues. Soliciting to dentists can be done in the same manner as it is to physicians.

Soliciting the Support of Other Healthcare Professionals

Nutrition counselors can benefit from strong relationships with other healthcare professionals. High on this list are nurses, physical therapists, exercise physiologists, psychologists, and social workers. Often, these professionals learn of a patient's nutritional needs in the course of their caregiving, opening the door for referrals. They may also have stronger relationships with physicians and can, therefore, provide an indirect system of referral.

Frustration among nutrition professionals often arises when other health professionals "practice" nutrition. Rather than dealing with these people as competition, challenge yourself to form alliances with them. They are often unaware of the complexity of the nutrition field and the skills required to effectively change eating behaviors. Much of your promotion to this group will take the form of education on who nutrition professionals are, what the practice can offer, and how nutrition benefits your clients.

You might promote your services through:

- Professional meetings;
- Inservices;
- Department meetings;
- In-house/professional newsletters;
- Paycheck stuffers;
- Bulletin boards;
- Open houses;
- Services offered to employees as a benefit or at a discount;
- Incentives for referring clients;
- Advertisements and promotions in institution's cafeteria;
- Displays in lobby and employee lounges;
- Ads or coupons on cafeteria cash register tape;
- Buttons or magnets;
- Testimonials from staff members;
- Games and competitions; and
- Cooking demonstrations.

Networking and liaisoning are important techniques for forming alliances with healthcare professionals. Networking, as you will recall from the previous discussion, is a process of communicating and sharing information with others. As a liaison, you become a link between two people or organizations, speaking out on behalf of one organization, while strengthening support for your own organization and your profession. Acting as a board or committee member is a good way to build alliances with other healthcare professionals and, in the process, heighten the power base of the organizations involved.

An example of liaisoning is the instructor who developed a nutrition counseling program with the local dentistry association. Dentists referred patients who needed nutrition counseling, and dietetic students provided the counseling at a modest cost in a clinic setting. Thus, the students gained exposure to counseling experience, and dentists became big supporters of nutrition services and the university's dietetic program. The instructor had provided a needed link between two organizations and expanded her own network greatly in the process.

Chapter 8

Worksite Nutrition Programs—Planning and Promoting

LEARNING ABOUT WORKSITES

In order to promote worksite nutrition services, it is important to have a fundamental understanding of the opportunities presented by this market. Healthcare costs have been among the most affected by rising costs in our inflationary environment. Some national leaders believe that the nation's competitive position is threatened by health costs, which have risen to 11 percent of the United States gross national product (Wall Street Journal, 1989). What can be done about escalating healthcare costs? Most would agree that prevention is better than the cure. Yet only a small percent of healthcare dollars are dedicated to prevention of illness. Rather, Americans spend their healthcare dollars treating illness.

Who stands to gain the most by taking a proactive stand to prevent illness? The answer is employers. They are in the most assailable position. They pay over half of these rapidly inflating healthcare bills through insurance programs, workers compensation, disability coverage, sick leave, and tax-supported state and federal health programs.

In addition to the dollars directly allocated to healthcare costs, employers suffer the burden of indirect costs, such as the cost of absenteeism, replacement, retraining, reduction in productivity, and low morale. The psychological price of interrupted services, coworker and family grief, and decreased morale must be paid as well.

With such a lucrative payoff, why aren't more employers launching health promotion programs? Two reasons are commonly expressed:

1. Business people want to be able to measure the results of their investments. Cost/benefit data is difficult to obtain, primarily because it requires many years of tracking to be certain of the results and all the factors that impact the results cannot be controlled. "Nonetheless, some companies have estimated the savings of health promotion programs as high as 2.7 million [dollars] annually." (Berry, 1981)
2. Healthcare bills are so high that most companies are not willing to spend any additional money on prevention.

Fortunately, money doesn't have to be an obstacle. Programs can be offered for payment in the following ways:

- 100 percent paid by employer/organization;
- 100 percent paid by employee/member; or
- Employer/organization and employee/member share a percentage of cost.

Some employers pay nothing by offering their endorsement and the convenience of a location. Others pay nothing, but absorb the cost of offering programs on company time. Many financial arrangements can be made to suit the needs of individual employers or organizations and their employees or members.

Not only do employers have the most incentive to offer health promotion programs, but the worksite offers a unique opportunity to increase participation and compliance. "The degree of voluntary participation at the worksite has run 90-95% in several surveys, while it averages only 30% for similar community programs offered free." (Berry, 1981)

Let's look at the primary benefits of worksite nutrition programs.

Potential Benefits to Employees/Members The potential benefits to employees/members are:

- Reduced illness/health risk factors;
- Feeling better physically and psychologically;
- Convenience of nutrition management programs in the workplace;
- Potential to harness social support and social influence from coworkers and management for behavior change;
- Opportunities for follow-up monitoring and reinforcement; and
- The availability of a daily eating situation that offers healthy selections.

Potential Benefits to Companies/Organizations The potential benefits to companies/organizations are:

- Reduced absenteeism;
- Reduced injury;
- Reduced healthcare expenditures;
- Reduced disability payments;

- Reduced cost of retraining;
- Higher productivity;
- Improved employee morale;
- Better employee relations; and
- Ability to attract employees.

Potential Benefits to the Worksite Nutrition Practice The potential benefits to the worksite nutrition practice are:

- Opportunity to reach a large segment of the population quickly;
- Broadens the base of referrals for all areas of the practice;
- Can be more lucrative; and
- Opportunity to be a more effective supporter and facilitator of change if you harness the social support and influence from among coworkers and management and take advantage of the opportunities for follow-up monitoring and reinforcement.

In 1983, in her article, "The Consulting Nutritionist in an Employee Health Office," Miriam C. Seidel, R.D., wrote: "The time is ripe for nutritionists to market their expertise in the corporate setting." (Seidel, 1983) The authors believe that this is still true. Why has so little progress been made? Has resistance from business and industry been the primary obstacle?

The truth is that very little has been done by nutrition practitioners to market services to worksites. Employers and other organizations rarely know what service options are available to them. In fact, employers have made the initial contact in the majority of the worksite nutrition service contracts performed to date. Only in recent years have healthcare institutions begun to consider wellness programs a viable business opportunity. Only in the last few decades has nutrition care received the respect it deserves. Gaining the respect of potential users can be a slow process. Perhaps a good analogy is prenatal care.

> At one time, women carried children for nine months with no medical contact whatsoever. Many women died in childbirth, miscarried, or gave birth to premature and defective babies. This was generally accepted as a fact of life. Medical researchers proved that women and children could be saved through prenatal care. At first, only the affluent could afford the care and many felt it was an unnecessary luxury. Now prenatal care is offered to all pregnant women, with few exceptions. Through education, pregnant women became dependent on prenatal care.

Similarly, with the aid of research, nutrition practitioners are and will continue to lead a movement to standardize professional nutrition care at the worksite. Obviously, this will take time to evolve. Recognizing that permeating this market requires advanced skills in marketing, selling, business planning, and relationship management can be very intimidating to nutrition practitioners. The challenge to pioneer virgin territory lies ahead.

The information in this section is based on the limited experiences of other worksite pioneers and available information on selling healthcare services. It is offered to assist you in building nutrition practices in the worksite setting. Keep in mind that the information presented in all chapters of this book applies to worksite practices as well. Although the types of nutrition services offered in the worksite are similar to those offered in institutional outpatient nutrition practices, the methods of acquiring and maintaining business differ to some degree. In this section, only the issues unique to worksites are discussed.

Determining Potential Worksite Services

The most important thing to remember is that the prospective worksite clients you are approaching expect you to respond to their needs and to address their business concerns. Never lose sight of the fact that the nutrition concerns you address are a means to an end. The end is addressing business concerns. What nutrition services should be considered? That decision must be your own, but the choices are numerous. Joseph, et al. (Joseph 1986) state:

> Education programs that focus principally on fundamental scientific concepts in nutrition will not easily succeed in the corporate classroom...Companies are seeking programs that can produce healthier lifestyles among participants, that are compatible with other programs such as physical fitness and Employee Assistance Programs (EAPs), and that are good for both employee and public relations.

The most common services currently provided to worksites are:

- Weight control programs:
  - Classes;
  - Competitions; and
  - Self-help programs.
- Cafeteria and point of purchase programs:
  - Modified menu choices;
  - Informational handouts;
  - Labeling foods with nutrient content;
  - Providing healthy foods in the vending machines; and
  - Games and promotions.
- Seminars and workshops on various nutrition topics:
  - Cholesterol reduction;
  - Nutrition and hypertension; and
  - U.S. dietary guidelines.

- Nutrition analysis and screening.
- Individual counseling/executive in-office counseling.

Note that very few counseling services are presently offered at the worksite. Most services are educational in nature. Some options for providing nutrition counseling services include support groups and group counseling programs that deal with chronic medical conditions (heart disease, hypertension, diabetes, weight management, family nutrition, etc.).

Refining Your Targets

Worksite is in itself a target market. Yet it is prudent for you to consider the best use of your time and your money. You want to focus your selling activities on the worksites that will have the greatest interest in your services.

What kinds of organizations are most likely to buy nutrition services for their employees? The findings of a recent study of the frequency of worksite health promotion activities was reported by Jonathan E. Fielding, M.D., M.P.H. and Philip V. Piserchia, M.S. In their article *Frequency of Worksite Health Promotion Activities,* they reported:

> The first National Survey of Worksite Health Promotion Activities surveyed a random sample of all private sector worksites with 50 or more employees, stratified by number of employers, geographic location, and type of industry. The 1,358 completed interviews constituted a response rate of 83.1 percent. Of responding worksites 65.5 percent had one or more areas of health promotion activity with slightly more than 50 percent of activities initiated within the previous five years. Overall prevalence by type of activity included health risk assessment (29.5 percent), smoking cessation (35.6 percent), blood pressure control and treatment (16.5 percent), exercise/fitness (22.1 percent), weight control (14.7 percent), nutrition education (16.8 percent), stress management (26.6 percent), back problem prevention and care (28.5 percent), and off-the-job accident prevention (19.8 percent). Mean number of activities across all worksites was 2.1 and for worksites with activities, 3.2. Activity frequency increased with worksite size, was highest in the western region (2.34) and lowest in the northeast (1.96), and varied considerably by industry type. The majority of worksites paid the entire cost of these activities. (Fielding and Piserchia, 1989)

Table 8-1 provides additional details. It has been adjusted with permission from the American Journal of Public Health to show only those variables that relate directly to worksite nutrition programs.

Fielding and Piserchia drew the following conclusions from this information:

> Compared to results of statewide surveys performed during the five years prior to this survey, this national survey suggests large prevalence increases in overall health

TABLE 8-1 Frequency of Health Promotion Activities by Stratifying Variables

[PREVALENCE IN PERCENT AND STANDARD ERROR (SE)]

Variables	% total worksite	Any activity	Health risk assessment	Blood pressure control	Weight control	Nutrition education
Worksite	50.2	55.2	18.5	8.8	8.6	9.3
<100 employees		(2.8)	(2.0)	(1.7)	(1.7)	(1.7)
100–249	30.5	71.0	34.6	19.0	14.2	20.4
		(2.8)	(2.4)	(1.8)	(1.9)	(2.3)
250–749	12.9	80.4	41.1	24.0	22.5	21.9
		(2.7)	(2.9)	(2.7)	(2.5)	(3.0)
750+	6.6	87.6	66.1	48.8	47.9	47.7
		(3.9)	(5.4)	(5.8)	(5.8)	(4.9)
Region						
Northeast	23.6	62.9	26.8	15.6	11.0	16.3
		(3.8)	(3.0)	(2.6)	(1.7)	(2.9)
North central	25.4	67.0	33.5	17.1	16.4	19.2
		(2.6)	(2.8)	(2.1)	(2.4)	(2.8)
South	32.6	61.8	25.7	16.4	14.1	16.1
		(3.3)	(2.0)	(1.6)	(1.7)	(1.9)
West	18.4	73.4	33.9	17.0	17.9	15.3
		(4.0)	(3.9)	(2.5)	(3.9)	(2.8)
Industry type						
Manufacturing	29.4	65.1	30.1	18.2	11.0	10.9
		(3.2)	(2.9)	(2.0)	(1.7)	(1.7)
Wholesale/retail	15.7	60.0	14.4	14.3	11.5	15.9
		(4.6)	(2.9)	(3.1)	(3.4)	(3.1)
Utilities/	3.6	77.9	42.6	17.5	13.7	17.0
transportation/		(6.3)	(9.6)	(6.0)	(7.2)	(6.6)
communications						
Financial/real	6.2	60.1	31.4	13.5	20.3	19.7
estate/insurance		(6.7)	(5.9)	(4.0)	(4.5)	(6.1)
Service	37.5	70.7	35.3	17.9	20.1	23.6
		(2.4)	(2.3)	(1.7)	(2.2)	(2.4)
Other (includes	7.5	51.3	21.5	9.1	4.5	5.1
construction, fishing,		(6.1)	(4.1)	(2.6)	(1.6)	(1.6)
& mining						
All worksites		65.5	29.5	16.5	14.7	16.8
		(1.7)	(1.7)	(1.1)	(1.2)	(1.3)

promotion activity, smoking cessation, nutrition education, and stress management; smaller increases were found in exercise/fitness; and no increase noted in weight control. Although methodological differences between surveys and lack of information on the life cycle of health promotion activities make any statements of trends tentative, the fact that greater than 50 percent of the activities were in place for fewer than five years lends support to growing prevalence of these activities.

Employees at the 750+ worksites are at least twice as likely to have each type of activity as employees in <100 worksites, with prevalence ratios of about 5:1 for blood pressure control and treatment, weight control and nutrition education; 4:1 for stress management; and 3:1 for health risk assessment, exercise/fitness and off-the-job accident prevention. The increased likelihood of large worksites having one or more activities may be due to increased likelihood of dedicated personnel, benefits and health staff.

No consistent rank order of prevalence exits among industry types although worksite size may be a confounding variable.

ARA's research on this topic revealed that:

- Public service organizations and organizations where fitness was critical to the job performance of employees (police, fire fighters, athletic club personnel) were more likely to contract for nutrition services.
- Size may also impact which services are offered and for what period of time. If you are looking for service contracts that will be offered on an ongoing basis for an extended period of time, larger organizations may be a more formidable target.
- Organizations with self-insured medical benefit plans could receive direct dollar savings from wellness programs. Consequently, wellness programs are very appealing to them.
- Management is a popular target for your efforts because business people often believe that the greater the salary of the employee, the greater return on their investment in health.

A study by Forke and Hunt (Forke and Hunt, 1986) that ignored size of organization suggests that an organization is more likely to offer nutrition services if management's concern for employee welfare is high. Companies who provided "in-house" assistance to employees experiencing personal problems and who provided several (greater than two) other health programs (fitness centers, health education, etc.) were more likely to provide nutrition programs. In this study, cost and other resources were the most common reasons that companies did not have worksite nutrition programs.

In order to identify these target organizations, certain sources of information may help:

- The Dun and Bradstreet Listing is a fairly good reference for determining size.
- Most chambers of commerce provide information on:

  - Demographics by county and city;
  - Community health organizations;
  - Competition;
  - Market forces;
  - Type of businesses/organizations;
  - Number of employees in these organizations; and
  - Contact people in these organizations (usually at least three key officers).
- You might network with local health clubs, insurance companies, physicians, and occupational health organization, to identify organizations with a high concern for employee welfare or fitness centers.

Market research may be helpful in determining which worksites to target. Market research might be done through focus groups, telephone interviews, or questionnaires. Only through a careful analysis of your worksite market and its needs can you finalize your service package. Your final service package will depend greatly on what your target market needs and wants and what you can afford to offer.

A sample proposal for a worksite nutrition survey follows (see Fig. 8-1), along with the actual survey (see Fig. 8-2).

The most crucial point in administering your surveys is to contact the appropriate people. Contacting the CEO, human resources director, or industrial nurse will provide you with the greatest amount of information. However, if other health programs are currently in place, the director of such services may have more knowledge of the organization's health goals and the nutritional needs of employees. Therefore, they may be more influential in selling your services to administration.

In some smaller towns and cities, every major industry may be contacted with ease. In fact, determining which CEOs would most likely be interested in nutrition programs could be aided by networking and by consulting with your institution's administrators. Most healthcare institutions have board members who are CEOs of local businesses. Their board memberships demonstrate their interest in health, and they may be able to direct you to other organizations with such interests.

PROMOTING TO WORKSITES

It would be nice to believe that there is such demand for your services that people will be lining up outside your office. The likely reality is that you will need to demonstrate the initiative to contact prospective clients and use effective selling techniques to develop business. Your efforts to gain individual clients and support from physicians will most likely be a process of promotion. Dealing with worksite organizations requires a sales process. The best results are obtained in marketing-oriented practices that actively sell and support new business continuously.

PROPOSAL FOR WORKSITE NUTRITION SERVICES SURVEY

Background

Cyville Nutrition Center is in the process of establishing nutrition programs that could be offered as part of a worksite benefit package. In developing such programs, the practitioners must understand the nutrition interest of key decision makers of organizations whose business they will solicit. This study will focus on the kinds of nutrition programs and features thereof that various organizations would purchase as employee benefits.

Objectives

The principal objectives of this study are:

1. To determine which nutrition services are of interest to employers.
2. To determine what benefits employers recognize in offering nutrition services.
3. To determine certain basic characteristics of organizations that would purchase nutrition programs for their employees.

Methodology

An announcement of the study accompanied by the questionnaire will be sent to key decision makers in 500 organizations within the community. The recommended source list will be the Dun and Bradstreet Listing and The Chamber of Commerce.

The completed questionnaires will be returned in pre-posted envelopes to Cyville Nutrition Center. Completed questionnaires will be turned over to marketing professionals for editing, coding, tabulation, and analysis.

Upon completion of the study, marketing professionals will produce a written report of findings, conclusions, and recommendations.

Expected Findings of the Survey

This survey will offer information on the level of interest of various organizations in:

- Purchasing nutrition services;
- Using nutrition services to address specific needs; and
- Various features of the services.

In addition, the survey will determine the characteristics of the organizations as a whole and then by the following characteristics:

- Type of organization;
- Number of employees; and
- Current use of health services.

Responsibilities

Marketing consultants have developed a draft of a questionnaire as part of this proposal.

FIGURE 8-1. Sample proposal for survey of worksite nutritional services market.

Cyville Nutrition Center will edit these drafts and make any suggested changes by (date).

Cyville Nutrition Center will print and mail the surveys to the 500 organizations.

Once the surveys are returned to the Cyville Nutrition Center, they will be forwarded to marketing consultants. Questionnaires will be edited, coded, and tabulated upon receipt by them.

If all of the above dates are met, our marketing consultants will be able to issue a report on the results of this study by (date).

FIGURE 8-1. *(Continued)*

NUTRITION SERVICES MARKET SURVEY FOR WORKSITE DECISION MAKERS

Cyville Nutrition Center is in the process of developing nutrition programs that will address many critical business concerns. The following questionnaire has been designed to determine which nutrition programs worksites are interested in offering as part of their employee benefits programs.

Please answer each question honestly, and feel free to make any comments that might help us understand how Cyville Nutrition Center's nutrition programs can best meet your needs. When you finish, return your questionnaire in the pre-posted envelope to Cyville Nutrition Center.

This survey is completely anonymous. You will not be asked for your name or any identification that will associate you or your organization with your responses.

1. How interested are you in using nutrition services programs to:

	Very Interested	Somewhat Interested	Not too Interested	Not at all Interested
A. Reduce absenteeism?	[ ]	[ ]	[ ]	[ ]
B. Reduce injury?	[ ]	[ ]	[ ]	[ ]
C. Reduce healthcare expenditures?	[ ]	[ ]	[ ]	[ ]
D. Reduce disability payments?	[ ]	[ ]	[ ]	[ ]
E. Improve employee relations and employee morale?	[ ]	[ ]	[ ]	[ ]
F. Reduce cost of turnover?	[ ]	[ ]	[ ]	[ ]

FIGURE 8-2. Sample questionnaire for surveying the desire of decision makers for nutritional services in the worksite.

G. Reduce the cost of retraining?	[ ]	[ ]	[ ]	[ ]
H. Increase productivity?	[ ]	[ ]	[ ]	[ ]
I. Improve your ability to attract employees?	[ ]	[ ]	[ ]	[ ]

J. Other/specify____

____

2. Below are a list of nutrition services. Please indicate your level of interest in the following services at your worksite by checking the appropriate box. Assume that in all cases your organization would decide who participates, the schedule, whether services are offered on or off company time, and who will pay for the services (employee/member, organization, or shared).

	Very Interested	Somewhat Interested	Not too Interested	Not at all Interested
A. Computerized Nutrition Analysis —1 to 7 days of diet regimen are analyzed by computer. Two sessions (1 hour and 1/2 hour) would be scheduled to gather data, interpret information, and recommend dietary changes.	[ ]	[ ]	[ ]	[ ]
B. Individualized Nutrition Counseling— A series of four counseling sessions are offered with the same counselor at the worksite, by appointment, each week for four weeks on a designated weekday. A personalized nutrition analysis is conducted. Dietary changes would be recommended, taking lifestyle and nutrition problems into account. Counsel to help employees make changes	[ ]	[ ]	[ ]	[ ]

FIGURE 8-2. *(Continued)*

	Very Interested	Somewhat Interested	Not too Interested	Not at all Interested
in eating habits is included.				
C. Nutrition Education Workshops—Participants would choose from a series of topics which workshops they would attend. Workshops are from ½ hour to 1 hour in length. Group sizes range from 7-35 members.	[ ]	[ ]	[ ]	[ ]
D. Group Nutrition Counseling—The opportunity is offered for co-workers with common nutrition concerns to join together in groups of 6-12 members to work on incorporating new eating habits into individual lifestyles. The group is guided by a nutrition counselor. One individual session of 1: hour is a prerequisite for this series of six to eight sessions, approximately 1-week apart.	[ ]	[ ]	[ ]	[ ]
E. Nutrition Fair—This is an inspiring 1-day series of displays, demonstrations, and activities designed to increase nutrition awareness.	[ ]	[ ]	[ ]	[ ]
F. Nutrition Displays and Handout Materials—These	[ ]	[ ]	[ ]	[ ]

FIGURE 8-2. *(Continued)*

health promotions encourage healthier eating choices and can be made available in high-traffic areas, breakrooms, or the cafeteria.				
G. Consulting Services for the Cafeteria—Services are offered to provide healthier food choices in the cafeteria and vending machines. Foods may be labeled with nutrient content.	[ ]	[ ]	[ ]	[ ]

3. If you are interested in workshops, how interested are you in the following nutrition topics?

A. Heart-healthy eating/ cholesterol reduction	[ ]	[ ]	[ ]	[ ]
B. Weight management	[ ]	[ ]	[ ]	[ ]
C. Nutrition and cancer	[ ]	[ ]	[ ]	[ ]
D. Food safety (pesticides and radiation)	[ ]	[ ]	[ ]	[ ]
E. Low-sodium diets	[ ]	[ ]	[ ]	[ ]
F. Low-calorie cooking	[ ]	[ ]	[ ]	[ ]
G. Nutrition quackery	[ ]	[ ]	[ ]	[ ]
H. Nutritionally healthy children	[ ]	[ ]	[ ]	[ ]
I. Healthy eating on-the-go	[ ]	[ ]	[ ]	[ ]
J. Nutrition and allergies	[ ]	[ ]	[ ]	[ ]
K. Nutrition and PMS/ osteoporosis	[ ]	[ ]	[ ]	[ ]
L. Fiber and the digestive system	[ ]	[ ]	[ ]	[ ]
M. Nutrition and stress management	[ ]	[ ]	[ ]	[ ]

What other topics are you interested in?

____

____

4. How important are each of the following factors in selecting a nutrition service program?

FIGURE 8-2. *(Continued)*

	Very Important	Somewhat Important	Not too Important	Not at all Important
A. Your relationship with the provider	[ ]	[ ]	[ ]	[ ]
B. Services provided on location	[ ]	[ ]	[ ]	[ ]
C. Employee interest	[ ]	[ ]	[ ]	[ ]
D. Flexibility of scheduling	[ ]	[ ]	[ ]	[ ]
E. Credentials of a registered dietitian	[ ]	[ ]	[ ]	[ ]
F. Family participation	[ ]	[ ]	[ ]	[ ]
G. Other/specify	[ ]	[ ]	[ ]	[ ]

____

5. If you are interested in providing workshops, seminars, or individual and group counseling, are adequate facilities available?

   ☐ Yes ☐ No

6. Are dining facilities provided at the worksite?

   ☐ Yes ☐ No

7. Which of the following arrangements for payment would you consider? Check as many as apply.

   ☐ Employee/member pays all
   ☐ Organization pays all
   ☐ Organization and employee/member each pay a percent of cost

Comments ____

____

8. What is the approximate number of employees at your location(s)?

   ☐ Below 1000 ☐ 3000-3999
   ☐ 1000-1999 ☐ 4000-4999
   ☐ 2000-2999 ☐ 5000 and over

9. What is the approximate number of employees you would consider for participation in nutrition service programs?

   ☐ Below 100 ☐ 600-1000
   ☐ 100-299 ☐ Over 1000
   ☐ 300-599

10. What health or wellness programs are currently offered at your worksite? Check as many as apply.

   ☐ Physical fitness ☐ Smoking cessation

FIGURE 8-2. *(Continued)*

- ☐ Stress management
- ☐ Substance abuse
- ☐ First aid
- ☐ Weight control
- ☐ Hypertension control
- ☐ CPR
- ☐ Nutrition
- ☐ None
- ☐ Other (please indicate) ______________________

11. Type of organization?
- ☐ Services
- ☐ Retail/sales
- ☐ Manufacturing
- ☐ Construction
- ☐ Wholesale
- ☐ Transportation
- ☐ Communications
- ☐ Public relations
- ☐ Public administration
- ☐ Public service
- ☐ Community
- ☐ Healthcare
- ☐ Other (please indicate) ______________________

12. Comments: ____

____

____

____

____

FIGURE 8-2. *(Continued)*

The Sales Approach

The first decision to be made regarding the sales process is who will do the selling? This may be the most critical question in the process. Since the expectations of corporations and companies are high, they demand sophistication of both programs and selling skills. Be sure the person or persons chosen are both skilled and properly prepared for the assignment. Often, the marketing department will take on this role.

It may be appropriate for several representatives from your practice to be involved in the sales process. If so, designate a contact person through whom all communication will flow. Also, be sure that all representatives are skilled and properly prepared for the assignment. It is often helpful to include the person who will deliver the services if a contract is signed. If trust, credibility, and rapport are established with the nutritionist during the sales process, the final decision is often favorably influenced. Also, if the nutritionist is involved in the process, he or she will have a first-hand knowledge of the decision makers, their expectations and concerns, how services were developed to address needs, and the contractual obligations. This is an important advantage as you approach service delivery. Be sensitive to overpowering your audience with too many representatives from your practice.

Who Is Your Competition?

Remember, you are often not competing against other nutrition programs for worksite health dollars. More likely, the competition is other health promotion programs and benefits. Three studies that examined the frequency of various health promotion programs in the worksite setting showed that nutrition ranked sixth or seventh behind CPR, first aid, drug and alcohol abuse, hypertension, physical fitness, stress management, and smoking cessation (Glanz, 1986). Therefore, you will most likely be forced to present the relationship of nutrition to other aspects of wellness in your sales presentation (Joseph, 1986). Your competitors may include fitness centers, health clubs, physical therapists, exercise physiologists, physicians, and chiropractors.

If you are competing against another contractor—possibly other institutional practitioners, private practitioners, or commercial nutrition businesses—you need to know early in the process. What you know about your competitors may alter your selling strategy.

How Do You Compete?

The rules for competing are as basic to this business as they are to any other business:

- If at all possible, *be the first* to get to the market.
- Distinguish your products and services by offering something unique that addresses a recognized need.
- Know your competitive advantages and disadvantages, and educate prospective clients, where appropriate.
- Take advantage of the reputation of your practice and your institutional affiliations.
- Get distinguished physicians or other business executives to recommend your services.
- Meet the organization's/user's needs.
- If you are a registered dietitian, emphasize the value.
- Create trust, credibility, and strong relational ties with key decision makers.
- Network with those who influence key decision makers (e.g., chamber of commerce).

- Launch an aggressive marketing campaign.

Being affiliated with an institution with a strong reputation is an advantage. ARA's focus groups with prospective clients from business and industry indicated that the *name* of a reputable community institution was highly influential.

Critical Elements of the Sales Process

Before we review each step in the sales process, let's focus on some issues that will affect all phases of the sales process. Consider this:

- Consistently emphasize the benefits of worksite nutrition programs. Remember, you are marketing to two groups: the organization and the employees. Therefore, you must focus on the value of your services to each group. A list of potential benefits to companies/organizations and employees/members appears in Chapter 7.

  Once you know what your clients perceive as benefits, emphasize these "hot buttons" throughout the sales process. For instance, during an interview with the CEO of a particular company, a nutrition counselor learned that the CEO had recently had bypass surgery and was following a low-fat diet. She asked him questions about his recovery and the impact his medical condition had on his work and the organization. She used heart disease prevention as her example throughout her presentation and addressed the CEO's need for help to adjust his eating patterns in the workplace. She also offered him a free nutrition analysis and consultation to further his interest. By using his situation as an example, she was able to establish the value to the organization of preventing heart disease and other medical conditions. Her nutrition programs are now an integral part of health promotion in that company.
- Be aware of the psychological aspects of selling and use them to your advantage. Keep in mind that decisions are based on both rational and emotional motivators. Rational motives reflect a desire to sound reasonable and rational. Generally, people want to appear as though their decisions are based on logic and reason. Rational motivators are usually meaningful only to the extent that they represent underlying, emotional issues. Rationalizations are often used to justify behavior, not explain it. Rationalizations disguise the true feelings of the individual.

  The emotional issues are those that ultimately motivate behavior. Emotional issues are those issues that surround how a person feels. Emerging from each issue are two related aspects. The first is the issue as it relates to the organization, and the second is the issue as it relates to the individual personally—their day-to-day worklife, career, reputation, and so on.

  The more secure an individual tends to be, the more rational their decision making is. This means that you must:

  - Tune into the verbal and nonverbal messages your prospective clients send. The importance of listening with both your eyes and ears cannot be overemphasized.
  - Show interest in and sensitivity to their feelings. By doing so, you may discourage the need for rationalizations that will disguise the feelings motivating the decisions.
  - Probe for understanding and verification. Assume nothing.
  - Tailor your presentation and the service and product offerings to clients' specific needs.
  - Most importantly, build trust, credibility, and rapport. How your prospective clients feel about you and other members of your sales team will help determine success or failure.
  - While it's true that prospective clients will listen carefully to your message, their interpretation may not be as you would expect. Prospective clients will scan your messages with these questions in mind:
    - "Are these people I want to work with?"
    - "Am I comfortable working with them?"
    - "Do these people have integrity?"
    - "Can I trust them?"
    - "Have they demonstrated a commitment to understand and address our needs?"
    - "Would they fit in with our organization? Will our employees/members accept them?"
    - "Will their presence enhance or diminish my image?"
  - Having a saleable package of products and services won't mean much if your prospective clients do not feel trust, credibility, and rapport with you and other members of your sales team.
- Too often, the strength of past and ongoing successes is overlooked. It is important to build on your successes to sell future business. Be sure to use such accomplishments (results) during your presentation.
- Get an autopsy. If the prospective client decides to terminate the sales process at any time, follow up on the rejection with either a telephone call or a brief meeting. Understanding what influenced your prospective clients' decisions will aid you in improving your sales technique, tailoring services to their needs, and increasing your sensitivity to worksite problems. The tough part here is listening to criticism without being defensive. Encourage prospective clients to "tell it like it is."

Keep these points in mind as you progress through all stages of the sales process.

Stages in the Sales Process

The sales process usually entails six basic stages:

1. Generating leads;
2. Getting a foot in the door;
3. Information gathering;
4. Information giving;
5. Determining and resolving basic issues and objections; and
6. Commitment.

While the order of these stages is important, there will be considerable overlap within the stages. These stages are also not intended to reflect the number of contacts you will have with prospective client organizations. That will vary from organization to organization. Certain factors will influence the time you need to invest in the selling process. Among them are:

- The prospective client's knowledge of your services;
- The prospective client's interest in your services when the selling process begins;
- The degree of influence your liaison has in the organization;
- Politics;
- Number of people involved in the decision-making process; and
- The organization's decision-making process.

Prospective clients enter the sales process at different stages. Some already have an interest in your services, and they may telephone you to request a presentation of services. Others may not perceive the value of your services; therefore, you will have to seek out certain prospective clients and educate them about the benefits.

Current worksite providers have indicated that the average number of contacts with prospective clients before a contract is signed is seven.

Note also that the sales closure rate on similar types of healthcare services is only 1 in every 20 prospective clients contacted. In other words, only 5 percent of all the organizations you approach are likely to accept your proposal for nutrition services. Many practitioners now realize that they quit too soon in their efforts to sell nutrition to worksites.

Generating Leads

The first stage of the sales process is generating leads. By identifying prospective clients with the greatest potential to buy, you narrow your potential market. Most leads are generated through networking. The following sources of information may help you generate leads:

- Local newspapers;
- Local health clubs;
- Health education organizations;
- Insurance companies (some discount insurance rates to organizations with wellness programs);
- Physicians' offices;
- Occupational health organizations (e.g., Council on Alcoholism);
- Professional organizations for human resources (e.g., American Society for Personnel Administrators—national and local chapters);
- Board members and major contributors to healthcare institutions;
- Publications received by CEOs, Human Resource Managers, and Industrial Nurses; and
- Executive management clubs and associations (Rotary Club, young president organizations, country clubs, etc.).

Getting Your Foot in the Door

Aim your initial contact at acquiring a personal meeting with key decision makers in the organization. Although you may be referred to someone in a lower position in the company's hierarchy, try to make your first contacts with key decision makers. If decision makers refer you to another contact person, use that reference when dealing with your sales audience. Also, offer to send copies of your documents to decision makers who are not present at your presentation.

A face-to-face discussion is considered the most successful sales approach. However, since business people will seldom make themselves available for a meeting without an appointment, the initial contact will probably be indirect. Methods such as general or targeted telephone and mailing campaigns are possibilities. You may choose to invite a group of human resources directors to participate in a focus group, where you can assess their needs while stimulating their interest. Figure 8-3 provides a sample letter of introduction.

You might follow up on your letter of introduction with a phone call such as this:

Jane: Hello Ms. Anyname. My name is Jane Doe. I'm a registered dietitian representing Abbott Nutrition Center. We are now offering nutrition programs at worksites. Our programs are designed to address many of the human resources management challenges presented by the changing workforce.

I sent you correspondence and two brochures last week, outlining our worksite programs. Have you had a chance to look them over?

Mary: No, not really. I remember opening the materials, but I haven't had much time to review them.

ABBOTT NUTRITION CENTER
111 N. FIRST STREET
MONMOUTH, IL 61462
Phone: (999) 123-4567

Date

Mary Anyname
Human Resources Director
XYZ Corporation
XYZ Plaza
XYZ, IL 61463

Dear Mary:

Do you intend to reduce healthcare expenditures, absenteeism, and the costs of sick leave, injury, disability, replacement, and retraining? Do you aim to increase productivity and compete for the best employees in your market, while improving employee morale?

Many companies are improving these key result areas by offering nutrition services at their worksites. Abbott Nutrition Center offers a variety of programs to fit the specific needs of your organization and employees. Such programs include computerized nutrition analyses, weight management programs, nutrition workshops, and group and individual counseling. Our nutrition counselors are registered dietitians who have made nutrition for active, working people their specialty.

Abbott Nutrition Center has been serving individuals with nutritional concerns for the past two years. We are now excited to be offering our services to worksites throughout Warren and Knox counties.

I am anxious to tell you more about the programs we offer and how your organization will benefit by them. I will telephone within the week to schedule a meeting with you. If you have questions you would like answered before that time, I welcome your call.

We are looking forward to serving you.

Sincerely,

Jane Doe, R.D.
Director

FIGURE 8-3. Sample letter of introduction to key worksite decision makers.

Jane: Given how busy you are, maybe we ought to get together over a lunch hour—my treat. That way, I'd have the opportunity to meet you and learn about some of the specific human resources challenges you are facing. Perhaps I could suggest programs that might assist you in meeting your challenges.

Mary: Well I don't know. I'm pretty busy right now.

Jane: Well, you have to eat sometime. And I'm sure if you take me up on my offer, you'll consider it time well spent.

Mary: OK. How about next week?

Many organizations have industrial nurses and either a part-time or full-time physician on staff. In these cases, nutrition practitioners report that the endorsement and, sometimes, the written approval of these individuals is essential. Be sure to obtain their endorsement and approval early in the process. Without it, you may waste valuable time. You can expect that some staff physicians will require an interview process and screening of credentials.

If there is no physician on staff, the endorsement of a well-respected, highly visible physician from your community is recommended. Figure 8-4 is an example of the type of endorsement that is useful in the sales process.

Tips for Keeping Your Foot in the Door Continually work on relationship building. Nurture relationships by building trust, credibility, and rapport. How? Consider these helpful hints:

- First and last impressions will be very important, since people seek evidence to support what they already believe.
- Dress professionally.
- Be on time.
- Establish consistent contact.
- Prepare for your meetings in advance so that details are fresh in your mind.
- Be sure you arrive with the information you said you'd have.
- Build and maintain the self-esteem of those representatives you meet. Everyone wants to feel important, admired, and respected and treated as though their feelings matter.
- When you are communicating with prospective clients, give them your undivided attention. Listen. Be responsive to their needs.
- Convey respect. Encourage prospective clients to feel that you have a genuine interest in getting to know and help them.
- Know where you stand with prospective clients. Invite them to give you feedback, and receive it openly. Keep checking back to see how they are feeling about the process.
- Answer questions directly. Say, "I don't know," if you don't. Ensure prospective clients that you will get answers to questions you are not readily prepared to respond to.
- Treat confidential information appropriately.
- Close each sales call by summarizing client's needs and emphasizing the corresponding value of your services. Gain a commitment, whether it is another meeting, a survey of participation, the opportunity to prepare a proposal, or the actual sale.

Bayview Cardiovascular Specialists
345 Sunrise Boulevard
Bayview, CA 32146
(413) 999-6543

June 6, 1989

Joseph Jones
Human Resource Director
XYZ Corporation
XYZ Plaza
Bayview, CA 32146

Dear Joseph:

If you are interested in reducing:

- Healthcare expenditures;
- Absenteeism and the costs of sick leave;
- Injury;
- Disability; and
- Cost of replacement and retraining; or, if you are interested in improving:
- Productivity;
- Employee morale;
- Employee relations; and
- Your ability to attract employees; consider the worksite nutrition services offered by Bayview Hospital. You won't be sorry.

Recently, I attended "Cooking for Your Heart's Content," sponsored by the Bayview Hospital Nutrition Center. The foods prepared in this healthy cooking program were not only delicious, but the calories, fat, cholesterol, and sodium content were well within dietary recommendations. I found this program to be an outstanding support to the Surgeon General's recent report on nutrition and health.

I recommend all the nutrition programs available through Bayview Hospital to my patients and colleagues. They are beneficial to all who have an interest in improving their health by improving eating and cooking habits.

Jane Doe, R.D., Director of Nutrition, will be contacting you upon my recommendation to survey your interest in the program.

If you would like to discuss this with me further, please feel free to contact me at the above address and telephone number.

Sincerely,

Brian G. Kelly, M.D.
Medical Director
Cardiovascular Specialists

FIGURE 8-4. Sample physician letter of recommendation.

Information Gathering
Once you have obtained an audience with a key decision maker, be prepared to listen, and arm yourself with open-ended questions that will enable you to probe for the needs, wants, expectations, and resources of your prospective clients. This information allows you to tailor your service offerings to meet client needs and affords a greater chance for a successful outcome. Also, armed with this information, you will be in a position to display greater confidence in your discussion with prospective clients.

Information gathering must take place early in the process because you must have an understanding of needs, wants, expectations, and resources before you can tailor your package of service offerings. However, information gathering is not a one-step process. At each stage in the process, important information may be disclosed and data formerly gathered must be verified. In fact, as you provide information to your prospective clients, it is critical that you gather data on their reactions to the information.

Critical Questions to Ask Before you make a formal proposal and, in some cases, before you make a general presentation of services, you will need the answers to certain questions that have been organized into three categories:

- Understanding the organization;
- Organization's needs and expectations; and
- Employee health profile.

The questions follow by category.

Understanding the Organization

- What is the name of the organization and its purpose or type of business it pursues?
- Is the organization centralized or decentralized?
- At what location(s) would services be delivered?
- What is the employee or member population at each location?
- What is the approximate number of employees/members you would consider for participation in nutrition service programs?
- What are the employee/member demographics?
- Is the organization or any part of the organization unionized? If so, would unionized workers be considered for nutrition service programs? If so, does the union need to be consulted at any point regarding these services?
- Is there a worksite eating facility? Is it vending, cafeteria, or dining room? If appropriate, would adjustments to current menus be considered?
- What are the general job responsibilities of the potential recipients of the nutrition services?
- What are the optimum times to meet with the employees/members?

- Will programs be provided to all employees/members or specific segments of the population only?
- What facilities are available to conduct programs?
- In which services are you interested?
- Are there multiple shifts?
- Do you know of other organizations with nutrition programs? What results have they recognized?
- How did you learn about our nutrition programs?
- Will there be incentives for the employees/members to use programs—bonus programs, contests, cost of services paid upon goal attainment, and so on?
- Do you have a wellness program or fitness center? If so, what programs are offered and what benefits of wellness programs are recognized?
- Who will make the final decision on contracting for services? Who will influence the decision?
- Are other healthcare service providers being contacted?
- Is the organization affiliated with HMO/PPO?
- Is there a possibility of workers' compensation or insurance reimbursement?

Organization's Needs and Expectations

- What are your perceptions of how nutrition services would be provided?
- What/who was the driving force behind seeking nutrition services?
- What do you expect nutrition services to do for your employees/members? (for example, reduce absenteeism, injury, healthcare expenditures, disability payments, cost of turnover, or cost of retraining; increase productivity; improve morale; or attract employees)?
- What problem(s) or need(s) would you like nutrition programs to address?
- Who will pay—organization, employee/member, or shared?
- Is there employee interest? May we survey employees/members?
- What is your expectation at this point about who will market the programs within your organization?
- How will billing be handled—payment up-front or payroll deductions?
- How often would you like to offer these programs (a one-time offering or on an ongoing basis)?
- Will services be provided on work time or personal time?
- Have there ever been nutrition programs offered? By whom? Why the change?
- Are there preset budgetary expectations?
- Is there an industrial nurse/physician on staff? Will they work with us?
- Will attendance be voluntary or mandatory?
- How will our success be measured?
- Would programs be open to families?

- What support staff will be available from the organization (for example, administrative, promotion, marketing, communication)?
- Time frame for implementation?
- Who will the organization coordinator be?
- What is your anticipated start date?

Employee Health Profile

- Within the context of your organization, what are your major concerns regarding your employees'/members' health?
- How do you perceive that improved health can enhance job performance?
- What is the rate of absence due to illness?
- What are the primary reasons for absence, disability, or injury? What is the rate of long-term absence due to injury or chronic illness?
- What changes have been experienced in the general health of employees over the past years?
- What health-related improvements are anticipated?
- What health-related hazards are anticipated?
- Are there other wellness programs already implemented? How can our efforts be integrated with current activities?

Sources of Information. Interviewing all key decision makers, individually, to gather the answers to these questions is ideal. Often, decision makers will respond differently to these questions, particularly regarding expectations. Since the decision will be based on how your product and service package will meet each decision maker's individual expectations, knowing those expectations is critical. Also, the interview process enables you to begin building rapport with each decision maker and to respond to their individual questions and concerns.

If you cannot negotiate for individual interviews, work toward a meeting of all decision makers. Since less information will be volunteered in this setting, you must probe skillfully and tactfully for the information you need.

Keep in mind that there are a variety of other sources for information. Consider talking to current employees/members, such as receptionists, office managers, nurses, or human resources professionals, if it is appropriate. Other sources of information include annual reports, internal reports, newsletters, and employee communications (ADA, 1986).

Employee/Member Participation Questionnaires If prospective clients show a strong interest, you may want to ask for the opportunity to survey the employees/members to determine employee/member interest in your programs prior to developing a proposal. It is important to collect this information before your proposal so that you can make projections more accurately, regarding:

- The actual participation;
- The resources you will need;
- The most appropriate programs;
- Direct costs; and
- Appropriate fees.

Some practitioners have chosen to conduct a survey in order to generate more interest in their programs. Keep in mind that if prospective clients are not interested, it is usually because they do not perceive that your programs will address their business concerns. If this is the case, employee/member interest will probably not alter their position. Participation surveys absorb a great deal of time and money. Because you want to spend your time and money in the most productive way, survey only if prospective clients are seriously interested in your services.

Some guidelines to follow are:

- Design a survey or questionnaire targeted at obtaining the information you and the client organization need in order to make appropriate decisions. Questionnaires must be designed so that they predict what people *will do*. They should be written in an easily understood fashion that employees can identify with.
- Determine how surveys will be disseminated. The company may offer some support staff to aid in this process. You may need to distribute surveys in a variety of ways to get a large enough return. Some possibilities include tables in lobbies and cafeterias or near time cards, paycheck inserts, employee communications, and staff meetings.
- The cost of doing the survey and any related participation should be included in your proposed fee. Some organizations will agree to pay for a survey of employee member participation whether or not they contract for your services.
- Determine how the surveys will be retrieved and how the data will be consolidated. Confidentiality is an issue. You may suggest that the questionnaires be returned to you in a self-addressed, postage-paid envelope. You may also pick them up from a locked box at the worksite, or, if the human resources department is trusted and willing, they might collect and tabulate the materials for you.
- If organizations want to roll up the data themselves, emphasize the importance of confidentiality. Again, your objective in using a survey or questionnaire is to learn what employees/members *will do*. If employees or members are placed in a position where perceived expectations of peers or management may influence their responses, the data may be distorted. Also, legal ramifications may become an issue if employees/members are asked to divulge information about their medical history.
- Because health promotion programs are usually voluntary, management usually wants a 30-percent participation level before they willingly buy into a program. Keep this in mind as you interpret the data and present it to your prospective client organizations.

- Tabulating and interpreting the data may be difficult. It takes time and specific expertise. There are marketing agencies available that specialize in performing these services.
- Determine any conflicts that might arise as a result of the survey. (A particular employer surveyed employees about opening a fitness center, but the employees were more concerned about day care and parking. Thus, the survey was a point of aggravation.)

A sample proposal for a worksite participation questionnaire follows (see Fig. 8-5), along with the sample questionnaire (see Fig. 8-6).

Another method of conducting a needs assessment is through a representative committee. Encourage organization representatives to invite employees/members from different divisions and hierarchial levels so that you hear the interests of a majority of the employees/members (Alford, 1986). This committee can be conducted like a focus group. It is recommended that the CEO or other key executives not be involved in the focus group meetings. Their presence often intimidates, and the open communication you encourage may be stifled (Mullis, 1986). This method works best if employees/members know what will be discussed and have the opportunity to discuss the issues with those they represent in advance.

Employees/members will be interested in the company's motives in providing such programs. If you have this information, include it along with instructions at the beginning of the questionnaire. It may help your survey population to be more open in answering your questions. Reassurance that nutritional information collected about any individual is as confidential as any other medical data will aid the employees' decisions to participate in your programs.

Information Giving

Information giving and information gathering are stages in the sales process that are very much intertwined. In some cases, they even occur simultaneously.

Keep these information-giving tips in mind:

- The more you know about the prospective client organization, the greater your opportunity to close the sale *if* you use the information to your and your client's best advantage.
- It isn't easy to find the right balance between holding back on information until you gather the data you need while still providing enough information to keep the client interested in pursuing your services. Take a look at how one nutrition practitioner handled this:

  RD: I'm delighted that you have set aside time to discuss our worksite nutrition programs. I mentioned to you on the telephone that many of our programs are designed to address some of the human resources management challenges of this decade. Specifically, programs like ours have resulted in

PROPOSAL FOR WORKSITE PARTICIPATION QUESTIONNAIRE FOR XYZ CORPORATION

Background
XYZ Corporation and Seaville Nutrition Center have been discussing the opportunity to offer nutrition programs as part of the employee benefit package. To determine the potential level of employee participation in various nutrition service programs, it was decided that a survey should be conducted. This study will focus on the kinds of nutrition programs that would be of the greatest interest to employees and the bearing that certain features will have on determining employee participation. While certain features cannot be changed, others will be adjusted if the survey results indicate a need to do so.

Objectives
The principle objectives of this study are:

1. To determine participation levels in various nutrition programs.
2. To discover how features of the service would encourage or discourage employee purchase of such services.

Methodology
An announcement of the study will be published in the employees' newsletter.
A questionnaire will be distributed at employee meetings during the week of (date) and collected at the close of those meetings. Completed questionnaires will be turned over to Seaville Nutrition Center for editing, coding, tabulation, and analysis. A return of approximately 300 questionnaires (75 percent) is anticipated. Upon completion of the study, Seaville Nutrition Center will produce a written report of findings, conclusions, and recommendations.

Expected Findings of the Study
This survey will offer information on the interest of employees of XYZ Corporation in:

- Various nutrition services;
- Various nutrition topics;
- Using nutrition services for specific needs;
- Times that would be most convenient to participate; and
- Involving family members in worksite nutrition programs.

All answers would be analyzed for the review of corporate decision makers and the entire employee group.

FIGURE 8-5. Sample proposal for worksite participation questionnaire.

Responsibilities

Seaville Nutrition Center has developed a draft of a questionnaire as part of this proposal.

XYZ Corporation will edit these drafts and make any suggested changes by (date).

Seaville Nutrition Center will print and deliver the surveys to XYZ Corporation by (date).

XYZ Corporation will distribute and collect questionnaires at staff meetings during the week of (date). Then they will be sent to Seaville Nutrition Center.

Questionnaires will be edited, coded, and tabulated upon receipt by Seaville Nutrition Center.

If all of the above dates are met, Seaville Nutrition Center will be able to issue a report on the results of this study by (date).

FIGURE 8-5. *(Continued)*

WORKSITE PARTICIPATION QUESTIONNAIRE

The following questionnaire has been developed by Seaville Nutrition Center upon the request of XYZ Corporation. The purpose of this survey is to determine if there is interest in various nutrition programs that XYZ is considering as a part of their employee benefits program.

Your feedback will determine whether nutrition services should be provided at your worksite. It will also determine which services are in demand and how they should be provided.

When you finish, please place this questionnaire in the box in the cafeteria labeled "Nutrition Questionnaires," or return it to the Human Resources Department. All questionnaires must be returned no later than (date).

This survey is completely anonymous. You will not be asked for your name or any identification that will associate you with your responses.

FIGURE 8-6. Sample questionnaire for surveying worksite interest in various nutrition programs.

1. How interested are you in the following nutrition topics or concerns?

	Very Interested	Somewhat Interested	Not too Interested	Not at all Interested
A. Weight management	[ ]	[ ]	[ ]	[ ]
B. Nutrition and heart disease/high cholesterol	[ ]	[ ]	[ ]	[ ]
C. Nutrition and high blood pressure	[ ]	[ ]	[ ]	[ ]
D. Nutrition and cancer	[ ]	[ ]	[ ]	[ ]
E. Nutrition and food allergies	[ ]	[ ]	[ ]	[ ]
F. Nutrition and osteoporosis	[ ]	[ ]	[ ]	[ ]
G. Food safety (pesticides & radiation)	[ ]	[ ]	[ ]	[ ]
H. Healthy cooking methods	[ ]	[ ]	[ ]	[ ]
I. Healthy eating on-the-go	[ ]	[ ]	[ ]	[ ]
J Nutrition myths	[ ]	[ ]	[ ]	[ ]
K. Nutritionally healthy children	[ ]	[ ]	[ ]	[ ]
L. Nutrition and stress management	[ ]	[ ]	[ ]	[ ]
M. Sports nutrition	[ ]	[ ]	[ ]	

What other topics are you interested in?

____

____

____

2. Assume that the opportunity to have a computerized nutrition analysis of your current diet was made available to you. Assume that a nutrition counselor would meet with you at the worksite to gather data, interpret the information, and make recommendations to address your nutrition needs. This service would cost you $ and your employer would pay the remaining cost of $. The service would be available to you by appointment, two designated weekdays between 8:00 A.M. and 5:00 P.M. Full payment must be made upon enrollment, or a payroll deduction can be arranged. Would you purchase this computerized nutrition analysis service?

Definitely Would Purchase	Probably Would Purchase	Probably Would Not Purchase	Definitely Would Not Purchase
[ ]	[ ]	[ ]	[ ]

FIGURE 8-6. *(Continued)*

Please indicate the reason(s) you might not be interested. Check as many as apply.

☐ No need for nutrition services
☐ Nutrition services available to me elsewhere
☐ Lack of time
☐ Available schedule inconvenient
☐ Not a priority
☐ Money
☐ Not comfortable receiving services at the worksite
☐ A computerized analysis isn't personal enough for me
☐ Other/specify______________________________

____

____

3. Assume that a series of nutrition education workshops were made available to you. You would select from a series of workshops which ones you would attend. They would range from 1/2 hour to 1 hour in length. The size of the group would be 7-35 members. They would be provided at your worksite during your lunch hour on designated weekdays between Noon and 2:00 P.M. Lunch will be provided and included in the cost. The workshops will cost you $ and your employer will pay the remaining cost of $. Full payment must be made upon enrollment, or a payroll deduction can be arranged. Would you participate in these nutrition education workshops?

Definitely Would Purchase	Probably Would Purchase	Probably Would Not Purchase	Definitely Would Not Purchase
[ ]	[ ]	[ ]	[ ]

Please indicate the reason(s) you might not be interested. Check as many as apply.

☐ No need for nutrition services
☐ Nutrition services available to me elsewhere
☐ Lack of time
☐ Available schedule inconvenient
☐ Not a priority
☐ Money
☐ Not comfortable discussing these issues with coworkers
☐ Uncomfortable in groups
☐ Want individual attention to my needs
☐ Other/specify______________________________

____

____

4. Assume that you are given the opportunity to join a group of coworkers, with common nutrition concerns, to work on incorporat-

FIGURE 8-6. *(Continued)*

ing new eating habits into your lifestyle. The group would be guided by a nutrition counselor. One individual session of 1 hour will be a prerequisite for the series. An individualized nutrition analysis will be conducted at that time. A series of eight sessions will be offered at the worksite, one each week for 8 weeks for 1 hour between Noon and 2:00 P.M. on a designated weekday. The size of the group would be between 6 and 12 members. Lunch would be provided and included in the cost. This series will cost you $, and your employer will pay the remaining cost of $. Payment must be made upon enrollment, or a payroll deduction can be arranged. Would you participate in a nutrition counseling group?

Definitely Would Purchase	Probably Would Purchase	Probably Would Not Purchase	Definitely Would Not Purchase
[ ]	[ ]	[ ]	[ ]

Please indicate the reason(s) you might not be interested. Check as many as apply.

☐ No need for nutrition services
☐ Nutrition services available to me elsewhere
☐ Lack of time
☐ Available schedule inconvenient
☐ Not a priority
☐ Money
☐ Not comfortable discussing these issues with coworkers
☐ Uncomfortable in groups
☐ Want individual attention to my needs
Other/specify______________________________

	Very Interested	Somewhat Interested	Not too Interested	Not at all Interested
5. How interested would you be in participating in a nutrition fair at your worksite? (A nutrition fair is an inspiring 1-day series of displays, demonstrations, and activities to increase your nutrition awareness.)	[ ]	[ ]	[ ]	[ ]

Please indicate the reason(s) you might not be interested. Check as many as apply.

☐ No need for nutrition education
☐ No time to participate
☐ Not a priority
☐ Don't feel comfortable discussing these issues at the worksite
☐ Other/specify______________________________

FIGURE 8-6. *(Continued)*

6. Please rank your preference of the nutrition programs discussed above. Place a "1" next to your first choice, a "2" next to your second choice, etc.
   - ☐ Computerized nutrition analysis
   - ☐ Nutrition education workshops (1/2-1 hour)
   - ☐ Group nutrition counseling sessions (series of eight)
   - ☐ Nutrition fair

7. How important is each of the following benefits in encouraging you to use a nutrition service?

	Very Important	Somewhat Important	Not too Important	Not at all Important
Improved overall health and decreased health risks	[ ]	[ ]	[ ]	[ ]
Feeling better	[ ]	[ ]	[ ]	[ ]
Improving your appearance	[ ]	[ ]	[ ]	[ ]
An ongoing support system	[ ]	[ ]	[ ]	[ ]

8. If nutrition services were open to family members, would anyone other than yourself participate?
   ☐ Yes ☐ No
   If yes, indicate the total number of family members participating in each service. (Do not include yourself.)
   - ☐ Computerized nutrition analysis
   - ☐ Nutrition education workshops (½-1 hour)
   - ☐ Group nutrition counseling sessions (series of eight)
   - ☐ Nutrition fair

9. Check your preference for the scheduling of nutrition services programs:
   - ☐ Immediately before work
   - ☐ During a scheduled meal period
   - ☐ Immediately after work
   - ☐ Other/specify________________________________

FIGURE 8-6. *(Continued)*

reduced healthcare expenditures, reduced disability payments, reduced cost of retraining, higher productivity, improved employee morale, better employee relations, and an improved ability to attract employees. Do any of these issues coincide with your organization's goals and objectives?

Joe: Of course! What organization wouldn't want to achieve those results?

RD: I'm sure you're right that some of these issues have a universal quality, but each organization has its own priorities and I could be of more service to you if I understood your organization's priorities.

Joe: Well, last year we went through a union campaign. The union didn't get in, and we've been trying to overcome the low morale and resulting problems ever since.

RD: Sounds like a difficult situation. Specifically, what resulting problems are you referring to?

Joe: The characteristic ones, I guess...high absenteeism, low morale, low productivity. Sometimes I think we underestimated the time it would take to recover. We still haven't rebuilt the trust. I know you said your nutrition programs could help, but I'm not sure I understand the connection.

RD: I'm pleased to have the opportunity to explain. Our services may help you to speed up the healing process and improve company results. You see, nutrition programs have a direct benefit on individual employees and their families and an indirect benefit to your organization. Showing employees that you care about their health and that you are willing to make an investment in their wellness makes an important statement about the company's concern for employee welfare. How do you feel about your comprehensive physical that the company provides free of charge?

Joe: It's great. I probably wouldn't get one otherwise. And they really push me, if I let it go too long.

RD: How does that make you feel?

Joe: I don't know (pause) I guess I feel like somebody notices I make a difference around here.

RD: That's what I'm talking about. We all like to feel appreciated. If employees begin to make positive changes in their eating habits, they will look better and feel better. As morale improves and as health improves, so will the attendance records of your employees. As attendance and morale improve, usually productivity does too. The National Dietitians Organization published some statistics I'd like to review with you...Here they are. This article indicates that in 1989, in a study of six worksites with comprehensive nutrition programs of six months or more in duration, overall employee attendance improved 6 percent. It's difficult to know if the primary catalyst was a sense of belonging and appreciation or improved health. I'm going to leave this article with you so that you can refer back to it and share it with others who will be involved in this decision.

Joe: Let's see—6 percent...(pause) that would mean about $50,000 annually to us. That's pretty impressive! But what's the cost associated with those savings?

RD: That depends on the nutrition program you select. We would help you design a program that would meet your organization's specific needs. Once determined, you make the decision as to who will pay what share of the expense.

Joe: Oh, so we don't necessarily have to foot the whole bill ourselves?

RD: That's right. We offer a variety of services that can be delivered in many different ways. Also, there are several different payment programs, ranging from the employees paying 100 percent of fees to the organization paying 100 percent of fees to any shared percentage in between. I'm sure we can find a program your organization could afford. The important thing is that we design a program that will deliver the results you want. To do that, I need to know more about your needs and your organization. Do you currently provide wellness programs of any kind?

Clearly, educating prospective clients on your programs before they understand the value of the programs to themselves places you at a disadvantage. Once you have established a perception of value, prospective clients are more open to listening with interest. This practitioner created interest early in the conversation by introducing the potential benefits of worksite programs and by asking good probing questions. She responded to Joe in a very general way, consistently emphasizing the importance of both tailoring programs to organizational needs and the need for more specific information to enable her to recommend appropriate programs.

When Joe revealed his skepticism, stating that he didn't see how nutrition programs could improve morale, productivity, and absenteeism, she did not seem threatened. Instead, she took advantage of the opportunity to educate the client, providing factual and statistical support for her conclusions. To establish more credibility, the practitioner used the personal example of Joe's sense of appreciation for the annual physical to emphasize how the organization's interest in his health improved his morale.

Once you are satisfied that you have gathered enough information to discuss specific elements of program design, you may suggest or the client may request a brief presentation of your services. This presentation is another opportunity for you to educate. One practitioner made this presentation of services:

RD: As I explain our programs and how they work, I want to invite you to jump in at any time with comments or questions. Or, if I get into areas you are not interested in, let me know.

Sue: Okay.

RD: Let's begin with a brief overview of why people seek nutrition services. There are three primary reasons: to learn what and how they should eat, to get help to incorporate changes into their lifestyle, and for ongoing support.

We address the first need—nutrition knowledge—through education. Most providers stop at education, but most people want and need more. For most of us, knowing what we should do isn't enough. For those who want help to incorporate changes into their lifestyles and ongoing support, we provide counseling services.

Sue: I can really relate to what you're saying. I know what *I should do* and occasionally I get real committed, until I stop paying attention. Sounds like I could use some counseling myself.

RD: You aren't alone Sue. The good news is: help is available and we have a strong track record of success. Our nutrition counselors are trained to consider environment, culture, social and psychological influences, needs, personal preferences, and motivation in assisting clients to incorporate new eating patterns into their lifestyles. We offer education and counseling on both an individual and group basis. Virtually any area of nutrition could be addressed through either individual or group programs. I have a comprehensive listing of our most popular requests. Weight management, cholesterol reduction, nutrition and cancer, stress management through nutrition, dining out, preventing weight gain with smoking cessation, label reading, and guided supermarket tours are usually the hot buttons. But each workforce is different, and we encourage users to have input into the selection of topics.

Sue: How do they provide input?

RD: There are several ways: a survey can be used, or a committee of representatives could be formed, or sometimes we hold open meetings or conduct interviews with representatives. We would have to determine the most appropriate method for gathering employee input later in this process.

Most importantly, we would survey your employees for very specific reactions to specific service offerings. You would make the final decision on the services, based on their feedback.

In the area of education, we normally survey:

A computerized nutrition analysis and screening with recommendations. This is a one time service offering. The discussion takes about one hour.

A series of three or four individual sessions. The first session is an hour; all follow- up sessions are a half hour.

A series of nutrition workshops of a half hour to one hour, usually working with anywhere from 12 to 50 members.

A nutrition fair.
In the area of counseling, we normally survey:
A series of three or four individual counseling sessions.
Individual executive counseling sessions in the executives' offices. The timing and frequency are based on the individual's needs.
A series of 68 group counseling sessions usually with anywhere from 6 to 12 group members with common nutrition concerns.
I have a brochure here that describes these services in detail.

Sue: Thank you. I will review it a little later.

RD: I'm sure cost is an important consideration. The services may be offered at full cost to employees, full cost to your organization, or a shared percent by each. Some employers set the program up at full cost to employees; however, they offer the opportunity to participate on company time. That is another choice you will make. Some employers extend this low-cost benefit to families of employees. It's a great way to build morale. Since morale is one of the primary needs you'd like to address, let's focus on some features we can build into your package of nutrition services. To ensure morale improves...

Confine your delivery of information to what the prospective client wants to know. There is a temptation to convince them that you are an expert in nutrition or to offer information you *want* to share. Don't waste their time. This may be important to you, but it's not likely to be important to them. Tailor your information to your clients' agenda and abandon yours.

Recognize the intangible nature of services. Selling services is not like selling a product. A product can be seen, touched, and, in some cases, heard. Since people tend to trust what they can experience through their senses, it is much easier to gain trust and confidence regarding a product than it is with a service. Successful service selling involves overcoming the intangible nature of the service.

The use of a portfolio is strongly suggested. Portfolios help a prospective client overcome the intangible nature of services by examining the scope of your work and establishing credibility. They are also used in the sales process to:

- Highlight your products, services, and programs;
- Demonstrate what you do and what you represent;
- Demonstrate your credentials when unknown to the client;
- Offer a vision and insight into your work; and
- Demonstrate your creative ability.

The following items are suggested for your portfolio:

- Business cards;
- Samples of products (cookbooks, incentives, contests);

- Brochures;
- Sample articles you have published;
- Professional educational materials;
- Statistical support for worksite programs;
- Media work;
- Resumes of previous experiences with worksites;
- Letters of reference from other worksites;
- Letters of recommendation from physicians;
- Sample menus;
- Computerized nutritional analysis; and
- Supporting photos.

Care should be taken in developing your portfolio. Make choices that emphasize the results recognized by worksites. Make choices that enhance the image and professionalism of your practice. The portfolio can be presented as a case of materials or other types of visual displays—posters, tapes, videos, or slide presentations. You may want to consider a leather binder or case, since your packaging will create an important first impression. Make your selections carefully regarding:

- Quality of paper;
- Color;
- Design;
- Format;
- Layout; and
- Printing (*thumbs down to photocopying*).

Be sure that any supporting photographs are current, clear, and of a professional quality.

If employee feedback is solicited through a questionnaire or meetings, you must consider how you will present the results of your findings. In some cases, worksite decision makers will prefer that you present the results at the proposal presentation. In other cases, decision makers will want to know what you learned from the employee/member feedback and what services you would be interested in offering prior to a formal proposal presentation. Be sensitive to the varying decision-making processes of each organization.

Drafting the Proposal Written proposals are expected. Most business clients will want to see a description of services, fees, and other arrangements proposed in writing. A well-written proposal will:

- Enable you to create and clarify expectations;
- Form the basis on which further discussion and negotiation can proceed;
- Help to overcome the intangible nature of services; and
- Enhance your professional image with business clients.

Proposals must be tailored to the individual needs of prospective client organizations. Standardizing proposals saves time, but often leads to lost opportunities. The general rules of thumb on writing proposals are to be brief, include key information only, and elaborate in your presentation.

Some thoughts to keep in mind when writing proposals include:

- Proposals can be deadly if they are:
  - Too long;
  - Detailed;
  - Dry or boring;
  - Not colorful;
  - Covering more information than the client wants;
  - Not individualized; or
  - Unexciting or unenthusiastic.
- Rather than lowering your price to obtain the business, alter the services.
- Not every opportunity is a good opportunity. Do not be afraid to say "no." Good references are critical to selling to worksites. You don't want negative references. Good reasons to say "no" include:
  - A poor reputation;
  - A lack of cooperation;
  - A lack of involvement or commitment;
  - A poor credit rating;
  - Little or no profit potential;
  - Inadequate facilities;
  - Low participation; and
  - Unwillingness to survey participation, if your dollar return is based on participation.
- Don't try to solve problems in a proposal. State what will be done.
- Offer lump sums rather than itemized costs. Tell them what is included in your fee, but don't break it down. Lump sums discourage haggling.
- If possible, include references or testimonies with your proposal.
- Suggest a method of payment that protects your interests if participation wanes. (For example, full pay at the first session or payroll deduction.)
- Create realistic expectations by addressing the assumption that some drop-outs will occur once the initial enthusiasm of new programs wears away.
- Only propose services that can be conducted on site.
- Be sure the assumptions upon which your price is based are stated clearly. Note that if the assumptions do not hold, your plan may not either.

To guide your efforts in proposal writing, a basic outline follows. For a sample proposal, see Figure 8-7.

PROPOSAL FOR WORKSITE NUTRITION SERVICES PROGRAM FOR XYZ CORPORATION

Objectives

The objections of this program are:

1. To provide nutrition services to XYZ Corporation that will:
   a. Improve morale; and
   b. Reduce absenteeism.
2. To provide nutrition services to employees that will:
   a. Reduce illness/health risk factors;
   b. Enable them to feel better;
   c. Be conveniently located at the worksite;
   d. Have the potential to harness social support and social influence for behavior change; and
   e. Offer opportunities for follow-up, monitoring and reinforcement.

Key Assumptions

Key assumptions are:

- Morale will improve as a result of demonstrating to employees and their families that the corporation cares about and is willing to make an investment in their employees' wellness.
- Absenteeism will improve as a result of:
  Improved employee health;
  Employees feeling better; and
  Improved morale.
- Service delivery would begin within 75 days. If not, the prices and other terms and conditions may vary.
- At least 80 percent of the 25 executives who indicated in the employee participation survey that they "would definitely use" the executive-in-office services will use the counseling service.
- At least 80 percent of the employee population indicating that they "would definitely attend" the nutrition education series (450) will enroll in at least three programs in the series.
- Over 35 percent of the employee population will participate in the nutrition services program.
- At the end of the 12 weeks, the need for additional and follow-up services will be evaluated.

Proposed Services

Proposed services include:

- Executive-in-office counseling program; and
- Nutrition education series.

FIGURE 8-7. Sample proposal for a worksite nutrition services program.

Provision of Services

Executive-In-Office Counseling Service

Seaville Nutrition Center will:

- Provide nutrition counseling services to 20 executives in their own offices by appointment on Mondays between 12:00 P.M. and 6:00 P.M. and Tuesdays and Thursdays between 8:00 A.M. and 6:00 P.M. for a period of 8 consecutive weeks.
- Provide an initial counseling session of approximately 1 hour to analyze nutrition history, nutrition needs, lifestyle, and food consumption. 30-minute follow-up sessions will be provided during the following 7 weeks.
- Provide an optional computerized analysis of a 3-day food consumption record to allow for more specific recommendations on nutrient excesses and deficiencies, at an additional fee. (Each executive will make their own choice regarding this option.)

Nutrition Education Series

Seaville Nutrition Center will:

- Provide a 55-minute nutrition workshop each week for 12 weeks at 12:00 P.M. and 1:15 P.M. on Fridays.
- Offer the following topics in the following order, based on employee demand indicated in the Employee Participation Survey:
  - Weight management
  - Nutrition and heart disease/high cholesterol
  - Nutrition and high blood pressure
  - Nutrition and cancer
  - Nutrition and food allergies
  - Nutrition and osteoporosis
  - Food safety (pesticides and radiation)
  - Healthy cooking methods
  - Healthy eating on-the-go
  - Nutrition myths
  - Nutritionally healthy children
  - Nutrition and stress management
- Encourage active participation. Some workshops include food tastings and food preparation demonstrations.
- Educate up to 50 participants in each session.
- Supply accompanying nutrition posters and handout materials for displays in the cafeteria for all 12 topics.
- Request audiovisual equipment at least 10 days in advance of the need.

XYZ will:

- Provide a conference room or classroom that will comfortably accommodate 40 participants seated in a U-shape.
- Arrange the room in the U-shape seating arrangement at least 2 hours prior to each session.
- Provide audiovisual equipment as requested by the dietitian for each presentation.

FIGURE 8-7. *(Continued)*

Both Services

Seaville Nutrition Center will:

- Involve physicians in prescribing a dietary regimen, if a medical condition exists.
- Provide one consistent registered dietitian to deliver services for the 12-week period.
- Provide documentation of services for recipients seeking insurance reimbursement.
- Conduct a preview session for all executives and employees 2 weeks before the enrollment deadline to create some excitement and to ensure that the programs are understood. The dietitian will be available after the session to respond to questions and discuss individual concerns.
- Provide various professionally printed instructional materials and informational handouts for use in sessions throughout the 12-week period.
- Protect the confidentiality of all medical and nutritional information specific to each employee.

XYZ will:

- Enroll employees in the programs on a "first come, first served" basis no later than 45 days prior to the first session. Substitute employees from a waiting list as cancellations occur.
- Notify Seaville Nutrition Center 40 days prior to the first session of the final enrollment for planning and billing purposes.
- Offer company time to employees to use the services.
- Designate an internal coordinator to enroll the employees in the programs, disseminate all pertinent information, schedule appointments during the times designated by the dietitian, and set up displays.
- Report any changes in the schedule to the dietitian at least 24 hours before the scheduled appointment.

Employees will:

- Schedule their own appointments.
- Cancel any appointment that cannot be met 24 hours in advance.
- Obtain a physician referral with a prescription for any special nutrition needs.
- File for reimbursement with his or her insurance company, if applicable.
- Arrange for payment at the time of enrollment.

Cost

The cost of providing nutrition services will include:

- The dietitian's time to:
  - Prepare and present the preview session and nutrition education series;
  - Prepare and review computerized nutrition analysis;
  - Prepare for nutrition counseling;
  - Counsel 20 executives;

FIGURE 8-7. *(Continued)*

  - Coordinate activities; and
  - Provide phone contact with participants.
- Professionally printed materials (surveys, brochures and handout materials, etc.) and workshops supplies.
- Expenses.

Initial employee participation survey cost: $250.

Executive-in-office counseling program cost:

  - XYZ Corporation will guarantee payment for 20 executives at a basic cost of $14,750.
  - If more than 20 executives enroll in the program, $590 will be charged for each additional participant.
  - For each computerized nutritional assessment requested, an additional $25 will be charged.

Nutrition education series cost:

  - The cost of this service is $15.00 per participant, per session, based on a guarantee of 40 participants per presentation/80 participants per topic: $14,400. No additional charge will be assessed by Seaville Nutrition Center for the 41st to 50th participants attending any presentation.
  - XYZ Corporation and employees will each share 50 percent of the cost of this service. XYZ Corporation will pay the fees for the difference between those attending and the 40 participants guaranteed, if participation drops below 40.
  - The cost for 12 sets of posters, displays, and demonstration materials in the cafeteria will be paid by XYZ Corporation: $1,000.

Payment

Employees participating in the nutrition education series will either pay cash or authorize payroll deduction at the time of enrollment. These fees will reimburse the Company for 50 percent of the advance payment.

Final enrollment information must be offered in writing 40 days prior to the first session. An invoice will be issued upon notification to XYZ Corporation for:

  - The initial survey;
  - The basic cost of the executive-in-office counseling;
  - Computerized nutritional assessments;
  - The basic cost of the nutrition education series; and
  - The 12 sets of nutrition display materials.

Services will not commence until payment of this invoice is received. All payments will be made within 30 days of billing. Late fees will be charged at a rate of 1 1/2 percent on any balance extended beyond 30 days.

Monitoring

Seaville Nutrition Center will:

FIGURE 8-7. *(Continued)*

- Provide a weekly list of employees who participated in the various nutrition services.
- Provide general statistics on executives participating in the executive-in-office counseling program (such as average change in cholesterol, blood pressure, weight, etc.).
- Provide workshop evaluations to participants and ask them to complete them during the last 10 minutes of each session. These will be tabulated, and the results will be presented to the program coordinator and key management the following week.
- Provide program evaluations to participating executives and the time to complete them at the end of the last session.
- Not discuss specific information relative to any employee's medical record.

XYZ Corporation will:

- Notify the dietitian immediately if the company or its employees feel that adjustments in service delivery could improve the program in any way.
- Track attendance, comparing current trends to results up to 12 months after the nutrition services program is delivered.
- Measure employee morale through observation and the written evaluations designed to assess employee reactions to the nutrition services program. (XYZ will be asked to participate in the design of the evaluation.)

References

References and testimony of the results of nutrition services programs will be provided upon request.

FIGURE 8-7. *(Continued)*

PROPOSAL OUTLINE

I. Objectives
   A. State company/organization and employee/member needs as you understand them
   B. State benefits of your service offerings to the company and the employees
II. Key Assumptions
   A. Participation
   B. How will services impact results?
   C. How long will prices, terms, and conditions remain constant?
III. Proposed Products and Services
   A. What services?
   B. What products?
IV. Provision of Products and Services

A. Where provided?
B. When provided? (start date, completion date, times)
C. How provided?
D. To whom?
E. By whom?
F. What are the responsibilities of each party? (facilities, information dissemination, etc.).
G. How will you address cancellations?
H. What necessitates an interruption in service?

V. Monitoring Service Delivery
A. How will you monitor?
B. How will they monitor?

VI. Cost
A. Fees—company/organization
B. Fees—employee/member
C. Expenses—phone calls, room charge, audiovisual aids, giveaways, administrative costs, catered meals, travel, etc.

VII. Payment
A. Arrangements
B. Penalties for late payment
C. Price increases

VIII. Testament
A. References
B. Testimony
C. Articles with statistical support

Presentation of the Proposal Before presenting the proposal, you may want to send or deliver professional looking copies to each person who is involved in the presentation. Allow a reasonable amount of time for perusal of the information gathered and the proposal itself.

The proposal should be presented enthusiastically, professionally, and in your own words. Most importantly, be prepared. Determine which visual aids will have the most impact. The visual presentation is as critical as good oral communication. Plan what information or data is best presented visually through overheads, charts, or handouts.

A suggested order for your presentation follows:

- *Introduction*—A brief overview stating the purpose of the meeting. It is helpful to refer to previous discussions, especially those that lend support to the proposal. Summarize the prospective client's needs as you understand them. Highlight how your program will address these needs.

- *Explanation* of how the program works—An explanation of the products and services, distribution plan, price and payment plan, and promotional strategies.
- *Discussion of benefits*—The benefit section is the most important because this is your opportunity to focus specifically on what is important to decision makers in terms of the need being satisfied.
- *Summary of the proposal*—A discussion of the proposal, giving a concise summary of key points. Be sure to expound on those points that you feel warrant further information. Restate how the service program will address the organization's needs.
- *Closing*—The closing section establishes the next step in the process. A commitment should be made at this point, whether it is for the company to further consider the proposal or for you to make adjustments as a result of the discussion. Time commitments can be established during the closing.

Recognize that each decision maker has a very individualized approach to decision making. Since differing responsibilities means different agendas and benefits, be sure that your presentation takes into account the needs and concerns of each decision maker present.

For example:

> To answer your question, John (CEO), programs like the one we're proposing have impacted the cost of absenteeism and retraining as much as 50 percent in some organizations. At the same time, Paul (HR Director), the statement that this type of investment makes to your employees about their employer's commitment to good health has improved morale in other companies. I'm sure you will experience similar results. I've brought survey results along to substantiate this.

During your presentation, your audience will most likely ask you to respond to questions and you may be faced with objections or resistance. Do not regard objections and concerns as criticism; rather, use them as an opportunity to market yourself and your programs. Consider ways to turn concerns into reasons to support the program.

Determining and Resolving Basic Issues/Objections

Throughout the sales process, decision makers will identify issues and concerns that may prevent you from closing the sale. Some of these issues can be easily addressed. Others are unresolvable. Some are surfaced openly. Others remain unspoken obstacles. Prospective clients are often reluctant to discuss sensitive issues or feelings. Your success depends on your ability to bring these underlying issues to the surface. You do this by exploring every lead and clue that prospective clients offer you. You want to seize every opportunity to surface thoughts, values, attitudes, and feelings.

How do you do this?

- Receive feedback openly. Don't respond defensively.
- Build trust, credibility, and rapport.
- Listen openly and consistently.
- Use all the interviewing techniques available to you. Probe; ask effective questions.
- Tactfully confront, when necessary, to clarify conflicting or contradictory messages.

Once these issues and concerns are surfaced, you have an opportunity to respond to them. You will close the sales where you can overcome them. At this time, review Table 8-2. As you review the chart, you will notice three columns. From left to right, the first column identifies the objection. The second indicates some of the common ways prospective clients present these objections. The third column suggests some possible approaches for overcoming the objections. It is important that you anticipate prospective client objections. Make choices and develop business strategies that will enable you to address their concerns and overcome their objections.

Commitment

Once the prospective client has all the information to make a decision, you must await an answer. It is common for the decision-making process in organizations to drag on far beyond your expectation or the timetable agreed upon by both parties. In order to discourage a lengthy decision-making process, consider these suggestions:

- Once you have offered all important information and surfaced and resolved the prospective client's concerns and issues, ask them how much time they will need to make a decision. Establishing a date often sets the pace for the decision-making process.
- If you have any time constraints that may affect their commitment, let them know before you ask for a decision date.
- Getting an appointment on that date to discuss the final decision may add additional momentum.
- Stay in close touch during the decision-making period. Be available to clarify any issues or to answer questions. Also, your calls are a subtle reminder that the clock is ticking and the decision-making process must go forward.

If acceptance of the proposal is not gained immediately, don't assume that the client will decide not to contract with you. Follow up in timely fashion. It is critical that you learn the concerns or issues that are obstacles to making the commitment. Sometimes they are concerns you can easily address.

Once you've gained the commitment, be sure to review your understanding of

TABLE 8-2 Common Objections to Worksite Nutrition Programs and Ways of Overcoming Them

Objections	How the objections show up	Ways to overcome the objections
Cost	• We can't afford it. • Our employees are low income. • Time away from the job is going to cost too much.	• Nutrition services are a low-cost benefit that will return your investment in the long run through reduced absenteeism, injury, healthcare expenditures, disability payments, and cost of retraining and through improved employee relations and morale. • Services do not have to be paid for by the organization. If interest is high, employees may be willing to pay for the services. Or the organization and the employee may share the costs. • Services can be offered at convenient times—off the clock. • Some insurance companies will offer reduced rates as incentives for participating in certain wellness programs.
Time	• There is too much time involved in these services. • Time on the clock is too costly. • Nobody is going to want responsibility for coordinating and administering this program—it would take too much time.	• Services can be delivered off the clock during meal periods, immediately before or after work shift, or we can piggyback meetings. And certain programs can be repeated to reach multiple shifts. • The majority of the administration can be handled by our Nutrition Center for an additional and minimal fee.
Liaison's perception of employee/member interest	• We tried seminars on health topics about 10 years ago and nobody came. • I really don't think there will be interest...most of our people are older."	• Research shows a considerable increase in interest and awareness of nutrition nationally during that period of time.

TABLE 8-2 *(Continued)*

Objections	How the objections show up	Ways to overcome the objections
Liaison's perception of employee/ member interest *(Continued)*	• If the food in the cafeteria is any indication, they don't care what they eat. • Men don't do the cooking anyway. They won't be interested.	• Since you are ready to contract for our services if employee interest is high, let's survey your employees." • Employees have input into our package of service offerings. All programs are voluntary, and employees select the topics for any seminars we offer. • Including families often sparks and supports employee interest. • You may be surprised to learn that 42 percent of the participants attending current programs are men.
Too much change and disruption	• If we get people stirred up about nutrition, we'll probably have to change our menu again in the cafeteria. • Trying to get employees back to work on time, after a meeting during lunch or before work, is too difficult.	• We can be flexible to provide the least disruption. The following can be tailored to suit the organization's needs: — The services offered. — The length of the session. — The schedule. — Repeating services for multiple shifts. — Meals can be served in conjunction with sessions. • As long as nutritional foods are available, no change would be necessary in your cafeteria. Instead, you may want to heavily merchandise nutritional food choices and label foods with nutrient content. The most you could do to support employee nutrition concerns in your cafeteria would result in little or no disruption.
Inability to influence key decision makers	• I think your services are exactly what we need, but I'll bet you can't convince my boss of that. • You've got my vote, but I wouldn't think of approaching my boss about this; he'd laugh me right out of the office.	• Explore the objections with the subordinate. • Arm the liaison with information that enables him or her to respond to the decision maker's objections. • Network with those who can influence the key decision maker.

TABLE 8-2 *(Continued)*

Objections	How the objections show up	Ways to overcome the objections
Inability to influence key decision makers *(Continued)*		• Be sensitive to your liaison's position, ask permission to contact the decision maker directly. • If possible, take both the decision maker and the liaison to lunch. • Emphasize the benefits of your services from the decision maker's perspective. • Sometimes a survey of employee interest may be persuasive to a decision maker.
Employee relations concerns	• I'd like to offer executive services, but that may be too sensitive an issue with our lower level employees. • I'd like to survey the employee interest, but morale is so low around here that I'm afraid the survey will stir things up again.	• A graduated benefits package that offers additional benefits for executive levels is a common practice. You may want to talk to some representatives of organizations that do this. Or we'd be happy to provide some references from our client list. • Opening nutrition services to employees can be a morale booster. Nutrition programs have a direct benefit on individual employees and their families and an indirect benefit to your organization. Showing employees you care about their health and that you are willing to make an investment in their wellness makes an important statement about the company's concern for employee welfare.
Credibility	• How do I know you are the right person to provide these services? • Can you quantify the results of your programs? • What proof do you have that your programs make a difference?	• Use every tool available to overcome the intangible nature of the services you offer. Offer your track record of results. Use a portfolio, and be sure to include: — Written references — Physicians' recommendations — Articles you've published — Statistics published on worksite programs. Encourage prospective clients to contact current or former clients directly.

TABLE 8-2 *(Continued)*

Objections	How the objections show up	Ways to overcome the objections
No responsibility	• Nutrition and fitness aren't our responsibility. Each person has to make their own choices about those issues. • We offer health insurance. That's all we have a responsibility to do.	• You may not feel a responsibility to provide nutrition services, but it may be to your advantage. Nutrition services are a low-cost benefit that will return your investment in the long run through reduced absenteeism, injury, healthcare expenditures, disability payments, and cost of retraining and through improved employee relations and morale.
Liability	• What happens if you give out poor advice here at the worksite and an employee's health is affected by it? • Who is liable for damages if you give out the wrong information?	• Our practice carries liability insurance against such legal issues. However, to date, no suits have ever been brought against an outpatient nutrition counselor. • We take full responsibility for the information and counseling we provide. We take great care to offer the most up-to-date information and, where applicable, follow physicians' instructions to the letter. • Most of the information we provide is usable by any adult to improve health. However, we do make a thorough inquiry into special health conditions so that we guard against misinformation.
Hiring a part-time dietitian	• Rather than pay your fees, it's probably cheaper to hire a dietitian to work on our payroll and we'd have more control. • If nutrition is so important to company results, why not look for a dietitian to work on staff in our fitness center?	• At first glance, a dietitian on staff may appear cheaper; a closer look may prove otherwise. Consider this: —A dietitian on staff would be entitled to benefits and additional taxes and other payroll costs must be paid. This increases their salary cost by 30 to 50 percent as compared to our flat rate. — With an employee, you pay for break periods and some downtime. You'll have to commit to a given number of hours, whether the dietitian is consistently needed or not. With our practice, you only pay for services actually rendered.

TABLE 8-2 *(Continued)*

Objections	How the objections show up	Ways to overcome the objections
Hiring a part-time dietitian *(Continued)*		— The dietitian you hire will have to develop many of the materials and program we are offering you. The development of a single program can take a couple of months. This cost is significant. — No dietitian has expertise in all areas of nutrition. We subcontract a specialist when necessary, to meet your needs. — The high visibility we have enjoyed in this community, particularly with the media, will maximize the public view of your commitment to employee welfare. • I assume you want control to ensure that your needs are met. I stand to lose as much, or more, than a dietitian on staff, if your organization's needs aren't met. Dissatisfied customers are damaging to my reputation and my business. • A 45-day cancellation notice can be included in our contract. This is satisfaction guaranteed.
Single dietitian practice	• What happens if you get sick? • What happens if you decide to dissolve your practice?	• I have arranged to subcontract work that cannot be postponed when I am sick or unable to provide services for any reason. Another dietitian cannot easily substitute for individual or group counseling sessions. So, we would postpone those. I would encourage you to interview the dietitian who would substitute for me. She has excellent credentials and a great deal of experience in delivering worksite programs. • I have only missed two days of work in five years. I encourage you to contact references from other worksites I service. They will assure you that services have never been interrupted for any reason.

TABLE 8-2 *(Continued)*

Objections	How the objections show up	Ways to overcome the objections
Single dietitian practice *(Continued)*		• You may experience cancellations for good reasons from any provider, regardless of size. But an institution as large as ours is not likely to dissolve its outpatient nutrition practice.
Prefers private nutrition practitioner	• The private nutrition practitioner is less expensive because they have very little overhead. • The private practitioner can offer more flexibility in her programs; she doesn't have to follow stamped-out hospital programs.	• Overhead may or may not be less. It depends on the parties involved. One reason costs are often lower is reduced quality. You may want to request a review of the support materials, for example. Often, they are photocopied and unprofessional. This will affect the credibility the recipient will feel for the dietitian providing the service. Because private practitioners do not have the pool of resources available to them that our nutrition center does, the quality of all services may be compromised.
	• With an institutional practice, we are just a little fish in a sea of clients. The private practitioner thinks our business is important, and she'll give us all the attention we need.	• Our services are tailored to the needs of each client. Programs are not standardized. We have a pool of resources to draw upon in adapting services that the private practitioner does not have. We encourage you to contact current worksite clients. They will assure you of our commitment to serve your needs and of our flexibility. • Because of the number of worksite clients we have serviced, we have a strong track record of success and references to substantiate our capabilities. Also, our experience has trained us to organize an effective service package. We built our worksite business on each client's individual needs. • Our institution's name carries instant credibility. When your employees hear our name associated with your nutrition services, it is a statement of quality. • Most private practices are small; if your dietitian is sick or the business folds, you may suffer an interruption in service.

the terms of the agreement and then consult your legal counsel. Your lawyer should draft a contract or letter of agreement representing the terms. Then you will present the contract to your prospective client contact. They may request adjustments to the agreement. Be sure to review the requested changes with your legal counsel before agreeing to them.

Occasions arise when you are asked to begin services before the agreement is signed. This is not recommended. If this request is made, contact your legal counsel for advice.

Refer to Chapter 6, "Administrative Considerations in Establishing the Practice," for additional information on contracts.

After the Sale

Effective salespeople have learned that follow up is part of every sale. Obviously, a show of appreciation is in order for starters. You might say:

> You've made the right choice. We are really enthused about the opportunity to provide services to your organization, and we'd like to thank you for having the confidence in us to award us the business.

Research shows that people often experience "buyer's remorse" immediately after an expensive purchase. This means once the commitment is made, people commonly second guess their decision. For this reason, you want to maintain contact. Continue building rapport, and address any doubts your prospective clients may experience. Whenever possible, give credit to the organization in talk shows, radio spots, and magazine and newspaper articles for their commitment to employee welfare. Organizations generally appreciate free publicity.

If the final decision isn't favorable, you still want to leave your prospective client with a positive feeling for your practice and your services. Thank the prospective client for the opportunity to discuss the provision of services with them.

> We have really enjoyed exploring this opportunity to serve you. Also, we've developed a great deal of respect for you and your organization in the process. We hope that if you consider providing nutrition services in the future, you will consider Lander's Nutrition Center. We want to thank you for the opportunity.

As mentioned earlier, it is critical for you to learn why you were not selected. Try to surface those factors that influenced the decision-making process. It is difficult to probe for "more" potentially negative feedback or to sound sincerely enthusiastic and appreciative of the opportunity to pursue worksite nutrition services when you are feeling the disappointment associated with the rejection. Keep in mind, however, that it is critical that you rise to the occasion. Consider your investment in this potential sale as collateral. That prospective client contact may refer other opportunities to you.

Resources to Support Worksite Nutrition Programs

Throughout this chapter, emphasis has been placed on the importance of providing statistics and the results of worksite experience to prospective clients. Obviously, when you are just starting out you must rely on the experiences of other practices. You will find a list of references at the end of the text that may be of assistance to you in getting worksite nutrition programs started.

Part 4

Conclusion

Chapter 9

Monitoring Performance

TRACKING RESULTS

Managing an efficient nutrition counseling practice requires constant evaluation of your efforts to meet goals and objectives. A system of monitoring, set in place as you begin your practice, will allow you to make such an evaluation on a regular basis with ease. At least you will have organized data upon which to base decisions.

Establishing measures of performance and maintaining a monitoring system are among the most important responsibilities you will undertake because they measure your success as a service provider and enable you to respond to problems before they escalate. They also provide a method for comparing effectiveness and revenue potential of various services. Results of evaluations serve as a catalyst for improvement of services.

As outpatient nutrition services have expanded, very little has been done to develop tools that assess the value of services and productivity of outpatient nutrition practitioners. Therefore, you may be forced to develop or adapt measurement tools that meet your needs. Six measures that you must develop for daily, weekly, and monthly evaluation of your practice are:

1. Client satisfaction;
2. Satisfaction of administration;
3. Satisfaction of referral agents;
4. Quality control;
5. Growth and financial progress; and
6. Cost/Benefit Analysis.

How you establish your system of monitoring will depend on the goals and objectives of your practice. The following discussion of each type of monitoring will provide you with a variety of possibilities.

Client Satisfaction

Not enough emphasis can be placed on the importance of ensuring client satisfaction. Why is client satisfaction so important? Repeat business, business reputation, referrals, sales, and profits rely heavily on client satisfaction.

Before you can measure satisfaction, you must know what factors are important to your clients. Keep in mind that the factors may vary significantly between clients in individual and group programs. Usually, this information is gathered during your market research. Initially, this is the only information you have on the criteria you will use to measure success. Experiences may indicate the need to expand your list of criteria.

As mentioned earlier, clients consider nutrition expertise a given. Clients measure effectiveness in two primary ways—results of the counseling effort and the manner in which counselors relate to them. They are concerned with the answers to questions like:

- "How will this counselor affect my ability to make changes?"
- "Do I trust this counselor?"
- "Am I comfortable talking with this counselor?"
- "Can I understand what I'm hearing?"
- "Are my problems understood?"
- "Am I being treated as an individual with individual needs?"

Evaluating client satisfaction means evaluating success as clients do. Expertise must always be a goal, but there's more to it. Clients want nutrition counselors to focus on behavior change rather than dietary regimens, strategies for behavior change rather than expertise, and applicability rather than quality of information.

Knowing where your counselors and your practice stand with your clients is an ongoing process. The following suggestions are offered to assist your counselors in generating the consistent flow of information needed.

Surface expectations early in the process. Clients' expectations are as varied as the number of clients. Nutrition counselors are not likely to meet expectations if they don't know what the expectations are. Clients seek counseling with some expectation of the counseling process and how nutrition care will be provided. They will begin to note discrepancies between the counselor's behavior and their expectations at the first session. Surfacing these expectations enables nutrition counselors to either work toward meeting those expectations or to help clients adjust to more realistic expectations.

Invite clients to give feedback, and receive it openly. Keep in mind, though, if nutrition counselors become defensive, clients are not likely to share their feelings again. Counselors must show their openness to feedback. For instance:

> My role is to help you to make changes in your eating behaviors. Since everyone is different, I want to adapt my approach to best meet your needs and I need your input to do that. As we work together, I'd like you to share your thoughts and feelings about the way I approach your nutrition care—not just the pleasant feelings either. I need to know how you are feeling about the process as we go along.

Encourage clients to set realistic goals, broken down into incremental steps. Goals become a measuring stick for clients, and they communicate clients' expectations of the results of nutrition counseling to the counselor. A comparison of results to the goals provides direct feedback.

On an ongoing basis, check with clients to see how they are feeling about the counselors and the process. A counselor might say:

> Mary, I'd like to take a few minutes before we close to find out whether our sessions are meeting your needs. What has helped you the most in our meetings? What could I do to be more helpful to you?

Common questions nutrition counselors use to do this include:

- "How do you feel about the counseling process?"
- "How would you like to alter the counseling process to make it more productive for you?"
- "You said you are 'disappointed with your results.' What were your expectations?"
- "How have you benefited by the counseling process so far?"

It can be difficult to ask questions like these if the counselor's "gut" reaction is that things aren't progressing as they should be. Sometimes, counselors are just not sure they want to hear the answer. That is when it is most important to hear the answer. Like it or not, counselors can only be successful if they know what the problems are. You and your counselors cannot respond to problems that are never surfaced.

Tune in to nonverbal messages, as well as the verbal ones. Nutrition counselors must concentrate not only on the explicit meaning of the message, but also on the implicit meaning—unspoken words and undertones that may be far more significant. Ideas for more objective assessments of client satisfaction follow.

For groups, a group discussion of the education or counseling process may net the most information because clients feel more comfortable expressing themselves in a group. Such discussions should not be delayed until the last session. Use all available opportunities to gather both verbal and nonverbal feedback. Then, techniques and presentations can be altered to meet the needs of the group before participants are lost.

If clients are hesitant to criticize the nutrition counselor in a face-to-face conversation, surveys may provide more feedback. These surveys can be done in the form of follow-up phone calls, mailings, or handouts provided immediately before or after a session, usually by a third party. A third party ensures anonymity of those clients who are timid. Not only are clients often more honest in their evaluation of a counselor to a third party, but a more accurate summary of the information may be obtained. Research suggests that service providers who conduct their own evaluations with customers have a tendency to skew the data. They tend to hear the messages they agree with more strongly than those they disagree with.

When preparing client satisfaction surveys, choose questions that answer the ultimate question:

"Is this practice meeting the needs and expectations of its clients?"

Use open-ended questions to encourage clients to provide comments and constructive criticisms. The following list of questions may help you prepare satisfaction surveys that relate to your services and programs. Remember, this is just a list and does not illustrate survey format.

If you ask a question, be prepared to respond to the comments/criticisms with actions.

CLIENT SATISFACTION SURVEY QUESTIONS

1. Rate the counselor on the following characteristics and please make comments.
   - Putting you at ease
   - Understanding your needs and problems
   - Encouraging you to set your own goals
   - Aiding you in planning behavior changes
   - Supporting your plans
   - Offering encouragement
   - Tailoring dietary recommendations to your individual needs
   - Answering your questions accurately
   - Meeting your nutrition needs
   - Speaking clearly and using terms you understand.
2. Were you satisfied with the accessibility of the counselor by telephone? If not, why?
3. Was the information provided on the services before you enrolled in a service program adequate?
4. Was the physical counseling setting appropriate? If no, what changes would you suggest?

5. How much time elapsed between the day you made the appointment and the first nutrition counseling session?
6. Was this lapse: Too long? Too short? Adequate?
7. How would you improve the process of making appointments?
8. Rate the following with regard to the receptionist:

    - Courteous
    - Helpful
    - Able to provide all the information you needed
    - Responsive to your needs
    - Adaptable to unforseen circumstances
    - Available when you called.

9. How often did you wait beyond your scheduled appointment to be seen by the nutrition counselor in the waiting room? How long did you wait (give shortest to longest time)?
10. Was your session ever canceled? If yes, was the reason explained? Were you given enough notice? Would you have preferred seeing another counselor instead of rescheduling?
11. Were you informed of the counseling fees prior to the first session?
12. What improvements would you suggest in the handling of payment? (You may want to list the options.)
13. Rate the following characteristics of the location and give any suggestions for improvement:

    - Parking
    - Convenience
    - Safety
    - Lighting
    - Temperature
    - Seating
    - General comfort.

14. List the various program topics and ask for comments on each.
15. Was the counselor/dietitian:

    - Well prepared
    - Easy to understand
    - Able to facilitate discussion
    - Courteous?

16. What suggestions do you have for improving the counselors effectiveness?
17. Which handouts did you find most helpful? Why?
    Which handouts did you find least helpful? Why?

18. Was the number of participants in the group: Appropriate? Too many? Too few?
19. Is there a day and time that would have better suited your schedule? If yes, please note.
20. Was the sequence of the topics appropriate? What changes would you suggest?
21. Was the length of the program: Appropriate? Too long? Too short?
22. What other topics would you have wanted to discuss?
23. What help did you receive in obtaining reimbursement from your insurance company?
24. Are there other ways we might have assisted the reimbursement process?
25. Would you recommend this program to a friend? Why or why not?
26. What improvements could we make to better serve you?

You might consider developing a "customer report card" of key measures. (Albrecht, 1988). The report card would be a list of key service factors upon which you want clients to evaluate the practice.

A system for automatically following up on clients who miss individual sessions and those who drop out of group programs should be in place. This practice can prevent permanent loss of a client, as well as provide information on problem areas. The questions on the previous pages can be used for follow-up on drop outs, as well as for clients who finish programs.

A suggestion box can be placed in your waiting room as another means of gathering feedback.

For groups, written evaluations completed at the end or immediately after the session are useful. If at all possible, ask that they be completed during a session, rather than after a session or through mailing. The return on mail evaluations is no better than the return on market surveys. Provide at *least* two opportunities to evaluate (one mid-session and one at the end), even when asking for written evaluation. Follow-up calls to those who do not complete group programs are imperative.

Keep records of attendance, participation in other programs, continuation of individual sessions, and referrals of other clients. Indirectly, client satisfaction can be determined through use of your services.

Worksite Client Satisfaction

Worksite practitioners must monitor client satisfaction in much the same way as all other nutrition practitioners. Yet certain interests of sponsoring worksite organizations can be a little different. A primary difference is that worksite nutrition programs serve the needs of two lords—users (those who use your services) and sponsoring organizations. Remember that the benefits to each lord are very different. The needs of both must be served in order for your practice to be successful. Understand how both the user and the sponsoring organization will measure success or failure, and consistently monitor those areas of performance. Ask:

- "How will you (the worksite administrators) judge our effectiveness?"
- "Can you make any suggestions for improving our program at your worksite?"
- "What feedback have you received that would help us better meet your needs and the needs of your employees?"

Summary progress reports presented to your liaison on an on-going basis will maintain consistent contact. Don't assume that "no news is good news." Keep checking back with your organizational liaison to learn how they are perceiving service delivery, receiving any feedback with appreciation. Don't be defensive.

Inform the worksite client liaisons early in the process of your intention to have participants evaluate services. Explain that you will share all information with them. Evaluation throughout the service delivery period enables you to make adjustments to your approach and to your service programs. Some clients are inclined to create their own evaluation. It is to your advantage if you can present the information to the client, rather than the other way around. That way you have the opportunity to present resolutions along with criticism. You also have the opportunity to highlight positive results and feedback.

Referring Agent Satisfaction

Referring agents, such as physicians, are more difficult to obtain feedback from because their time is limited. Nonetheless, their satisfaction is of utmost importance to the growth and maintenance of the practice. Your best indicators of their satisfaction may be continued referrals, response to counselors' recommendations, organizational clients to whom the physician recommended your programs, and word of mouth.

A common complaint among the physicians who participated in the focus groups conducted nationally was the lack of feedback from nutrition counselors. By providing more feedback to the physicians, you may be able to gain more from them. Any feedback done by phone or in person allows you the perfect opportunity to ask for an evaluation in return, and it serves as a consistent reminder of your support. Silence is not golden in the marketing arena.

Written evaluations/surveys sent through the mail will seldom be returned. Therefore, personal contacts with the physician or his or her staff are recommended. Visiting the office at convenient times, phone calls, luncheons with groups of physicians, and networking are all ways to reach the referring agents and to determine their level of satisfaction. You might even ask referring agents to speak at various programs, and speak to them before or after the event.

If you are marketing to organizations for worksite nutrition programs, ask a variety of referring agents for letters of endorsement. This will help you determine which agents support your efforts and in what ways.

If you are providing nutrition counseling in the physician's office, a feedback mechanism should be set in place prior to beginning such services. Ask for a regularly scheduled meeting. As a member of the office staff, nutrition counselors may also gain feedback through office meetings, conversations with office support staff, and medical record notes from the physician regarding nutrition counseling. A brief questionnaire could be attached to monthly reports. In the physician's office, the best indicator of satisfaction is the renewal of your contract.

Satisfaction of Administration

Experience shows that administrators get into the outpatient nutrition business primarily for two reasons:

1. Additional revenue; and
2. To attract patients and market other services.

You must understand what has motivated your administrators to support your practice. Ask for expectations to be outlined. Know what results are expected each week, month, and year. Monitor actual results against these targets. Know what reports are expected and when.

The satisfaction of administration will generally rest with the achievement of expected results. If results are not achieved, don't wait for someone to point this out. Instead, act quickly. Respond to the discrepancy with an action plan regarding how you intend to get results back on track. In general, relate to administration as a private practitioner would relate to a banker. (Administration will only support the practice as long as it continues to be a viable business venture or directly supports one.)

If marketing the institution is a primary purpose for administration's support, be sure you track referrals to other services and report the results to administration on an ongoing basis. You might also track the number of people new to the hospital who are using your services.

Obviously, there is more to monitoring satisfaction than tracking results. Create and take advantage of every opportunity to understand the perceptions of administrators. Keep in mind that they will be influenced by the perceptions of other formal and informal leaders within the institution. So keep your ears open and solicit input from employees and department heads throughout the institution.

Growth and Financial Progress

Your finance department or accountant will be able to help you set up a record keeping system that will meet the needs of your practice. Growth and financial progress should be tracked on a weekly, monthly, and yearly basis. Not only will you want to keep track of dollars, but also number of clients, number of sessions, and how time is spent. In relating these factors to your profits, you can determine changes you need to make in your practice to meet your financial goals. Another factor that institutional practices will need to look at is whether the practice refers clients to other programs within the institution.

Develop a record-keeping system that provides information you need to evaluate the progress and future of your business. In any case, records should be easy to understand and maintain.

Although administrators and other management staff may only ask for reports on a monthly basis, there are items that you must track on a more frequent time schedule so that you can react to the information before a month has passed. This is especially critical in start-up situations. For example, recording financial transactions as they occur seems only logical. Also, a weekly record of "no-shows" and dropouts allows you to follow up promptly, dealing with problems before they cause a greater loss of clients. Table 9-1 lists information you may wish to gather and the frequency with which it should be recorded.

TABLE 9-1 Frequency of Recording Various Data

Frequency	Information to record
As the event occurs	Follow-up phone calls Financial transactions Number attending any group session No shows to individual and group sessions
Daily	Number of new clients Number of returning clients Number of "no shows"
Weekly	Number of programs presented Ongoing participation in each program Income and profit from each service Expenses
Monthly	Cash flow Income statement Expense report Summary of activities
Annually	Cost/benefit analysis

If there is more than one counselor in the practice, each one will have a separate report for daily and weekly activities. If you are selling taxable products, you must record that income in a separate column, because you will report it to the state Department of Revenue for quarterly tax payments. Learn what information is desired on a monthly basis and organize your reporting accordingly. See Figure 9-1 for a sample of a practitioner's monthly report for a weight management program.

Your actual results must be compared to projections you have made so that you may identify the strengths and weaknesses and make necessary changes and

MONTHLY REPORT

Month of ________________________________

Marketing Programs

Number of times presented	________
Number of people attending	________
Time spent	________

Group Programs

Number of new classes started	________
Number of participants attending	________
Number of participants in ongoing classes	________
Time spent	________

Follow-up Programs

Number of sessions presented	________
Number of participants	________
Time spent	________

Revenue

Package program	________
Follow-up sessions	________
Extra individual sessions	________
Subtotal	________
Minus expenses	________
Profit	________

FIGURE 9-1. Sample monthly report form for a weight-management program.

improvements. Sample financial worksheets can be found in the Sample Strategic Plan in Chapter 4.

Since your promotional efforts are geared at growing your clientele and, in turn, your income, monitoring growth demands an evaluation of your promotional effectiveness. The questions to be answered in measuring promotional effectiveness are:

- Do the vehicles attract the clientele I have targeted?
- Are the vehicles attracting sufficient numbers?
- Could different messages, vehicles, placement, or timing increase business?
- Has the vehicle reached as many people as it is likely to reach? Is this an appropriate time to change vehicles?
- Are there less expensive ways of building the desired client flow?

Even advertising agencies find it extremely difficult to answer these questions. However, some measurements are typically used to evaluate advertisements.

Pretesting occurs prior to the ad's appearance in the media. One method of pretesting commonly used is a checklist. The checklist should include factors that you expect the ad to accomplish, such as attracting attention, arousing interest, and so on.

A consumer jury test can be conducted. In jury tests, clients or potential clients are asked to evaluate advertisements by comparing them to other ads. Or they may be asked questions regarding ads they have seen or heard, to determine the impact of the ad. The big disadvantage of pretesting lies in the setting; the ad will not be evaluated from its actual point of distribution (newspaper, radio, etc.). The jury may subconsciously think of the process as a test and pay more attention to details than the normal reader would.

During the course of the promotion, surveying clients and counting inquiries are the most common evaluation tools. Promotional efforts can be tracked by asking your clients how they learned of your services. You may also receive some feedback on the impact of ads by surveying your clients. Find out what they remember about the ad and why it affected them. Surveying can be done in the initial interview or as a part of the paperwork you ask them to complete (diet history, release form, etc.).

Other ways of tallying the number of clients drawn to your services through promotions is by coding coupons, registration forms, and so on. For instance, a practice promoted its weight management programs through direct mail, physicians offices, and posters with tear-off cards in the grocery store. The registration cards in each promotion were different colors. Therefore, all that was necessary to determine how many clients were drawn to the program was to count the different colored cards. You can use this data to determine which promotions afford you the greatest number of clients. Unfortunately, it is virtually impossible to determine what other behavioral and psychological factors have influenced the sale.

Posttesting can be conducted once promotion has been done. The evaluation measures used are recognition/readership tests and recall tests. Essentially, recognition/readership tests are surveys to determine whether the ad was read or heard. Recall tests determine (also through a survey technique) what people remember about a promotion. These methods will help you decide whether the ad was effective or not, but they will not give you information regarding the influence of the ad on the purchase.

If you contract an advertising agency, they will aid you in evaluating promotions. Marketing departments can also be of assistance. However, you will find that much of your promotion efforts are trial and error. More important than knowing that your promotion campaign is a success may be recognizing failures and remedying them.

When a promotion fails, it is difficult to know why it has failed. You may have the right vehicle, but timing and/or location may be wrong. Price may be wrong. Or the value of the service may not be clearly communicated. Sometimes it is worth your while to try the promotional vehicle again, altering some of the factors.

Cost/Benefit Analysis

As the pursuit of third-party payment for nutrition services has grown along with the need to demonstrate the value of nutrition services, cost/benefit analysis and cost effectiveness analysis have become an integral part of outpatient nutrition practice monitoring. The goal in cost/benefit analysis is to maintain or improve health outcomes at the lowest cost without compromising quality (Simko, 1989). Therefore, cost/benefit analysis requires monitoring of more than finances. It requires monitoring effectiveness in terms of health outcomes.

Three considerations must be made in developing a system of monitoring effectiveness:

1. What parameters will be measured?
2. What method of collecting and recording data will be used?
3. Who will the comparison group consist of?

Measurable health outcomes must be determined for each service you provide. Such parameters could include weight gain/loss, changes in blood cholesterol, hemoglobin levels, infant mortality, and so on. Once parameters have been chosen, a system for collecting the data and recording it will be necessary. Three resources that may aid you in collecting cost/benefit data are: 1) the skills training program developed by the Nutrition Services Payment System Committee of the ADA, available through state NSPS representatives (Dougherty, 1989), 2) *Costs and Benefits of Nutrition Services: A Literature Review* (Disbrow, 1989), and

3) *Effectiveness and Cost Effectiveness of Nutrition Care: A Critical Analysis with Recommendations* (Splett, 1991).

You can compare the results of your methodologies to the national statistics, a control group, or the results of other research using similar methodologies. In any case, a comparison group should be determined at the onset of data collection (Simko, 1989).

MONITORING AND ADAPTING TO CHANGING DEMANDS

Over time, health concerns change, some products/services become obsolete, new opportunities arise, and institutional goals mature. As these changes evolve, so must the practice. Periodic evaluation and continued market research are ways to stay informed of such changes.

Business plans are not set in stone. As actual revenues and expenses are compared to projections, some discrepancies will arise. Perhaps some services are seasonal, or perhaps new information in the media has caused an increase in demand for some services or products. The quicker that services can be adapted to consider this information, the greater the potential for success.

Although consumer-orientation is the driving force in the marketing concept, consumer demands are not the sole reason for adapting services. Managers must open their ears to the institution, referring agents, the staff, and the competition. Thus, market analysis and adaptation must be perpetual in the life of a successful outpatient nutrition practice.

Successful practitioners update their market research on a regular basis. They review current literature (both professional and lay) to be aware of changes in health, disease prevention and treatment, and health care delivery. They network to gain information on the competition and the possibilities for new clients and services. Just as being first with a product or service is an important marketing strategy at the onset of a practice, it is also important to the maintenance and growth of that practice.

Chapter 10

Conclusion

The word pioneer has been mentioned consistently throughout this text and rightly so. We applaud the outpatient nutrition practitioners who blazed these new frontiers. They demonstrated enthusiasm, innovation, a dedication to the nutrition profession, and the courage to take risks.

The pioneers interviewed during the research stage took issue with this view. Many said that the characteristic that spurred them into action was much more basic—a strong survival instinct. They had the vision to see the changes afoot. They recognized that inpatient career opportunities were shrinking, patients and clients needed and wanted more than the limited nutrition education provided in the inpatient setting, and the reputation of the profession was at stake because current approaches to nutrition care did not produce the expected results—eating behavior change. They ventured into these unchartered territories as a matter of survival.

Yet, like the pioneers who first explored our land 200 years ago, the casualties have been high. A small percentage of those first outpatient nutrition practices survived. It's no wonder, considering how ill-prepared they were.

The profession has learned much from these pioneers, and the beneficial knowledge has been shared through the chapters of this book. Today's outpatient nutrition practitioners have taken the blindfolds off, confronting their decisions about venturing into this business with a clear understanding of what is involved. The authors' intentions were to change attitudes for consideration, provide successful approaches, and stimulate nutrition practitioners to build profitable outpatient practices. Using the information contained in this book, coupled with business management skills and an entrepreneurial spirit, today's outpatient nutrition practitioners are moving the profession from the "pioneering stage" to the "homesteading stage." Pioneers forged forward, facing unanticipated opportunities and obstacles. The homesteaders learned from the pioneers. They took calculated risks and anticipated a prosperous and rewarding life. They knew that they had their work cut out for them, but they were prepared for the challenges they faced. Today's outpatient nutrition practitioners look to the future with insight into its opportunities. They can fortify themselves with the knowledge and skills to plant roots that will grow and prosper. They build nutrition practices with firm foundations. They will insist on and properly manage the necessary financial and nonfinancial resources. They will expand their own capabilities to meet the changing and intensifying consumer demand for nutrition services.

The business aspect of outpatient nutrition services may seem overwhelming at first glance. Overcoming the perceptions of low value and physician control may seem insurmountable. No pioneer in this business would say that building a profitable practice is easy. However, just like learning new eating habits, it is a stepwise process that can be accomplished with counsel, support, and perseverance. Pioneers who now run successful outpatient practices eagerly admit that the rewards are worth the long hours and hard work. Beyond the reward of satisfaction from building and growing a profitable outpatient practice, practitioners gain recognition from their institutions, their referral agents, and their professional peers. They have acquired new skills and an expanded knowledge base in having established a business, a feat outside the realm of nutrition. They have the pride of self-improvement.

Hopefully, this text has sparked a greater enthusiasm and a growing determination in you to stake your claim and homestead your outpatient nutrition practice.

Glossary

Some of the terms commonly used throughout this book that may need clarification follow.

Business plan refers to a document that outlines the financial expectations of a business or a single service. The business plan may include an outline of strategies to reach both financial and nonfinancial goals.

Client refers to recipients of nutrition education and counseling services.
Colleague refers to nutrition practitioners within the same practice.
Counselor refers to nutrition counselors.

Group setting refers to group counseling, support groups, and group education classes.

Individual setting refers to individual education and counseling sessions.
Institutional nutrition practitioner refers to all nutrition professionals providing nutrition education and counseling services in an outpatient practice associated with a health care institution. The term is not intended to serve as a title. Several states now regulate the practice of dietetics and nutrition counseling. Contact your state dietetic association in order to determine the licensure and advertising regulations of the state in which you intend to practice in an outpatient practice.

Marketing refers to the planning and managing of strategies to provide profitable services and/or products.
Market mix refers to the management of the four key areas of marketing decision making. The four key areas are: 1) product and service, 2) place, 3) price, and 4) promotion.
Market segment refers to a group within the population whose members share similar characteristics and buying practices.

Market share as it applies to nutrition practices, refers to the percent of the nutrition business a practice has gained within a specified market segment. (Usually, market share is measured in terms of potential dollars to be spent on nutrition services on an annual basis.)

Networking is the process of gathering information and obtaining support for the business through personal contacts, usually of an informal nature.

Nutrition counselor is used throughout the text as a generic term describing all nutrition professionals providing nutrition education and counseling. The term is not intended to serve as a title. Several states now regulate the practice of dietetics and nutrition counseling. Contact your state dietetic association in order to determine the licensure and advertising regulations of the state in which you intend to practice.

Nutrition practitioner refers to all nutrition professionals providing nutrition education and counseling services in an outpatient practice. The term is not intended to serve as a title. Several states now regulate the practice of dietetics and nutrition counseling. Contact your state dietetic association in order to determine the licensure and advertising regulations of the state in which you intend to practice in an outpatient practice.

Organizational client refers to any organization contracting for outpatient nutrition services to be delivered to members. The organization may be a special interest or community group. In this context, organization usually refers to a nonprofit group.

Packaged programs refers to the combination of a specified number of services or sessions for a combined price.

Practice refers to the business entity established to offer professional nutrition services.

Practitioner refers specifically to nutrition practitioners (*see* nutrition practitioner).

Private nutrition practitioner refers to all nutrition professionals providing nutrition education and counseling services in a private practice. The term is not intended to serve as a title. Several states now regulate the practice of dietetics and nutrition counseling. Contact your state dietetic association in order to determine the licensure and advertising regulations of the state in which you intend to practice in an outpatient practice.

Private practice refers specifically to the business entity established to offer professional nutrition services that is not affiliated with an institution.

Promotion refers to marketing and communication strategies designed to:

- Increase awareness of the services or products;
- Persuade current clients to use more of the services or products; and

- Persuade users of competitive services to use your services.

  The term advertising is often confused with promotion. Advertising is only one form of promotion.

Referral agents refers to those individuals or organizations, usually physicians, nursing staff, health care administrative staff, or health organizations, who refer clients to the practice.

Strategic planning is a process of assessing needs and developing strategies to reach organizational goals.

Survival kit refers to nutrition instruction and materials provided to the client by an inpatient dietitian for use until further instruction and counseling can be provided by an outpatient nutrition counselor.

Target market is a market segment that a business directs its services and products toward and, therefore, its marketing strategies.

Worksite refers to the physical location where employees or organizational members work and meet, respectively.

Worksite nutrition practitioner refers to all nutrition professionals providing nutrition education and counseling services in a worksite setting. The term is not intended to serve as a title. Several states now regulate the practice of dietetics and nutrition counseling. Contact your state dietetic association in order to determine the licensure and advertising regulations of the state in which you intend to practice in an outpatient practice.

You refers to the person or persons responsible for planning, establishing, and managing the outpatient nutrition practice.

FURTHER READINGS

Negotiating and Selling

Nierenberg, Gerard I. 1990. *The Art of Negotiating* (cassette and text). International Center for Creative Thinking. Mamaroneck, NY.

Nierenberg, Gerard I. 1987. *Fundamentals of Negotiating*. New York: Harper and Row.

Cohen, Herb. 1983: *You Can Negotiate Anything*. New York: Bantam Books, Inc.

Selling Skills

Fisher, Roger and William L. Ury. 1983. *Getting to Yes: Negotiating Agreement Without Giving In*. New York: Penguin Books.

Rackman, Neil. 1989. *Major Account Sales Strategy*. New York: McGraw-Hill Publishing Co.

Worksite Nutrition Programs

Seidel, Miriam C., R.D. 1983. Consulting nutritionist in an employee health office. *Journal of the American Dietetic Association*, Vol. 82, No. 4.

Berry, Charles A., M.D., M.P.H. 1981. Good Health for Employees and Reduced Health Care Costs for Industry. Health Insurance Association of America.

Journal of Nutrition Education (Supplement). 18(2): April 1986.

Why is Nutrition Important to Business? Washington Business Group on Health, Institute on Organizational Health, Office of Disease Prevention and Health Promotion, U.S. Dept. of Health and Human Resources.

Business and Health. Washington Business Group on Health, Box 33039, Washington, D.C. 20033.

Corporate Commentary. Washington Business Group on Health, 229 1/2 Pennsylvania Ave., Washington, D.C. 20003.

Corporate Fitness and Recreation. Corporate Fitness and Recreation, Brentwood Publishing Corp., 825 Barrington Ave., Los Angeles, CA 90049.

Employee Health and Fitness. American Health Consultants, 67 Peachtree Park Drive, NE, Atlanta, GA 30309.

Worksite Health Promotion. Health Education Quarterly (1982 special issue). Human Sciences Press, 72 Fifth Ave., New York, NY 10011.

Fielding, Jonathan E., and Philip V. Piserchia. 1989. Frequency of worksite health promotion activities. *Am J Pub Health*, MS, Vol. 79, No. 1.

Berry, M.W., W.J. Rinke, and H. Smickklas-Wright. 1989. Work-site health promotion: The effects of a goal-setting program on nutrition-related behaviors. *Journal of the American Dietetic Association* 89(7): 914–920.

Healthy People: The Surgeon General's Report on Health Promotion and Disease Prevention. DHEW Publ. No. (PHS)79-55071,1979.

National Report of Worksite Health Promotion Activities: A Summary. Office of Disease and Health Promotion, DHHS Publ. No. (PHS)88-129390, 1987.

Promotion Health Preventing Disease: Objectives for the Nation. Washington, D.C.: Department of Health, Education and Welfare, 1979.

Davis, M.R., K. Rosenberg, D.E. Iverson, T.M. Vernon, and J. Bauer. 1984. Worksite health promotion in Colorado. *Public Health Reports* 99:538.

National Heart, Lung, and Blood Institute. 1984. *Demonstration Projects in Workplace High Blood Pressure Control: Summary Report*. DHHS, Public Health Service, NIH Publ. No. 84-2119. Washington, D.C.: Government Printing Office.

The American Dietetic Association, the Society for Nutrition Education, and the

Office of Disease Prevention and Health Promotion. 1986. *Worksite Nutrition: A Decision-Maker's Guide*. Chicago: American Dietetic Association.

Shannon, B., M. Hendricks, P. Rollins, and R. Schwartz. 1987. A comprehensive evaluation of worksite nutrition program and weight control program. *Journal of Nutrition Education* 19:109.

REFERENCES

Akron City Hospital. *Policy and Procedure Manual.* Akron City Hospital, 525 E. Market St., Akron, OH 44309.

Albrecht, Karl. 1988. *At America's Service.* Homewood, IL: Dow Jones-Irwin.

Albrecht, Karl and Ron Zemke. 1985. *Service America!* Homewood, IL: Dow Jones-Irwin.

Alford, Margaret M. 1986. A guide for nutrition educators at the worksite. *J Nutr Ed* 18(1):S19–S21.

ARA Healthcare Nutrition Services. 1988. *Nutrition Counselor: Strategies for Results, Controlling the Pace of Counseling.* Philadelphia: ARA Services.

Bell, Linda Schaffer and Michele M. Fairchild. 1989. Development of a productivity index to increase accountability of ambulatory nutrition services. *J Am Diet Assoc.* 89(4):517–519.

Benefits represent significant part of compensation. *Benefits Today* 6(9) 1989.

Berry, Charles A. 1981. *Good Health for Employees and Reduced Health Care Costs for Industry.* Health Insurance Association of America.

Business bulletins. 1987. *Small Business Reports.* 12(5):16.

Cohen, Dorothy. 1972. *Advertising.* New York: John Wiley and Sons.

Consulting Nutritionists in Private Practice. 1988. *Nutrition Services Payment System: Resource Packet.* Chicago: The American Dietetic Association.

Cross, Audrey Tittle. 1988. Malpractice liability in private practice of nutrition. *J Am Diet Assoc* 88(8):946–948.

Direct Mail Advertising Association. 1965. *What People Think About Direct Mail.* Summary of A Consumer Attitude Study Conducted by A.C. Nielson Company.

Disbrow, Doris D. 1989. The costs and benefits of nutrition services: A literature review. *J Am Diet Assoc* 89(4):supplement.

Dougherty, Darlene A. and Carol J. Gilmore. 1989. President's page: Documenting the economic costs and benefits of nutrition services. *J Am Diet Assoc* 89(4):549–550.

Dunlap, B.J. 1986. Marketing in the health care arena: A preventive approach. *J Am Diet Assoc* 86(1):29.

Earl, Robert. 1988. Payment and reimbursement for nutrition care services: Guidelines for registered dietitians. *Clin Mgt* 4(3):9–12.

Fielding, Jonathan E. and Philip V. Piserchia. 1989. Frequency of worksite health promotion activities. *Am J Pub Heal.* 79:16–20.

Finn, Susan Calvert and Wolf Rinke. 1989. Probing the envelope of dietetics by transforming challenges into opportunities. *J Am Diet Assoc* 89(10):1441.

Forke, Donna and Shirley Hunt. 1986. Factors related to implementation of worksite nutrition programs. *J Nutr Ed* 18(1):S29–S31.

Glanz, Karen. 1986. *Nutrition Programs in the Workplace.* Prevention Leadership Forum. Washington, D.C.: Washington Business Group on Health.

Goldsmith, J. 1989. A radical prescription for hospitals. *Harv Bus Rev* 89:104.

Halling, James F. 1986. Marketing mind set: A concept mandated for success in dietetics. *Topics in Clin Nutr* 1(3):21-26.

Haschke, Marilyn B. 1984. President's page: Marketing in dietetics. *J Am Diet Assoc* 84(8):933.

Health care costs for businesses soared in 1988, manufacturers' survey shows. *Wall Street Journal.* A2. 1989.

Helm, Kathy King. 1987. *The Entrepreneurial Nutritionist.* New York: Harper and Row.

Hess, Mary Abbott. 1988. Reflections on the hundredth monkey: The new consciousness in dietetics. *J Amer Diet Assoc* 88:669.

Hysen, P. 1989. Business plans get results. *Food Mgt* 24:101.

Joseph, Hugh M., Janet Andelis, and Rozanne Kapitan. 1986. The business of providing worksite nutrition programs. *J Nutr Ed* 18(1):S16-S18.

Kernaghan, Salvinija G. and Barbara E. Giloth. 1984. *Working with Physicians in Health Promotion.* Chicago: American Hospital Publishing.

Koteski, D.R. and S. McKinney. 1988. Who does the public think should perform health care tasks? *J Am Diet Assoc* 88(10):1281.

Kotler, Philip. 1971. *Marketing Decision Making: A Model Building Approach.* New York: Holt, Rinehart and Winston.

Kotler, Philip. 1982. *Marketing for Non-Profit Organizations* (2nd edition). Englewood Cliffs, NJ: Prentice Hall.

Laumer, J. Ford and Robert C. Erffmeyer. *Researching Your Market.* Business Development Publication MT 8. U.S. Small Business Administration.

Laumer, J. Ford, J.R. Harris, H.J. Guffey, and R.C. Erffmeyer. 1988. *Researching Your Market.* Management Aid. U.S. Small Business Administration.

Lewis, R.C. 1984. Theoretical and practical considerations in research design. *The Cornell Hotel and Restaurant Administration Quarterly* 24:25.

Major, Michael J. 1986. Beating Burnout and Promoting Productivity. *Mod Off Tech* 60.

Mancuso, Joseph R. 1983. *How to Prepare and Present a Business Plan.* New York: Prentice Hall.

Maslach, Cristinia. 1982. *Burnout—The Cost of Caring.* Englewood Cliffs, NJ: Prentice Hall.

Monsen, Elaine R. 1989. For your information: Editor's outlook. *J Am Diet Assoc* 89(10):1429.

Moosbrugger, Mary C. 1986. Market research helps manage the risk of product development. *Prom Heal*:4-10.

Mullis, Rebecca M. and Darlene Lansing. 1986. Using focus groups to plan worksite nutrition programs. *J Nutr Ed* 18(1):S32-S33.

Murray, Janet, Barbara Shannon, and Laura Sims. 1986. Nutrition as a component of health promotion programs in the northeast. *J Nutr Ed* 18(1):S25-S29.

Murray, Nancy. Achieve TPR: methods and mechanics. 1985. *Clin Mgt.* 1(1):1-3.

Parks, Sara C. and Debra L. Moody. 1986. Marketing: A survival tool for dietetic professionals in the 1990s. *J Am Diet Assoc* 86(1):33.

Parks, Sara C. and Debra L. Moody. 1986. A marketing model: Applications for dietetic professionals. *J Am Diet Assoc* 86(1):37-43.

Policastro. *Developing a Strategic Business Plan.* Business Development Publication MP21. U.S. Small Business Administration.

Raab, Constance and Jeanne Tillotson (eds.) 1983. *Heart to Heart: A Manual on Nutrition Counseling for the Reduction of Cardiovascular Disease Risk Factors.* Washington, D.C., U.S. Government Printing Office.

Rose, James C. 1986. Effective financial management: An essential component of marketing. *Topics in Clin Nutr* 1(3):59-67.

Rose, James C. 1989. *How to Write a Business Plan. Hosp Food & Nutr Focus Special Report.* Rockville, MD: Aspen Publishers.

Ross Professional Development Series. 1989. *Linking Strategies for Dietitians Networking, Liaison Building, and Mentoring.* Columbus: Ross.

Ross, Susan. 1987. Adult learning theory: Application to weight- management. *Nutr News* 50(2):5.

Seidel, Miriam C. 1983. Consulting nutritionist in an employee health office. *J Am Diet Assoc* 82(4).

Shaw, Marvin E. 1971. *Group Dynamics: The Psychology of Small Group Behavior.* New York: McGraw-Hill.

Simko, Margaret D. and Martha T. Conklin. 1989. Focusing on the effectiveness side of the cost-effectiveness equation. *J Am Diet Assoc* 89(4):485-487.

Splett, Patricia L. 1991. Effectiveness and cost effectiveness of nutrition care: A critical analysis with recommendations. *J Am Diet Assoc* (Supplement): S1-S55.

The American Dietetics Association. 1988. Code of Ethics for the Profession of Dietetics. *J Am Diet Assoc* 88(12):1592-1593.

The American Dietetic Association. 1985. *Nutrition Services Payment System: Guidelines for Implementation.* Chicago: The American Dietetic Association.

The American Dietetic Association. 1986. *The Competitive Edge: Marketing Strategies for the Registered Dietitian.* Chicago: The American Dietetic Association.

U.S. Small Business Administration. *Marketing for Small Business: An Overview.* Business Development Publications MT2.

Vickery, Constance E. and Patricia Hodges. 1986. Counseling strategies for dietary management: Expanded possibilities for effecting behavior change. *J Amer Diet Assoc* 86(7):924.

Ward, Marcia. 1984. *Marketing Strategies.* Johnson City, NY: Marcia Ward.

Wellman, Nancy S. and Mary Kay Fox. 1990. President's page: The Midas touch. *J Am Diet Assoc* 90(9):1278-1281.

Zemke, Ron and Susan Zemke. 1981. 30 things we know for sure about adult learning. *Mag Hum Res Dir:* supplement entitled *Training.*

Zifferblatt, Steven M. and Curtis Wilbur. 1977. Dietary counseling: Some realistic expectations and guidelines. *J Amer Diet Assoc* 70:591.

Index

Administrative support staff, role of, 77
Administrators
  common objections to service, 133, 134-138
  monitoring satisfaction of, 312
  selling services to, 131-133
Adult learning, nature of, 6
Advertising, 214-224
  brochures, 216
  choice of methods, 214
  newspaper advertising, 217-220
  nutrition fairs, 223-224
  preview sessions, 214
  printed ads, 214-215
  promotion incentives, 220-223
  Yellow Pages listings, 215-216
American Dietetic Association, 7, 23, 190
American Hospital Association Guide, 36
AMI, 36
Assets, balance sheet analysis, 89
AUBER Bibliography of Publications of University Bureaus of Business and Economic Research, 37
Automobile accidents, non-owned automobile liability, 179

Bad debt, 82-83
Balance sheet analysis, 88-90
  assets, 89
  equity, 89-90
  liabilities, 89
Behavior change
  survival kit approach, 14
  time factors, 5
Billing statement, 188
  sample of, 189
Break even analysis, 90-93
  break even point, 90-91, 92
  in case study, 128-129
  fixed expenses, 91
  graphical representation, 93
  process of, 91-93
  variable expenses, 91
Brochures, 216
  examples of, 228-229
Burn-out, 202, 203
Business plan, 20
Business strategies
  in case study, 108-114
  innovation, 64-65
  location of service, 65-67
  positioning, 63-64
  price of service, 68-76
  promotion, 76
  scheduling, 78-79
  staffing, 76-78

Cancellation of appointments, handling of, 153
Capital expenditures, 84-85
Capitated plans, 193
Cash flow projections, 86-88
  and start-up costs, 87-88
  steps in preparation of, 87
Cash flow statement
  in case study, 120, 128
  and profit and loss statements, 88
Chart notes, SOAP system, 162
Claims-made policy, liability insurance, 179
Client information, record-keeping, 162
Clients
  assignment of clients to counselors, 175
  client satisfaction survey questions, 308-310
  concerns of, 5-6
  monitoring satisfaction of, 306-311
  orientation packet to, 151
  promotions to, 235-236
  reasons for using nutrition services, 9
Clinics, as location of service, 66-67
Code of ethics, for dietetics profession, 182-184
Communications, 153-155
  courtesy in, 154
  face-to-face communication, 155
  with physicians, 241-242
  telephone communication, 154-155
  of up-to-date information, 155
  written communication, 155
Community expense, 83
Community exposure, publicity, 212
Community facilities, as location of service, 67
Community needs, and strategic planning, 25
Compensation program, 175-176
  determining appropriate program, 175-176

Competition
analysis in case study, 103-106
analysis of, 55-56, 58
indirect competition, 56
nature of, 55
and pricing, 70
rules for competing, 261-262
and selling of worksite program, 260-261
strengths and weaknesses analysis, 56, 58-59
competitive advantages, 58
competitive disadvantages, 58
opportunities, 59
threats, 59
Comprehensive general liability, 179
Computer programs, nutrition evaluations, 28
Confidentiality, 158-159
Contests
ideas for, 223
promotion incentives, 222-223
Contracts, 180
Copayment, 75
Cost/benefit analysis, 316-317
resources to aid in, 316-317
Counseling
encouraging ongoing counseling, 158
ensuring sound counseling and recommendations, 157-158
group counseling, 13-14, 27
individual counseling, 13, 26
and nutrition service, 13
Coupons
example of, 221
promotion incentives, 220-221
Credit cards, for payment, 160

Databases, as information source, 38
Demand, and pricing, 69-70
Dentists, as referral source, 244
Depreciation, meaning of, 85
Desired return, and pricing, 70-71
Diabetes educator, job description, 163-174
Direct influence, nutrition service, 25
Direct mail, 224-226
advantages of, 224-225
best use of, 225
costs of, 226
disadvantages of, 225
sources for mailing lists, 225
Disciplinary action, establishment of, 176
Documentation, and reimbursement for services, 186, 188, 190
Dress code, 176

Education
group education, 26-27
individual education, 26
and nutrition service, 11, 13
Employment contracts, 174-175
Entrepreneurship, nature of, 15
Environmental interventions, nutrition service, 27
Equipment
cost of, 81
depreciation, 85
types needed, 81
Equity, balance sheet analysis, 89-90
Ethics, code of ethics for dietetics profession, 181-183
Executive summary, 139-141
example of, 140, 141, 143
features of, 139-140
Expenses, 84-85
capital expenditures, 84-85
expense worksheet, 116-119
fixed expenses, 91
inventory expenses, 84
matching to revenue, 85-86
period expenses, 84
variable expenses, 91

Financial analysis
balance sheet analysis, 88-90
break-even analysis, 90-93
in case study, 114-129
cash flow analysis, 86-88
monitoring financial progress, 313-316
profit and loss projections, 83-86
start-up costs
bad debt, 82-83
community expense, 83
equipment, 81
labor costs, 81
overhead, 80
professional fees, 82
program licensure fees, 81
promotional costs, 82
supplies, 81-82
training and education, 82
travel expenses, 82
in strategic plan, 144
Financial goals, 62
Financial officers, 16
Financial planning, 79-94
Fixed expenses, 91
Food products, 28-29
types of, 28-29
Food service director, 16
Fraudulent services, 7
Free products/services, valuation of, 29
Fringe benefits, 68

Gifts, promotion incentives, 222
Giveaways
promotion incentives, 221
types of, 222
Goal setting, 62-63
in case study, 107-108
financial goals, 62
nonfinancial goals, 62-63
Group programs
group counseling, 27
group education, 26-27
nutrition services, 13-14
Guidelines
assignment of clients to counselors, 175
for communications, 153-155

compensation program, 175-176
for confidentiality, 158-159
disciplinary action, 176
for dress code, 176
employment contracts, 174-175
for office policies and procedures, 158
for payment for services, 159-161
for personalization of services, 155-154
for personnel management, 163
policies related to delivery of service, 148-149
for productivity, 163, 174
for record-keeping, 161-163
reimbursement for services, 184-193
for scheduling of clients, 149-153
for sound counseling/ recommendations, 156-158
statement of philosophy, 148

Health care institutions, concerns related to nutrition, 6-7
Healthcare professionals, 244-245
liaisoning with, 244-245
networking with, 244-245
Hospital stay, decreased length of, 5
Hospitals, as location of service, 66

Income statement. *See* Profit and loss projections
Individual programs
individual counseling, 26
individual education, 26
Information gathering, sales process, 268-271
Innovation, value of, 64-65
Institutional practice, advantages of, 16-17
Insurance, liability insurance, 179
Intrapreneurship
and institutional practice, 16
nature of, 15
and nutrition services, 15-16
Inventory expenses, 84

Job description, diabetes educator, 163-174

Labor costs, 81
Lateness, and scheduling, 152
Legal agreements
components of binding agreement, 179
content of, 180-181
contracts, 180-181
letters of agreement, 180
proprietary rights, 181
verbal agreements, 180
Legal issues, professionals for, 177-178
Letters of agreement, 180
content of, 180-181
Liabilities, balance sheet analysis, 89
Liability, malpractice, 178-179
Liability insurance, 179
claims-made policy, 179
comprehensive general liability, 179
non-owned automobile liability, 179
occurrence policy, 179
professional liability, 179
terms related to, 179
Liaisoning, with healthcare professionals, 245
Libraries, information sources of, 36
Licensure fees, 81
Life cycle, of products/services, 61-62
Lifestyles, changes in, 6
Location of services, 65-67, 195
and appearance of facility, 66
in case study, 111
community facilities, 67
enhancement features, 65
hospitals, 66
physician's offices, 66-67
subletting in clinic, 67

Mail surveys, 37, 39
Malpractice, 178-179
elements of successful suits, 178
legal basis, 178-179
liability insurance, 179
steps for protection against, 178-179
Management strategies, in strategic plan, 144
Market analysis, 32-59
in case study, 99-106
questions addressed by, 32
researching target markets, 32-33
analysis of competition, 55-56
analysis of strengths and weaknesses, 56-59
community information resources, 36-37
examination of market forces, 41, 55
experience of nutrition practitioner, 33-35
marketing department, 35
networking, 36
professional marketing groups, 35-36
surveys, 37-41
Market forces
in case study, 102-103
study of, 41, 55
types of, 41, 55
Market segmentation, 29-31
basis of, 30
information required about, 34
requirements for, 33
selection of market segments, 60-61
types of market segments, 33
Marketing
definition of, 19
requirements for, 19-20
and strategic planning, 20-22
Marketing department, and market analysis, 37
Marketing mix, areas of, 24
Marketing strategies, in strategic plan, 143-144
Medline, 36
Mission statement, 23-24
in case study, 97
examples of, 23-24
nature of, 23
Mistakes, handling of, 157
Monitoring of performance
and adaptation to change, 317
administrator satisfaction, 312

Monitoring of performance *(Cont.)*
client satisfaction, 306-311
cost/benefit analysis, 316-317
financial progress, 313-316
referral source satisfaction, 311-312

Naming of practice, 209
Networking, 212-213
building strong networks, 212
with healthcare professionals, 244-245
learning about market through, 36
meaning of, 212
planning for, 212-213
Newspaper advertising, 217-220
example of ads, 219-220
Nomenclature, and reimbursement for services, 191
Nutrition counselors, role of, 77-78
Nutrition evaluations, 28
computer programs, 28
process in, 28
Nutrition fairs, 223-224
Nutrition services
clients, concerns of, 5-6
consumer reasons for use of, 9-10
direct influence, 25
education and counseling of, 11, 13, 26
environmental interventions, 25
free products/services, valuation of, 29
group programs, 13-14, 26-27
health care institutions, concerns of, 6-7
institutional practice, advantages of, 16-17
intrapreneurship and, 15-16
nutrition evaluations, 28
nutrition practitioners, needs and desires of, 7
outpatient versus inpatient providers, 11, 12
physicians, concerns of, 6
price setting, 8
product offerings, 28
public displays, 27
and referral agents, 10
specialized practice, 10-11
survival kit approach, 14

Occurrence policy, 179
Office policies and procedures, 158
Opportunities, in market analysis, 58
Orientation packet, for clients, 151
Outpatient nutrition managers, role of, 78
Outpatient service, 6
versus inpatient service, 11, 12
Overhead, 68
and financial analysis, 80

Package pricing, 72
Payment for services, 159-161
communication about payment policy, 160
fee schedule versus set fee, 159
forms of payment, 160
non-paying clients, 161
time for payment, 159-160
from worksite programs, 160-161
Per-head pricing, 72
Period expenses, 84
Personal interviews, 39, 41
Personalization of services, 155-154
ensuring feeling of, 156
Personnel management, 163
Philosophy statement, 148
Physicians, 237-243
attracting attention of, 238-240
communication with, 241-242
concerns related to nutrition, 6
describing services to, 237
involving in programs, 237-238
overcoming barriers raised by, 242-243
physician advocate, 240-241
as referral agents, 10
Physician's office, as location of service, 66-67
Physician's orders, and reimbursement for services, 191
Portfolios
items for, 283-284
packaging of, 284
Positioning, 63-64
in case study, 108-111
definition of, 24
example of, 63-64
nature of, 63
Press kits, 210
items in, 210
Preview sessions, 214
Price of service, 68-76
in case study, 113
and copayment, 75
cost and pricing, 68
factors in price setting, 68
competition, 70
cost, 68-69
demand, 69-70
desired return, 70-71
free services, valuation of, 29
negotiating price, 75
package pricing, 72
per-head pricing, 72
placing value on services, 8
price adjustments, 72-73
price reductions, 75
project pricing, 72
retainers, 72
time factor pricing, 71
unit of service pricing, 71
worksite pricing, 73-75
Printed ads, 214-215
Printed materials
choosing support materials, 207-208
types of, 28
Productive hours, 68
Productivity, maximization of, 163, 174
Products
food products, 28
printed materials, 28
related products, 29
selection of, 61-62
case study, 97-98, 106-107
Professional fees, 82

Professional liability, 179
Profit, 68, 91
Profit and loss projections, 83-86
  accounting equation of, 83
  components
    depreciation, 85
    expenses, 84-85
    revenue, 84
  matching expenses to revenue, 85-86
  preparation of, 86
Profit and loss statements
  in case study, 119-120
  and cash flow statement, 88
Program development, 206-208
  custom programs, 206
  and needs of clients, 208
  purchased programs, 206-207
  questions in selection of program, 207
Project pricing, 72
Promotion, 76
  advertising, 214-224
  and attention getting, 227-228
  to clients, 235-236
  cost of, 82
  decisions related to, 226-227
  direct mail, 224-226
  examples of, 113-114, 115
  features versus benefits, 230-232
  goals of, 76
  maximization of return on investment, 234
  monitoring success of, 315-316
  naming of practice, 209
  networking, 212-213
  publicity, 210-212
  questions in strategy development, 76
  to referral agents, 237-244
  sales calls, 224
  and target market, 227, 233
  targeting same service to different markets, 232
Promotion incentives, 220-223
  contests, 222-223
  coupons, 220-221
  gifts, 222
  giveaways, 221
Proposals, 284-292
  advantages of, 284
  negative elements of, 285
  outline for, 290-291
  presentation of, 291-292
  proposal for worksite nutrition services survey, 254-255
  survey proposal, 41, 42-43, 47-48
  for worksite nutrition services program, example of, 286-290
Proprietary rights, 181
  meaning of, 181
PTS Mars, 36
Public displays, 27-28
  sites for, 27
Publicity, 210-212
  community exposure, 212
  press kits, 210
  published articles, 210, 212
Published articles, as publicity, 210, 212

Rand McNally Commercial Atlas and Marketing Guide, 37
Record-keeping, 161-163
  client information, 162
  frequency of recording data, 313
  monthly reports, 314
  permanent records, 162-163
  reasons for, 162
  types of chart notes, 162
Referrals
  agents for, 10
  dentists, 243-244
  healthcare professionals, 243-244
  inpatient dietetic staff, 213
  monitoring satisfaction of, 311-312
  physicians, 237-244
Reimbursement for services, 184-193
  billing statement, 188, 189
  capitated plans, 193
  documentation requirements, 188, 191-192
  factors affecting reimbursement, 190-193
  information required by third party payers, 188
  introductory letter to insurance carrier, 185-186
  and nomenclature, 191
  and physician's orders, 191
  questionnaire for insurance carrier, 187
  setting reimbursement policy, 184, 186-190
  source of information related to, 190
Retainers, 72
Revenue
  matching to expenses, 85-86
  meaning of, 84
Rotation of staff, 200

Sales calls, 224
  nature of, 224
Sales process
  elements of, 262-264
  gaining access, 265-267
  generation of leads, 264-265
  information gathering, 269-272
  stages in, 264
Scheduling, 78-79
  in case study, 111
  sample schedule, 79
Scheduling of clients, 149-153
  and cancellations, 153
  communicating length of session to client, 150
  and completion of forms, 151
  and lateness of clients, 152
  minimizing unbillable time, 152
  and rescheduling, 153
  review of sessions with client, 150-151
  time needed per client, 150
  walk-ins, handling of, 150
Services
  selection of, 61-62
    case study, 97-98, 106-107
SOAP system, 162

Specialized practice, nutrition services, 10-11
Staffing, 76-78
  administrative support staff, 77
  burn-out, 202, 203
  in case study, 110-111
  concerns related to, 77
  and creating good impression for services, 204
  nutrition counselors, 77-78
  outpatient nutrition managers, 78
  rotation of staff, 200
  selection errors, types of, 200-201
  time splitting for inpatient and outpatient services, 200
  transferring dietian from inpatient to outpatient, 201-202
  and unrealistic expectations of staff, 202-203
Start-up activities
  checklist for, 194-195, 196-199
  choosing support materials, 207-208
  controlling impression of sessions, 205
  creating appearance of prosperity, 205-206
  employee selection and staffing, 195, 200-204
  program development, 206-208
  setting up facilities, 195
Start-up costs, types of, 87-88
Strategic planning, 20-22
  business description in plan, 142
  business plan, 20
  and community needs, 25
  components of process, 21-22
  executive summary, 139-141
  financial planning, 79-94
  goal setting, 62-63
  management strategies section, 144
  market analysis, 32-59
  marketing strategies section, 143-144
  mission statement, 23-24
  purposes of, 20-21
  selecting services/products, 24, 25-29, 61-62
  strategies, development of, 63-79
  target markets, 29-31, 60-61
  written plan, 133, 138-139
Strategic planning case study, 95-129
  background information, 95-97
  business strategies, 108-114
  financial analysis, 114-129
  goal setting, 107-108
  market analysis, 99-106
  mission statement, 97
  product/services selection, 97-98, 106-107
  target markets, 98-102
Supplies, 81-82
  categories of, 81
  cost of, 81-82
Surveys, 37-43
  cost effectiveness, 37
  definition of terms in, 41
  explanation to participants, 41
  focus groups, 37, 39
  mail surveys, 37, 39
  nature of questions, 40
  nutrition services questionnaire, example, 43-46, 50-54
  personal interviews, 37, 39
  survey proposal, 41, 42-43, 47-48
  telephone interviews, 37, 39, 40
  waste involved in, 40
  for worksite programs, 271-282
Survival kit approach, 14, 213

Target markets
  in case study, 98-102
  market segmentation, 29-31
Telephone communication, 154-155
  handling telephone coverage, 158
Telephone interviews, 37, 39, 40
Threats, in market analysis, 59
Time factor pricing, 71
Training and education expenses, 82
Travel expenses, 82

U. S. Small Business Administration, publication of, 37
Unit of service pricing, 71

Variable expenses, 91
Verbal agreements, 180

Walk-ins, handling of, 150
Where to Find Business Information: A Worldwide Guide for Everyone Who Needs the Answers to Business Questions, 36
Worksite programs
  benefits of, 247-248
  common objections to, 294-299
  common services provided, 249-250
  monitoring client satisfaction, 310-311
  payment for services, 160-161
  pricing for, 73-75
  proposal for worksite nutrition services survey, 254-255
  public displays, 27
  sales approach
    elements of sales process, 262-263
    follow-up after sale, 300-301
    nutrition services market survey for worksite decision makers, 255-260
    portfolio, use of, 283-284
    proposals, 284-292
    representative for program, 260
    stages in sales process, 264-273
    survey of employee/members, 271-283
    understanding competition, 261
    targeting organization for program, 250-253
Written communication, 155

Yellow Pages listings, 215-216
  example of, 216